METHODS IN MOLECULAR BIOLOGY

For further volumes:
http://www.springer.com/series/7651

Immunological Tolerance

Methods and Protocols

Edited by

Ashleigh S. Boyd

Associate Professor in Stem Cell Biology and Regenerative Medicine, Research Department of Surgical Biotechnology Division of Surgery and Interventional Science University College London (UCL), Royal Free Hospital, London, UK

UCL Institute of Immunity and Transplantation, Royal Free Hospital, London, UK

Humana Press

Editor
Ashleigh S. Boyd
Associate Professor in Stem Cell Biology and Regenerative Medicine
Research Department of Surgical Biotechnology
Division of Surgery and Interventional Science
University College London (UCL)
Royal Free Hospital
London, UK

UCL Institute of Immunity and Transplantation
Royal Free Hospital
London, UK

ISSN 1064-3745 ISSN 1940-6029 (electronic)
Methods in Molecular Biology
ISBN 978-1-4939-8936-2 ISBN 978-1-4939-8938-6 (eBook)
https://doi.org/10.1007/978-1-4939-8938-6

Library of Congress Control Number: 2018963826

This Humana Press imprint is published by the registered company Springer Science+Business Media, LLC, part of Springer Nature.
The registered company address is: 233 Spring Street, New York, NY 10013, U.S.A.

Preface

"Immunological Tolerance," the state in which the body is unresponsive to antigen, ensures the development of a "non-self" reactive T cell repertoire, as well as development of tolerogenic regulatory immune populations that protect us from disease. Continuing to understand how tolerance develops and, in the context of diseases such as autoimmunity and cancer, falters and breaks down will offer invaluable insight into how to manipulate these mechanisms to improve treatment of these diseases. This knowledge may also be applied to induce immunological tolerance in the setting of allogeneic transplantation as first described by Peter Medawar and Frank Macfarlane Burnet, who were awarded a Nobel Prize in 1960 for their seminal work in transplantation tolerance.

Since then the concept of immunological tolerance has blossomed into an entire, separate discipline in immunology, where advances have been regularly observed in small and large animal model systems but as of yet have largely failed to be replicated in the clinical setting. Yet, with recent advances in immunotherapy and techniques such as genome editing in concert with the isolation and characterization of novel subsets of tolerogenic cells, the prospect for harnessing the power of the immune system clinically to control unwanted responses to both self and foreign antigen now appears to be edging closer to reality than ever before.

With this in mind, I have developed this edition with a strong emphasis on techniques that can be used to understand or manipulate tolerance in human cells and to assess human disease in this setting directly. The chapters have been organized thematically into five parts. In Part 1, we focus on the isolation of tolerogenic cell types from stem cells, which are a self-renewing cell type responsible for producing and maintaining tissues in the body. While their biology in this respect is well established, different classes of stem cells and their progeny are now emerging as potential agents of immunomodulation, and we explore this capacity from both ex vivo isolated stem cells and laboratory-engineered stem cells (so-called induced pluripotent stem cells). Part 2 extends the premise of isolating tolerogenic cell populations for study and therapeutic utility by covering the ex vivo isolation of tolerogenic lymphocytic cells, including recently characterized B regulatory populations. In Part 3, we explore multiple methods to study the mechanisms underpinning tolerance, as well methods to induce tolerance through thymus progenitors which may be utilized in the future to reconstruct the thymus, the key site for central tolerance induction. How such methods of tolerance induction are invoked practically, as first envisioned by Medawar and Burnet, in context of transplantation, is considered in Part 4. Finally, Part 5 includes methods to assess the breakdown of immune tolerance in specific pathological conditions.

When I was asked to compile this special edition of *Methods in Molecular Biology* on "Immunological Tolerance" I was both honored and somewhat daunted by the task of covering the massive scope of the field. I have attempted to focus on what I consider to be important contemporaneous issues and methods, which I sincerely hope you will enjoy and find useful in your quest to further advance the field.

Finally, it would be remiss of me not to acknowledge my husband, Neil, for his steadfast support of my academic career (and in life in general), and to our daughter, Olivia, the light of our lives, who makes us realize what really matters in the end.

London, UK *Ashleigh S. Boyd*

Contents

Contributors

CHRISTINE M. BARBON • *IO Bioscience, Oncology IMED Biotech Unit, Astrazeneca, Gatehouse Park, Waltham, MA, USA*

PAOLA BONFANTI • *The Francis Crick Institute, London, UK; Great Ormond Street Institute of Child Health, University College London, London, UK; Institute of Immunity and Transplantation, University College London, London, UK*

ASHLEIGH S. BOYD • *Associate Professor in Stem Cell Biology and Regenerative Medicine, Research Department of Surgical Biotechnology Division of Surgery and Interventional Science University College London (UCL), University College London (UCL), Royal Free Hospital, London, UK; UCL Institute of Immunity and Transplantation, Royal Free Hospital, London, UK*

PETER BUTLER • *Research Department of Surgical Biotechnology, UCL Division of Surgery and Interventional Science, University College London (UCL), Royal Free Hospital, London, UK*

DALIA BURZYN • *Division of Immunology, Department of Microbiology and Immunobiology, Harvard Medical School, Boston, MA, USA*

RACHEL R. CASPI • *Immunoregulation Section, Laboratory of Immunology, National Eye Institute, NEI, NIH, Bethesda, MD, USA*

MASSIMILIANO CERLETTI • *UCL Research Department for Surgical Biotechnologies & Institute for Immunity and Transplantation, University College London, London, UK*

MELISSE CHEE • *Research Department of Surgical Biotechnology, UCL Division of Surgery and Interventional Science, University College London (UCL), Royal Free Hospital, London, UK*

JUN CHEN • *State Key Laboratory of Ophthalmology, Zhongshan Ophthalmic Center, Sun Yat-sen University, Guangzhou, China; Immunoregulation Section, Laboratory of Immunology, National Eye Institute, NEI, NIH, Bethesda, MD, USA*

SHERRIE J. DIVITO • *Department of Dermatology, Brigham and Women's Hospital and Harvard Medical School, Boston, MA, USA*

GUI JIE FENG • *European Cancer Stem Cell Research Institute, Cardiff University, School of Biosciences, Cardiff, UK*

EVA C. GUINAN • *Department of Radiation Oncology, Dana-Farber Cancer Institute, Boston, MA, USA; Department of Radiation Oncology, Harvard Medical School, Boston, MA, USA*

JOANNA HESTER • *Transplantation Research Immunology Group, Nuffield Department of Surgical Sciences, John Radcliffe Hospital, University of Oxford, Oxford, UK*

TIE ZHENG HOU • *UCL Institute of Immunity and Transplantation, University College London, London, UK*

KENNETH J. JANEC • *Department of Radiation Oncology, Dana-Farber Cancer Institute, Boston, MA, USA*

ROWAN H. KELNER • *Department of Radiation Oncology, Dana-Farber Cancer Institute, Boston, MA, USA*

MI-JEONG KIM • *Joslin Diabetes Center, Boston, MA, USA*

MYRA A. LIPES • *Joslin Diabetes Center, Harvard Medical School, Boston, MA, USA*

HuiJuan Lv • *Joslin Diabetes Center, Harvard Medical School, Boston, MA, USA*
Diane Mathis • *Division of Immunology, Department of Microbiology and Immunobiology, Harvard Medical School, Boston, MA, USA*
Claudia Mauri • *Division of Medicine, Centre for Rheumatology, University College London, London, UK*
Juan Bautista Menendez-Gonzalez • *European Cancer Stem Cell Research Institute, Cardiff University, School of Biosciences, Cardiff, UK*
Madhvi Menon • *Division of Medicine, Centre for Rheumatology, University College London, London, UK*
Kate Milward • *Transplantation Research Immunology Group, Nuffield Department of Surgical Sciences, John Radcliffe Hospital, University of Oxford, Oxford, UK*
Adrian E. Morelli • *Department of Surgery, T.E. Starzl Transplantation Institute, University of Pittsburgh Medical Center, Pittsburgh, PA, USA*
Hiromitsu Nakauchi • *Institute for Stem Cell Biology and Regeneration Medicine, Stanford University School of Medicine, The University of Tokyo, Tokyo, Japan*
Toshinobu Nishimura • *Institute for Stem Cell Biology and Regeneration Medicine, Stanford University School of Medicine, The University of Tokyo, Tokyo, Japan*
James E. Norton • *Department of Radiation Oncology, Dana-Farber Cancer Institute, Boston, MA, USA*
Elia Piccinini • *Institute of Biomaterials and Biomedical Engineering, University of Toronto, Toronto, CA, USA*
Omar S. Qureshi • *Celentyx Ltd, Birmingham Research Park, Birmingham, UK*
Khadir Raddassi • *Department of Neurology, Yale School of Medicine, New Haven, CT, USA*
David J. Roberts • *Nuffield Division of Laboratory Sciences, University of Oxford, Oxford, UK*
Neil P. Rodrigues • *European Cancer Stem Cell Research Institute, Cardiff University, School of Biosciences, Cardiff, UK*
Elizabeth C. Rosser • *Division of Medicine, Centre for Rheumatology, University College London, London, UK*
Lubaid Saleh • *European Cancer Stem Cell Research Institute, Cardiff University, School of Biosciences, Cardiff, UK*
David M. Sansom • *UCL Institute of Immunity and Transplantation, University College London, London, UK*
Thomas Serwold • *Joslin Diabetes Center, Boston, MA, USA*
Jessica Stolp • *Transplantation Research Immunology Group, Nuffield Department of Surgical Sciences, John Radcliffe Hospital, University of Oxford, Oxford, UK*
Panayotis Verginis • *Laboratory of Cellular Immunology and Immune Tolerance, Division of Immunology and Transplantation, Biomedical Research Foundation Academy of Athens, Athens, Greece*
Katerina Vlachou • *Laboratory of Autoimmunity and Inflammation, Institute of Molecular Biology and Biotechnology, Foundation for Research and Technology, Heraklion, Greece*
Amy Wagers • *Department of Stem Cell and Regenerative Biology, Harvard Stem Cell Institute, Harvard University, Cambridge, MA, USA*
Suzanne M. Watt • *Nuffield Division of Laboratory Sciences, University of Oxford, Oxford, UK*
Anna Wilson • *Research Department of Surgical Biotechnology, UCL Division of Surgery and Interventional Science, University College London (UCL), Royal Free Hospital, London, UK*

KATHRYN J. WOOD • *Transplantation Research Immunology Group, Nuffield Department of Surgical Sciences, John Radcliffe Hospital, University of Oxford, Oxford, UK*
MASAAKI ZAITSU • *Transplantation Research Immunology Group, Nuffield Department of Surgical Sciences, John Radcliffe Hospital, University of Oxford, Oxford, UK*
WEI ZHANG • *Nuffield Department of Women's Reproductive Health, University of Oxford, Oxford, UK*

Part I

Isolation of Stem Cells and Their Progeny for Immunological Tolerance Applications

Chapter 1

Isolation and Characterisation of Human Adipose-Derived Stem Cells

Anna Wilson, Melisse Chee, Peter Butler, and Ashleigh S. Boyd

Abstract

Recently, adipose-derived stem cells (ASCs), obtained from fresh human lipoaspirate, have shown promise as immunomodulatory agents having demonstrated immunosuppressive functionality both in vitro and in vivo. A number of researchers have described the isolation of ASCs through the enzymatic digestion of fat samples, followed by a number of purification steps, involving centrifugation and filtration. Here, we utilize a standard isolation technique, with the added purification of putative ASCs by fluorescence activated cell sorting (FACS). ASCs are an extremely valuable resource in clinical applications, including reconstruction, regeneration, and investigations into immune activity. This method could be used to isolate and purify ASCs for such downstream applications.

Key words Adipose-derived stem cells, Adipose stem cells, ASCs, Isolation, Characterization, Immunosuppression, Immunomodulation, Stromal vascular fraction, Collagenase, Lipotransfer, Lipoaspirate

1 Introduction

Similar to bone marrow-derived mesenchymal stem cells (MSCs), adipose-derived stem cells (ASCs) are multipotent adult stem cells which, as their name suggests, can be isolated from adipose (fat) tissue [1]. First identified in 2001, obtained via liposuction, ASCs were initially named processed lipoaspirate (PLA) cells [1]. Morphologically similar to fibroblasts, upon differentiation, ASCs can give rise to adipocytes, osteocytes, and chondrocytes. This plasticity may offer potential for their use in regenerative medicine as large numbers of these daughter cells can be generated from an easily isolated stem cell source. Furthermore, since aspirated fat is in plentiful supply from many plastic surgery procedures, such as liposuction and liposculpture, and the precursor cells can be purified by a variety of processing and enzymatic techniques to obtain the ASC-rich stromal vascular fraction (SVF) it is relatively straightforward to obtain ASCs [2–4].

Ashleigh S. Boyd (ed.), *Immunological Tolerance: Methods and Protocols*, Methods in Molecular Biology, vol. 1899,
https://doi.org/10.1007/978-1-4939-8938-6_1,

A further similarity between MSCs and ASCs is their promising immunomodulatory capacity [5–11], which has been observed to be either cell-contact dependent [6] or mediated by cytokines and trophic factors such as TNF-α, IFN-γ, IDO, PGE-2, and IL-17 [12–15]. In vivo, ASCs have been used for this purpose in spinal cord injury and neurodegenerative diseases [16, 17], allergic [10] and autoimmune diseases (for example, rheumatoid arthritis and inflammatory bowel disease) [18, 19], and in reducing Graft Versus Host Disease (GVHD) [20]. Clinical trials are bringing the use of injectable and implantable ASCs closer to becoming a reality for patients [21–24].

However, adipose-derived stem cells have proven problematic to identify in culture, and studies have been carried out to point to particular cellular markers, which may make them easier to recognize. Previous work has characterized ASCs based on their morphology [25–27], cell surface marker expression [28], and/or by assessing their ability to differentiate into specific lineages [29]. Once isolated, adipose stem cells have an even, round phenotype, in contrast to the irregular shape of endothelial cells. When cultured, they adhere to plastic and assume a fibroblast-like morphology within several days [30].

Rigotti's groundbreaking work showed positive characterization by flow cytometry of ASCs with respect to antibodies against CD105, CD73, CD29, CD44, and CD90. ASCs correlated negatively with CD31, CD45, CD14, and CD34 expression [28]. This characterization was echoed in another study which reported ASC positive expression of CD13, CD44, CD73, CD90, and CD105, but which did not express CD45, CD69, CD117, or HLA-DR [26]. These findings were consolidated by the International Society for Cellular Therapy (ISCT), who recently published guidelines for the identification of pluripotent and multipotent stem cells [27]. Herein, we isolated ASCs from human fat tissue using a combined approach of washing, centrifugation, and filtration followed by cell sorting based on their expression of the markers CD90, CD73, CD105, and CD44 and lack of expression for the markers CD45 and CD31. This method could be used to isolate and purify ASCs for downstream applications such as for regenerative medicine and reconstruction or for immune suppression studies.

2 Materials

All solutions should be prepared using ultrapure water and analytical grade reagents. Prepare and store all reagents at room temperature, unless stated otherwise. Diligently follow all waste disposal regulations when disposing of waste materials.

2.1 Isolation of ADSCs

1. Washing solution: Phosphate-buffered saline (PBS) (Sigma-Aldrich, Poole, UK), 1% penicillin/streptomycin liquid (P/S, Gibco, Life Technologies, Thermo Fisher Scientific, Paisley, UK).
2. HBSS solution: Hanks Balanced Salt Solution (HBSS, Gibco), 1% P/S (Gibco).
3. Tissue culture medium: Alpha-MEM (Gibco), 10% fetal bovine serum (FBS, cat#10091-148, Gibco), 1% P/S (Gibco).
4. Flow cytometry buffer: 50 mL PBS (Sigma)/0.25 mL FBS (0.5%, as before).
5. Collagenase type 1 (#17100017, Life Technologies, Thermo Fisher Scientific).
6. Beckton Dickinson 40 and 100 mm cell strainers, 15 and 50 mL Corning centrifuge tubes, 25 cm^2 tissue culture flasks, 0.2 mm syringe filters, 10 cc syringes, and weighing boats (all from VWR International, Lutterworth, UK).
7. Trypan Blue solution 0.4% (Thermo Fisher Scientific).

2.2 Culture and Expansion of ASCs

1. Washing solution: PBS (Sigma), 1% P/S (Gibco).
2. Tissue culture media: Alpha-MEM (Gibco), 10% FBS (Gibco), 1% P/S (Gibco).

2.3 Flow Cytometry

1. Flow cytometry buffer: 50 mL PBS/0.25 mL FBS (0.5%).
2. 5 mL polypropylene flow cytometry tubes (#352063, BD Biosciences).
3. 0.25% Trypsin-EDTA (1×), Phenol red (all Thermo Fisher Scientific).
4. Alpha-MEM, 10% FBS, 1% P/S (all Thermo Fisher Scientific).
5. Anti HLA-DR PerCP (#ab91333, Abcam, Cambridge, UK).
6. MSC Phenotyping Kit (Miltenyi Biotec, Oxford, UK).
7. 7-aminoactinomycin D (7AAD ThermoFisher Scientific).
8. Propidium iodide (PI, Sigma).
9. OneComp eBeads (#01-1111-42, eBioscience, Aachen, Germany).

2.4 Differentiation

1. Stempro adipogenic differentiation kit (Thermo Fisher Scientific).
2. Stempro chondrogenic differentiation kit (Thermo Fisher Scientific).
3. Stempro osteogenic differentiation kit (Thermo Fisher Scientific).
4. 12-well plates (VWR).

5. Cover slips (VWR).
6. ASC basic media (Alpha-MEM, 10% FBS, 1% pen/strep).
7. Paraformaldehyde 4% (Sigma Aldrich).
8. Isopropanol 60% (Sigma Aldrich).
9. Oil-Red-O (#ab150678, Abcam).
10. Alizarin Red (#ab142980, Abcam).
11. Alcian Blue 8GX (#ab145250, Abcam).

2.5 Fluorescence Activated Cell Sorting (FACS)

1. BD Biosciences flow cytometry tubes (as before).
2. 0.25% Trypsin-EDTA (1×), Phenol red.
3. Alpha-MEM, 10% FBS, 1% penicillin/streptomycin (all Thermo Fisher Scientific).
4. Flow cytometry buffer: 50 mL PBS/0.25 mL FBS (0.5%) (suppliers as before).
5. MSC Phenotyping Kit (Miltenyi Biotec).
6. Isotype control cocktail (Miltenyi Biotec).
7. Anti HLA-DR PerCP (Abcam).

3 Methods

All procedures should be carried out in a laminar flow hood, at room temperature, unless otherwise specified. We recommend processing human lipoaspirate within 24 h of collection, having stored it in sterile laboratory conditions at room temperature [29].

3.1 Adipose Tissue Harvest

Surplus fatty tissue can be collected following Coleman fat transfer procedures from adult human patients undergoing routine plastic surgery procedures. It is essential that local ethics approval is in place and all guidelines are followed. Patients are to be consented for the donation of surplus fatty tissue and its use in research, and provided with a patient information sheet. The procedures can be performed with or without the use of local anesthetic solution infiltration preoperatively. Fat can be harvested from the abdomen in six distinct areas, typically through a 2 mm-diameter cannula, into a 10 cc syringe. The fat filled syringes should then be centrifuged at 400 × *g* for 3 min to separate the oil, supernatant, and blood (Fig. 1), which can be poured off manually. Surplus fat is then collected.

3.2 Isolation of ASCs

From each patient, up to two samples of 5 g can be acquired. The process of ASC isolation is summarized in Fig. 1. Dispense each sample into a sterile specimen tube and wash three times with 20 mL PBS solution. Add 30 mg of collagenase type I (6 mg per

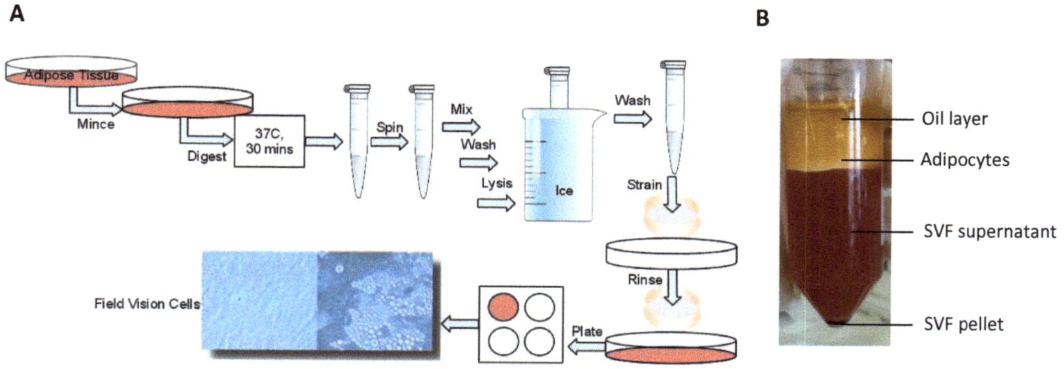

Fig. 1 Diagrammatic summary of the process of ASC isolation from adipose tissue and the appearance of the stromal vascular fraction (SVF). (**a**) Depiction of the steps involved in ASC isolation from lipoaspirate. (**b**) The stromal vascular fraction is first apparent following centrifugation of the aspirated fat

1 g adipose tissue, made up in 15 mL HBSS) to each sample. Shake the suspension and incubate for 2 h at 37 °C, 5% CO_2, 90% humidity. Immediately after this, centrifuge the sample at 300 × *g* for 5 min, and aspirate the supernatant. Resuspend the resulting pellet in complete culture media (Alpha-MEM, 10% FBS, 1% p/s), and combine both the samples into one tube, filtering sequentially through 100 μm and then 40 μm cell strainers. Centrifuge the samples again at 300 × *g* for a further 5 min, then aspirate the supernatant and resuspend the final pellet in 1 mL culture medium (*see* Fig. 1b to ascertain the appearance of the final cell pellet and SVF supernatant). Determine the cell number using the Trypan Blue assay. Incubate at 37 °C, 5% CO_2, 90% humidity in a 25 cm^2 culture flask.

3.3 Trypan Blue Cell Counting Protocol

With the cell pellet still in 1 mL of complete media, mix cells by pipetting up and down or vortexing. In a 96-well plate, pipette 90 μL of Trypan Blue solution into two adjacent wells. Pipette 10 μL of cells in media, into the first well and mix well. Then pipette 10 μL of cells from the first well into the second well, and mix well. Pipette 10 μL from the second well into the haemocytometer, and count cells. The resulting cell number represents a 1 in 100 dilution; therefore, the average number obtained should be multiplied by 10^6 in order to calculate the number of cells per 1 mL of media, i.e., per 10 g of fat.

3.4 Expansion of ADSCs In Vitro

Following the placement of ASCs into culture flasks in culture media (Alpha-MEM, 10% FBS, 1% p/s), allow them to adhere to culture plastic for 72 h. After this, wash cells twice with PBS, and replace culture media. Repeat after a further 48 h. At 7 days from isolation, the cells can be detached from the plate using trypsin, and counted using the Trypan Blue assay [31, 32].

3.5 Phenotypic Analysis of Putative ADSCs by Flow Cytometry

Following isolation, in culture putative ADSCs retain markers in common with other mesenchymal stromal/stem cells (MSCs), including CD90, CD73, CD105, and CD44 and remain negative for CD45 and CD31. Using these markers ADSCs can be immunephenotyped by flow cytometry. Control samples required include unstained controls, single stain controls, and isotype stain controls using the same cells as to be analyzed for test antibodies. Since as most cells emit low level auto-fluorescence, an unstained control is used to set up the photomultiplier (PMT) voltages on the flow cytometer to a level wherein the unstained cells should appear in the first quartile of a four decade logarithmic scale for each fluorochrome measured. Isotype controls are also required. They are used as a specificity control to distinguish specific from nonspecific binding. Together, these controls allow for the appropriate gating of the desired cell population. The following sections describe the process for antibody labeling and analysis of samples on a flow cytometer [33].

3.5.1 Flow Cytometry Cell Staining

1. Make up two aliquots of one million putative ADSCs each, in culture media.
2. Centrifuge tubes at 300 × *g* for 10 min. Then aspirate the supernatant.
3. Resuspend cells in 90 μL buffer.
4. Add 10 μL of MSC Phenotyping cocktail and 10 μL of Anti-HLA-DR PerCP to tube 1, and 20 μL of isotype control cocktail to tube 2.
5. Vortex to mix and incubate tubes for 10 min in the refrigerator.
6. Add 3 mL of flow cytometry buffer to each tube, then centrifuge at 300 × *g* for 10 min. Aspirate the supernatant.
7. To stain for cell viability, resuspend each cell pellet in 100 μL buffer containing 7AAD or PI (1:250 dilution). Vortex to mix and incubate tubes in the refrigerator for 10 min.
8. Add 3 mL of flow cytometry buffer to each tube, then centrifuge at 300 × *g* for 10 min. Aspirate the supernatant.
9. Resuspend each cell pellet in 400 μL flow buffer in preparation for acquisition.
10. Place all tubes on ice prior to acquisition on a flow cytometer.

3.5.2 Compensation for Flow Cytometry

Compensation is the process of subtracting the spectral spillover from one fluorochrome into the detector of another. Single stain controls can be used to set the instrument to compensate for this fluorescence spill over between channels. However, fluorescently conjugated beads (such as OneComp eBeads™, eBioscience) provide an alternative to cells in achieving this, and allow for a reliable and reproducible benchmark with the added advantage that they replace precious samples, enabling every cell to be retained for analysis.

1. Aliquot 500,000 cells each (or one drop of OneComp eBeads; except for in the "no stain" tube, for which cells should always be used) into five separate tubes. Label as "PerCP," "PE," "APC," "FITC," and "no stain." These tubes will be used as single stain controls and an unstained control.
2. Add 100 μL of flow cytometry buffer to each tube. Then add the following to the appropriate tube:
   (a) PerCP tube—add 10 μL CD73 Biotin antibody.
   (b) PE tube—add 10 μL CD105 PE antibody.
   (c) APC tube—add 10 μL CD73 APC antibody.
   (d) FITC tube—add 10 μL CD90 FITC antibody.
   (e) No stain tube—500 μL buffer only, no antibody.
3. Vortex to mix and incubate tubes for 10 min in the refrigerator.
4. Add 2 mL of flow cytometry buffer to each tube to dilute antibody, centrifuge at 300 × *g* for 10 min. Aspirate the supernatant.
5. Add 10 μL Anti-Biotin PerCP to the PerCP aliquot, mix well, and incubate in the refrigerator for 10 min. Then wash with 1 mL flow cytometry buffer, centrifuge at 300 × *g* for 10 min, and aspirate the supernatant.
6. Resuspend each pellet in 400–500 μL buffer, ready for flow cytometry, and store on ice. Process as soon as possible.

3.5.3 Acquisition and Analysis on a Flow Cytometer

The samples and controls should be acquired on a flow cytometer. Our samples were acquired using a MACSQuant 10 (Miltenyi Biotec, Germany) and MACSQuant Analysis software (Miltenyi Biotec) to identify progression of surface marker characteristics of isolated ASCs.

3.6 Differentiation

In order to show that isolated ASCs have stem cell potential, in common with MSC differentiation, ASCs can be induced to differentiate into three different cellular lineages namely adipocytes, osteocytes, and chondrocytes which together are referred to as the tri-lineages. This section describes the process for inducing differentiation toward each lineage.

3.6.1 Directed Differentiation

1. Determine cell number.
2. Make up differentiation media as per StemPro instructions for adipogenic, chondrogenic and osteogenic differentiation (Gibco, UK).
3. Sterilize cover slips by dipping them into 70% ethanol, then place into wells in 12-well plate.
4. Wash each well with PBS (1% penicillin/streptomycin).

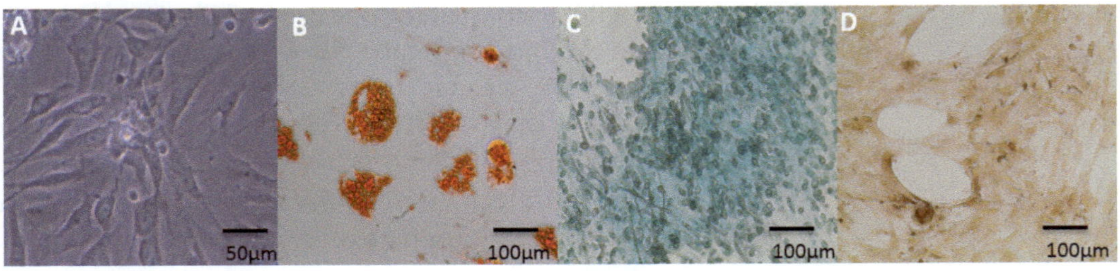

Fig. 2 Appearance of ASC in culture and following targeted tri-lineage differentiation. (**a**) Appearance of adipose derived stem cells (ASCs) in culture at day 7. Following isolation, ASCs were driven to undergo targeted differentiation to the tri-lineages (**b–d**). (**b**) Oil red O staining of lipid droplets generated via adipocyte differentiation of ASCs. (**c**) Alcian blue staining of chondrocyte nuclei following ASC chondrocytic differentiation. (**d**) Alcian red staining of osteoblasts following osteogenic differentiation of ASCs. Images captured on a EVOS XF light microscope and are representative of $n = 3$ independent experiments

5. Seed 30,000 cells per well and add 1.5 mL culture media. Incubate at 37 °C, 90% humidity, 5% CO_2.
6. For chondrogenesis, allow the cells to adhere for 2–3 h prior to changing the medium to chondrogenic differentiation medium. For adipogenesis, allow the cells to adhere for 24 h prior to changing the medium to adipogenic and osteogenic differentiation media, respectively.
7. Wash wells and replace differentiation media once per week, for 21–28 days, while monitoring cell growth and differentiation.
8. Staining for adipose cells can be performed at 21 days, and for chondrocytes and osteocytes at 28 days (as below; Fig. 2).

3.6.2 Phenotyping of Differentiated ASC–Derived Cells

In order to show that isolated ASCs have stem cell potential, in common with MSC differentiation, ASCs can be induced to differentiate into three different cellular lineages namely adipocytes, osteocytes, and chondrocytes. This section describes the process of staining the differentiated cells to show that they have become committed to the MSC/ASC tri-lineages (*see* Fig. 2).

Staining of ASC-Derived Adipocytes

1. Fix with 4% PFA for 1 h.
2. Mix three parts ORO with two parts distilled water.
3. Remove PFA, rinse with DI water.
4. Add 2 mL 60% isopropanol to each well and leave for 5 min.
5. Remove and add 2 mL ORO working solution, leave for 5 min.
6. Remove ORO, rinse with DI water.

Staining of ASC-Derived Osteocytes

1. Fix with 4% PFA for 1 h.
2. Aspirate and rinse twice with DI water.
3. Cover wells with Alizarin red solution, leave for 30 min.
4. Remove Alizarin red and wash 4× with DI water.

Staining of ASC-Derived Chondrocytes

1. Fix with 4% PFA for 1 h.
2. Aspirate and rinse twice with DI water.
3. Stain with 1% Alcian Blue solution for 30 min.
4. Rinse with DI water.

3.7 Fluorescence Activated Cell Sorting (FACS)

To isolate putative ASCs from lipo-aspirate, rather than simply to analyze surface marker expression, the cells should be stained in a similar manner as for flow cytometry analysis. The benefit of using FACS is that the cells can be separated based on their expression of ADSC markers and retained for downstream experiments.

Current ASC enrichment techniques include monolayer expansion and surface marker-based sorting. Cultured ASCs grown in monolayers are defined by their ability to adhere to plastic surfaces and fast proliferation rates; this method is yield-effective because non-adherent cell types, for example, erythrocytes and leukocytes, are washed away enabling more efficient proliferation of ASCs. The ideal solution would be to immediately isolate and characterize the ASCs, based on cell surface marker expression, such that a precise fraction of specific cells could then be re-injected into the operative site [34].

1. Determine cell number. If possible, use >ten million cells for cell sorting.
2. Perform staining as per flow cytometry protocol, amending the amount of antibody used; for example, use 25 μL of MSC phenotyping cocktail for every ten million cells stained.
3. Stain further samples to set compensation controls.
4. Place all samples on ice and acquire on flow cytometer as soon as possible following staining.

4 Notes

1. 5ccs of lipoaspirate provides sufficient volume of fat for isolation of ASCs, with relative ease in processing.
2. Washing is an essential first step in isolation of ASCs from lipoaspirate; the more thoroughly this is done, the better the adhesion of ASCs to tissue culture plastic will be.
3. During filtration of the SVF through cell strainers, it may prove helpful to aspirate some air through the cell strainer while pouring the digested fat to be filtered. This needs to be done slowly to prevent clogging of the cell strainers with large debris.
4. Exclude dead cells from analysis by staining with propidium iodide (PI) or 7-aminoactinomycin D (7AAD) in conjunction with their forward and side light scattering properties.
5. When ASCs are processed clumps of dead fat cells can arise which may cause line blockages during flow cytometry. We

therefore recommend filtering all cell suspensions through a 40 μm cell strainer.

6. It may be helpful to use a larger nozzle, for example 100 μm, when using the FACS machine with ADSCs, due to their adherent nature; in order to avoid blockages and damage to cells.
7. Flow cytometry gating strategy:
   (a) ASCs that have been cultured for 7 days prior to flow cytometry can be initially viewed on a plot with forward scatter versus side scatter as unstained cells. Cell debris should be eliminated and the main cell population can then be identified and gated.
   (b) Single stain controls should be run to establish compensation. We advise using OneComp eBeads, although ASCs can be used in conjunction. When running single stain controls, gates are set in order to ensure there is no spectral overlap between the peaks seen.
   (c) Once compensation settings have been applied, the ASC samples stained with the MSC Phenotyping Cocktail should be acquired next. Create plots to view each stain singly and in the following combinations: CD73 and CD90, CD90 and CD105, and CD73 and CD105. Cells that are double positive for CD73 and CD90 should be gated as a separate population and then viewed against CD105 in order to capture those cells which are positive for all three MSC markers.

Acknowledgments

This work was supported by the Restoration of Appearance and Function Trust (RAFT), with funding from the Kirby Laing Foundation.

References

1. Zuk PA et al (2001) Multilineage cells from human adipose tissue: implications for cell-based therapies. Tissue Eng 7(2):211–228
2. Doi K et al (2013) Stromal vascular fraction isolated from lipo-aspirates using an automated processing system: bench and bed analysis. J Tissue Eng Regen Med 7(11):864–870
3. Blaber SP et al (2012) Analysis of in vitro secretion profiles from adipose-derived cell populations. J Transl Med 10:172
4. Ong WK, Sugii S (2013) Adipose-derived stem cells: fatty potentials for therapy. Int J Biochem Cell Biol 45(6):1083–1086
5. Jeong SH, Ji YH, Yoon ES (2014) Immunosuppressive activity of adipose tissue-derived mesenchymal stem cells in a rat model of hind limb allotransplantation. Transplant Proc 46 (5):1606–1614
6. Nagaya R et al (2014) Mechanisms of the immunosuppressive effects of mouse adipose tissue-derived mesenchymal stromal cells on mouse alloreactively stimulated spleen cells. Exp Ther Med 7(1):17–22
7. Barone AAL et al (2013) Immunomodulatory effects of adipose-derived stem cells: fact or fiction? Biomed Res Int 2013:383685

8. Puissant N et al (2005) Immunomodulatory effect of human adipose tissue-derived adult stem cells: comparison with bone marrow mesenchymal stem cells. Br J Haematol 129 (1):118–129
9. Yanez R et al (2006) Adipose tissue-derived mesenchymal stem cells have in vivo immunosuppressive properties applicable for the control of the graft-versus-host disease. Stem Cells 24(11):2582–2591
10. Cho KS et al (2009) IFATS collection: immunomodulatory effects of adipose tissue-derived stem cells in an allergic rhinitis mouse model. Stem Cells 27(1):259–265
11. Bahrami B et al (2017) Adipose derived stem cells exert immunomodulatory effects on natural killer cells in breast cancer. Cell J 19 (1):137–145
12. Yoo KH et al (2009) Comparison of immunomodulatory properties of mesenchymal stem cells derived from adult human tissues. Cell Immunol 259(2):150–156
13. Gronthos S et al (2001) Surface protein characterization of human adipose tissue-derived stromal cells. J Cell Physiol 189(1):54–63
14. Caplan AI, Dennis JE (2006) Mesenchymal stem cells as trophic mediators. J Cell Biochem 98(5):1076–1084
15. Cui L et al (2007) Expanded adipose-derived stem cells suppress mixed lymphocyte reaction by secretion of prostaglandin E2. Tissue Eng 13(6):1185–1195
16. Kingham PJ et al (2014) Stimulating the neurotrophic and angiogenic properties of human adipose-derived stem cells enhances nerve repair. Stem Cells Dev 23(7):741–754
17. Ohta Y et al (2017) Intravenous infusion of adipose-derived stem/stromal cells improves functional recovery of rats with spinal cord injury. Cytotherapy 19(7):839–848
18. Gonzalez-Rey E et al (2009) Human adult stem cells derived from adipose tissue protect against experimental colitis and sepsis. Gut 58 (7):929–939
19. Lopez-Santalla M et al (2015) Human adipose-derived Mesenchymal stem cells modulate experimental autoimmune arthritis by modifying early adaptive T cell responses. Stem Cells 33(12):3493–3503
20. Mariani E, Facchini A (2012) Clinical applications and biosafety of human adult mesenchymal stem cells. Curr Pharm Des 18 (13):1821–1845
21. Missana MC et al (2007) Autologous fat transfer in reconstructive breast surgery: indications, technique and results. Eur J Surg Oncol 33 (6):685–690
22. Bernard RW, Beran SJ (2003) Autologous fat graft in nipple reconstruction. Plast Reconstr Surg 112(4):964–968
23. Coleman SR (2006) Structural fat grafting: more than a permanent filler. Plast Reconstr Surg 118(3 Suppl):108S–120S
24. Yoshimura K et al (2008) Cell-assisted lipotransfer for cosmetic breast augmentation: supportive use of adipose-derived stem/stromal cells. Aesthet Plast Surg 32(1):48–55 discussion 56-7
25. Fraser J et al (2007) Differences in stem and progenitor cell yield in different subcutaneous adipose tissue depots. Cytotherapy 9 (5):459–467
26. Deimling LI, et al. Interaction of human, canine and murine adipose-derived stem cells with different biomaterials. 5th European Conference of the International Federation for Medical and Biological Engineering, vol. 37, Pts 1 and 2, 2012. p. 1315.
27. Dominici M et al (2006) Minimal criteria for defining multipotent mesenchymal stromal cells. The International Society for Cellular Therapy position statement. Cytotherapy 8 (4):315–317
28. Rigotti G et al (2007) Clinical treatment of radiotherapy tissue damage by lipoaspirate transplant: a healing process mediated by adipose-derived adult stem cells. Plast Reconstr Surg 119(5):1409–1422
29. Bunnell BA et al (2008) Adipose-derived stem cells: isolation, expansion and differentiation. Methods 45(2):115–120
30. Kolle SF et al (2013) Enrichment of autologous fat grafts with ex-vivo expanded adipose tissue-derived stem cells for graft survival: a randomised placebo-controlled trial. Lancet 382(9898):1113–1120
31. Punshon G et al (2008) Assessment of the potential of progenitor stem cells extracted from human peripheral blood for seeding a novel vascular graft material. Cell Prolif 41 (2):321–335
32. Suga H et al (2008) Numerical measurement of viable and nonviable adipocytes and other cellular components in aspirated fat tissue. Plast Reconstr Surg 122(1):103–114
33. Maecker HT, Trotter J (2006) Flow cytometry controls, instrument setup, and the determination of positivity. Cytometry A 69A (9):1037–1042
34. Kanthilal M, Darling EM (2014) Characterization of mechanical and regenerative properties of human, adipose stromal cells. Cell Mol Bioeng 7(4):585–597

Chapter 2

Isolation of Murine Hematopoietic Stem Cells

Juan Bautista Menendez-Gonzalez, Lubaid Saleh, Gui Jie Feng, and Neil P. Rodrigues

Abstract

Bone marrow resident hematopoietic stem cells (HSCs) are responsible for the lifetime generation of the wide profusion of blood and immune cell types found in the body. In addition, therapeutically, in the context of bone marrow transplantation, HSCs have been successfully deployed to restore normal blood-forming capacity in patients being treated with high-dose chemotherapy for hematologic malignancies. The known ability of bone marrow transplantation to either restore or reset the immune system and to engender immune tolerance has suggested that HSCs may be applied therapeutically for a wider range of clinical conditions, including immunological/autoimmune disorders and allogeneic organ transplantation. Herein, we describe a flow-cytometry-based method to isolate mouse HSCs for continued experimental investigation into such therapeutic uses.

Key words HSCs, Tolerance, Transplantation, Flow cytometry, Cell sorting

1 Introduction

One of the key elements for successful allogeneic organ transplantation is efficient induction of immune tolerance. Treatment of recipients with a variety of immunosuppressive agents can induce immune tolerance by modulating T cell or B cell activity and effectively prevent acute rejection of transplanted organs [1] yet life-threatening complications, such as an increased risk of infections and malignancies can occur with prolonged use of immunosuppressive drugs. There is therefore an unmet clinical need to develop novel, alternative strategies to induce immune tolerance with tempered use of immunosuppressant drugs. In this vein, studies in mouse models (and larger animals) have demonstrated that allogeneic transplantation of bone marrow containing hematopoietic stem cells (HSCs) using mixed chimerism protocols allows for immune tolerance induction to solid organ transplantation and reduces the percentage of graft rejection by the host immune system [2]; in this setting transplanted allogeneic HSCs

Ashleigh S. Boyd (ed.), *Immunological Tolerance: Methods and Protocols*, Methods in Molecular Biology, vol. 1899,
https://doi.org/10.1007/978-1-4939-8938-6_2, © Springer Science+Business Media, LLC, part of Springer Nature 2019

generate donor T cells, which due to their development and education in the host thymus can ameliorate T lymphocyte responses and prevent immunogenicity toward transplanted allogeneic organs [3–5]. Furthermore, using bone marrow transplantation in the context of autoimmune disorders such as scleroderma [6] suggests that the therapeutic utility of HSCs may extend to the treatment of other autoimmune conditions or immunological disorders and beyond its hitherto largely restricted use in the treatment of hematological malignancies. To this end, further characterization and understanding of HSC biology will facilitate the expanded therapeutic use of bone marrow transplantation.

Mouse HSCs have been extensively characterized by different cell surface markers, and have defined the HSC population as Lin^- $c\text{-}Kit^+$ $Sca\text{-}1^+$ (LKS) $CD150^+$ $CD48^-$ [7–11]. CD150 and CD48 are members of the signaling lymphocytic activation molecule (SLAM) family markers that can also be used to characterize the different hematopoietic progenitor populations that comprise the LKS compartment [12].

Fluorescence activated cell sorting (FACS) technology allows the recognition and separation of cell populations based on parameters such as size, shape, and fluorescence intensity of the cell surface markers. Hence, by targeting cell-specific HSCs surface markers with antibodies (Ab) conjugated with fluorochromes, we describe a method, based on FACS, where we can detect and isolate purified as Lin^- $c\text{-}Kit^+$ $Sca\text{-}1^+$ (LKS) $CD150^+$ $CD48^-$ HSCs from mouse bone marrow (BM).

2 Materials

2.1 General Materials

1. Plastic-ware: petri dish, 1.5, 15, and 50 mL centrifuge tubes.
2. 70% ethanol.
3. Biological safety cabinet.
4. Centrifuge.
5. FACS buffer: phosphate-buffered saline (PBS) with 2% of fetal bovine serum (FBS).

2.2 Bone Marrow Isolation

1. Young adult C57/BL6 mice, typically 6–12 weeks old mice, are used for isolation of HSCs.
2. 10 mL syringes with 25-G needles (BD) to flush out the bone marrow from femur and tibia.
3. Dissection tools: Micro-dissecting scissors and forceps (Sigma).
4. 70 μm cell strainer (Miltenyi Biotec).
5. Ammonium chloride (NH_4Cl) (STEMCELL Technologies).

2.3 Pre-enrichment Using AutoMACS

1. Lineage biotinylated cocktail. 1 mL of lineage cocktail in FACS buffer includes biotin conjugated CD4 (3.25 μL), CD3e (6.25 μL), CD8a (6.25 μL), Grl (31.25 μL), Mac-1 (62.5 μL), B220 (62.5 μL), Ter119 (125 μL).
2. Microbeads: anti-biotin and c-kit microbeads are available from Miltenyi Biotec.
3. AutoMACS (Miltenyi Biotec).
4. CellTrick 30 μm (Sysmex UK).
5. Laboratory rotator.

2.4 HSC Staining

1. Fc block: purified anti-CD16/32.
2. Streptavidin conjugated with PerCP.
3. SLAM staining mix: includes c-kit-APC, Sca-1-PE, CD150-PE-Cy7, CD48-FITC, and (10 μL of lineage biotinylated cocktail for the c-kit enrichment protocol). All antibodies described in this protocol are available from BD Biosciences. Note that all antibodies should be titrated before use for optimal results.
4. Fluorescent minus one (FMO): include all the antibodies of the panel except the one that is being assessed. FMOs represent when the true positive expression of a cell surface marker begins in a multi-color panel. The use of FMOs gives information to set up the gates in the cell sorter where spill over from other fluorochromes is present.
5. OneComp beads (eBioscience): each drop of beads contains two populations; a positive population that will capture any mouse, rat, or hamster antibody and a negative population that will not react with antibody.

2.5 Flow Cytometry

1. FACS cell sorter (i.e., BD FUSION II ARIA, BD Biosciences).
2. Polystyrene FACS tubes (BD Biosciences).
3. 4′,6-diamidino-2-phenylindole (DAPI) (Molecular probes): use at 1/10000 dilution. When excited by a UV/Violet laser DAPI emits blue fluorescence upon binding to AT regions of DNA in dead cells.

3 Methods

3.1 Bone Marrow Isolation

1. Sacrifice mouse by cervical dislocation and dissect femurs and tibias from both legs (*see* **Note 1**). Remove as much flesh as possible and carry out the following steps under sterile conditions.
2. Immediately cut the ends from each bone and flush out the bone marrow into a petri dish using a 10 mL syringe with 25-G

needles filled with FACS buffer from either ends of the bone (*see* **Note 2**).

3. Prepare a single cell suspension by resuspending up and down the marrow through the 10 mL syringe. Filter the BM cells through a 70 μm cell strainer placed over a 50 mL centrifuge tube.
4. Centrifuge the BM cells at 500 × *g* for 5 min at 4 °C. Remove the supernatant using a glass pipette.
5. Resuspend the cell pellet in 1 mL of NH4Cl and incubate for 2 min at RT (*see* **Note 3**). Add 9 mL of FACS buffer to neutralize the lysis, and centrifuge at 500 × *g* for 5 min at 4 °C. Remove the supernatant using a glass pipette.

3.2 Pre-enrichment with the AutoMACS Separator

Pre-enrichment of hematopoietic progenitor and stem cells can be achieved either by depletion of lineage positive cells or by positive selection of c-kit positive cells.

3.2.1 Lineage Depletion Using Anti-Biotin Microbeads

1. Resuspend the cell pellet in 300 μL of FACS buffer containing 50 μL of biotinylated lineage cocktail per mouse.
2. Transfer into a 1.5 mL micro centrifuge tube and stain for 10–15 min at 4 °C.
3. Wash with 1 mL of FACS buffer and spin down at 500 × *g* for 5 min at 4 °C. Remove the supernatant using a glass pipette.
4. Resuspend the cell pellet in 300 μL of FACS buffer containing 40 μL of anti-biotin microbeads. Shake the microbeads vigorously prior to usage to ensure that the magnetic microbeads are well mixed.
5. Incubate for 15 min at 4 °C in the dark while rotating (*see* **Note 4**).
6. Wash the cells with 1 mL of FACS buffer and spin down at 500 × *g* for 5 min at 4 °C. Remove the supernatant using a glass pipette.
7. Resuspend the cell pellet in 1 mL of FACS buffer and filter the cells through a 30 μm strainer to prevent clogging of the magnetic column during the separation. Transfer the sample into a 15 mL centrifuge tube. Rinse the tube with 1 mL of FACS buffer and collect to obtain a final volume of 2 mL.
8. Place the tube into the AutoMACS rack. Label a 15 mL centrifuge tube for the negative population (−ve) and one for the positive population (+ve) (*see* Fig. 1) (*see* **Note 5**).
9. Initiate and clean AutoMACS prior to separation.
10. Select program *depletes*. Each separation has an average time of 15 min.

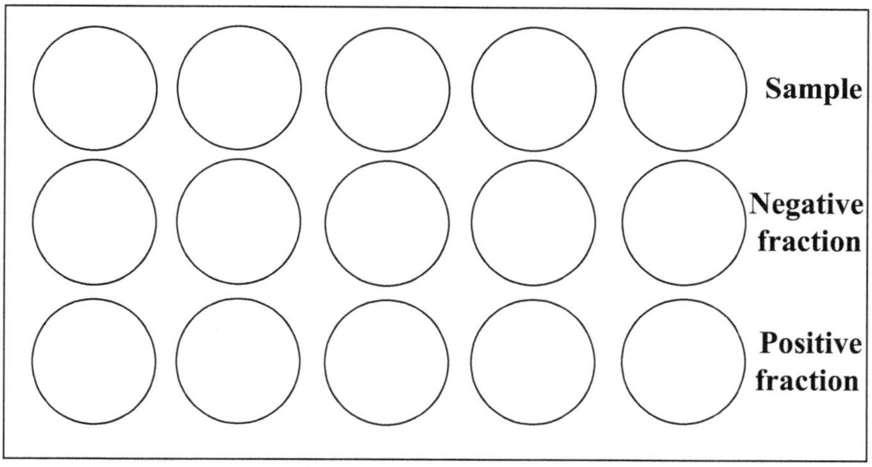

Fig. 1 AutoMACS rack schematics. Samples in a 15 mL centrifuge tubes are placed in the top raw (named sample). An empty 15 mL centrifuge tube is placed in the second raw to collect the negative fraction. An empty 15 mL centrifuge tubes is placed in the third raw to collect the positive fraction

11. Collect the tube containing 4 mL of the lineage negative population—This tube contains the HSCs. Separate 7 aliquots of 100 μL for FMOs, unstained and DAPI control Spin down at 500 × *g* for 5 min at 4 °C. Remove the supernatant using a glass pipette.

3.2.2 c-Kit Positive Enrichment Using Anti-c-Kit Microbeads

1. Resuspend the cell pellet in 300 μL of FACS buffer containing 20 μL of anti-c-kit microbeads. Shake the microbeads vigorously prior to usage to ensure that the magnetic microbeads are well mixed.
2. Incubate for 15 min at 4 °C in the dark while rotating (*see* **Note 4**).
3. Wash the cells with 1 mL of FACS buffer and spin down at 500 × *g* for 5 min at 4 °C. Remove the supernatant using a glass pipette.
4. Resuspend the cell pellet in 1 mL of FACS buffer and filter the cells through a 30 μm strainer to prevent clogging of the magnetic column during the separation. Transfer the sample into a 15 mL centrifuge tube. Rinse the tube with 1 mL of FACS buffer to obtain a final volume of 2 mL.
5. Place the tube into the AutoMACS rack. Label a 15 mL centrifuge tube for the negative population (−ve) and one for the positive population (+ve) (*see* Fig. 1) (*see* **Note 5**).
6. Initiate and clean AutoMACS prior to separation. Select program *posseld2s*. Each separation has an average time of 15 min.

7. Collect the tube containing 2 mL of the c-kit positive population. Separate 7 aliquots of 50 μL into 1.5 mL centrifuge tubes for FMOs, unstained and DAPI control. Spin down at 500 × *g* for 5 min at 4 °C. Remove the supernatant using a glass pipette.

3.3 HSC Staining

1. Resuspend the cell pellet in 50 μL of Fc block and immediately add 50 μL of SLAM staining mix or the appropriate FMO staining mix. Transfer into a 1.5 mL centrifuge tube and stain for 25–30 min at 4 °C in the dark.
2. While staining, prepare compensation beads for each antibody. Add 1 drop of beads into a 5 mL polystyrene FACS tube and add a previously titrated amount of antibody for a single stain. Stain for 20 min at 4 °C in the dark. Wash the cells with 1 mL of FACS buffer and spin down at 500 × *g*. Discard the supernatant and resuspend the beads in 200 μL of FACS buffer.
3. Wash the cells from **step 1** with 1 mL of FACS buffer and spin down at 500 × *g* for 5 min at 4 °C. Remove the supernatant using a glass pipette.
4. Resuspend the cell pellet in 100 μL of FACS buffer containing 1 μL of Streptavidin conjugated with PerCP (do not stain the FMO Streptavidin-PerCP tube in this step). Stain for 15 min at 4 °C in the dark.
5. Wash with 1 mL of FACS buffer and spin down at 500 × *g* for 5 min at 4 °C. Remove the supernatant using a glass pipette.
6. Resuspend the cell pellet in an appropriate volume of FACS buffer (typically 700 μL) and filter through a 30 μm strainer into a polystyrene FACS tube. Keep sample on ice until analysis.

3.4 FACS Sorting

In order to isolate purified HSCs from mouse bone marrow:

1. Add DAPI (1/10000) prior to sorting. Live cells are distinguished as DAPI negative.
2. Set up the plots (*see* Fig. 2), voltages and gates using the unstained tube and FMOs.
3. Compensate the spill over between fluorochromes using the compensation beads.
4. Finally, run the sample and sort purified HSCs in the desired medium as live cells (DAPI negative), Lin^- $c\text{-}kit^+$ $Sca\text{-}1^+$ $CD150^+$ $CD48^-$ (*see* Fig. 2) (*see* **Note 6**).
5. It is recommended to re-sort a fraction of HSCs to check the purity.

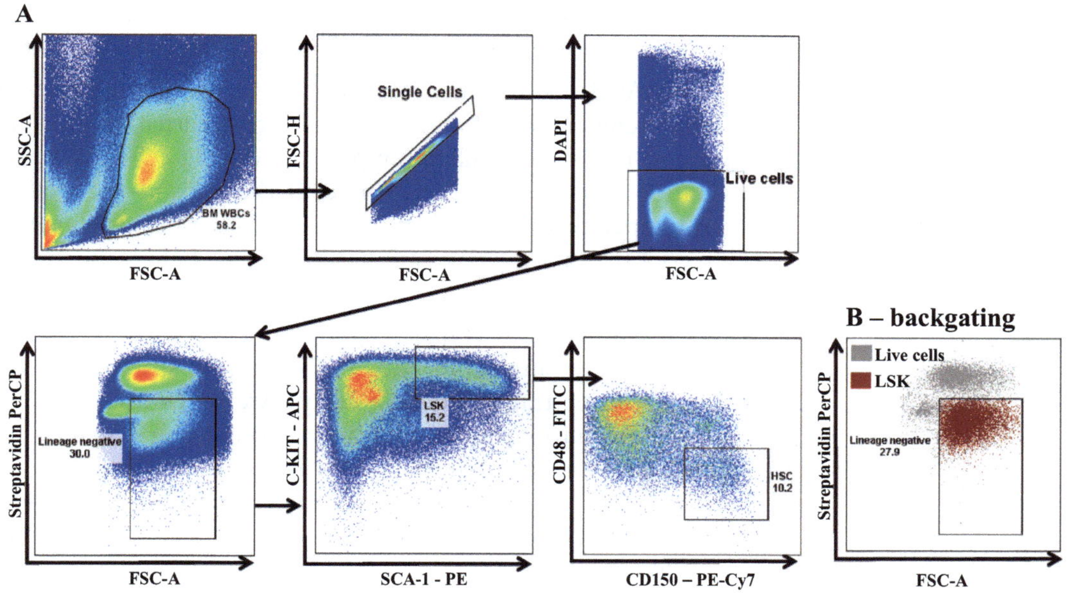

Fig. 2 Flow cytometry plots to isolate murine HSC after c-kit enrichment. (**a**) Bone marrow WBCs are gated based on their size (FSC-A) and granularity (SSC-A). To discard doublets, we select single cells employing FSC-A/H. Subsequently, live cells are gated as DAPI negative. Then, lineage negative cells from which LSK cells are selected as c-kit and Sca-1 positive. Finally, HSCs are gated as CD150 positive and CD48 negative. (**b**) To properly select the lineage negative gate, a backgating strategy is used. Overlap your LSK population with the live cells into the lineage/streptavidin plot to determine where the LSK cells reside

4 Notes

1. From one 8-to-12-week-old C57BL/6 mouse, we usually obtain 4000-to-6000 purified HSCs. To obtain more HSCs from a mouse, dissect the hip bones, spine, and other long bones (i.e., sternum, humerus, radius).
2. As an alternative method to flush the marrow out of the bones we have isolated the bone marrow crushing the bones using a mortar and pestle. Using this method, we have achieved higher number of total bone marrow cells. Place the clean bones in a mortar containing 10 mL of FACS buffer. Crush the bones using the pestle until bones resemble a homogeneous white pellet, while the red marrow is dispersed in the FACS buffer. Pipette up and down with a 10 mL pipette until all red marrow are dissolved in the FACS buffer and filter through a 70 μm strainer placed in a 50 mL centrifuge tube. Add 10 mL to the mortar, rinse, and collect the marrow into the 50 mL tube. Repeat this step three times.
3. Lyse the red blood cells for exactly 2 min—exceeding this time could lead to over lysis and loss of white blood cells. If after the 5 min centrifugation there is still a large red blood cell pellet present, repeat the lysis process for an extra 2 min.

4. It is important to shake the microbeads prior to usage to avoid aggregation of the magnetic beads in the bottom of the tube.
5. AutoMACS Pro 15 mL rack contains a cooling agent that under temperatures lower than 8 degrees turns into a solid state to maintain a chilled temperature during cell separation. Caution must be taken to not chill the rack in the freezer (or temperatures lower than 0 degrees) as samples may freeze. Precool the rack for at least 2 h in the fridge before use.
6. For RNA preparation, we isolate HSCs directly into 350 μL of RLT plus buffer (Qiagen) and extract RNA immediately (alternatively samples in RLT buffer can be stored at − 80 degrees). For transplantation assays, we sort HSCs directly into FACS buffer (containing or not containing BM support cells) and transplant into mice without centrifugation. We recommend to perform several tests to determine the accuracy of the cell sorter and count the number of cells after sorting.

Acknowledgments

This work was supported by the Life Science Research Network Wales, an initiative funded through the Welsh Government's Ser Cymru program, Leukaemia Cancer Society, Leukaemia Research Appeal for Wales and the Lady Tata Memorial Trust. JBMG was funded by a Ser Cymru Richard Whipp Studentship.

References

1. Ildstad ST, Shirwan H, Leventhal J (2011) Is durable macrochimerism key to achieving clinical transplantation tolerance? Curr Opin Organ Transplant 16:343–344
2. Leventhal J, Abecassis M, Miller J et al (2012) Chimerism and tolerance without GVHD or engraftment syndrome in HLA-mismatched combined kidney and hematopoietic stem cell transplantation. Sci Transl Med 4:124ra28. https://doi.org/10.1126/scitranslmed.3003509
3. Shizuru JA, Weissman IL, Kernoff R et al (2000) Purified hematopoietic stem cell grafts induce tolerance to alloantigens and can mediate positive and negative T cell selection. Proc Natl Acad Sci U S A 97:9555–9560. https://doi.org/10.1073/pnas.170279297
4. Zheng J, Umikawa M, Zhang S et al (2011) Ex vivo expanded hematopoietic stem cells overcome the MHC barrier in allogeneic transplantation. Cell Stem Cell 9:119–130. https://doi.org/10.1016/j.stem.2011.06.003
5. Fujisaki J, Wu J, Carlson AL et al (2011) In vivo imaging of T reg cells providing immune privilege to the haematopoietic stem-cell niche. Nature 474:216–220. https://doi.org/10.1038/nature10160
6. Sullivan KM, Goldmuntz EA, Keyes-Elstein L et al (2018) Myeloablative autologous stem-cell transplantation for severe scleroderma. N Engl J Med 378:35–47. https://doi.org/10.21430/M3SM4LTLH
7. Forsberg EC, Prohaska SS, Katzman S et al (2005) Differential expression of novel potential regulators in hematopoietic stem cells. PLoS Genet 1:e28. https://doi.org/10.1371/journal.pgen.0010028
8. Kiel MJ, Yilmaz ÖH, Iwashita T et al (2005) SLAM family receptors distinguish hematopoietic stem and progenitor cells and reveal endothelial niches for stem cells. Cell 121:1109–1121. https://doi.org/10.1016/j.cell.2005.05.026

9. Kiel MJ, Yilmaz OH, Morrison SJ (2008) CD150 cells are transiently reconstituting multipotent progenitors with little or no stem cell activity. Blood 111:4413–4414

10. Kim I, He S, Yilmaz ÖH et al (2006) Enhanced purification of fetal liver hematopoietic stem cells using SLAM family receptors. Blood 108:737–744. https://doi.org/10.1182/blood-2005-10-4135

11. Yilmaz ÖH, Kiel MJ, Morrison SJ (2006) SLAM family markers are conserved among hematopoietic stem cells from old and reconstituted mice and markedly increase their purity. Blood 107:924–930. https://doi.org/10.1182/blood-2005-05-2140

12. Oguro H, Ding L, Morrison SJ (2013) SLAM family markers resolve functionally distinct subpopulations of hematopoietic stem cells and multipotent progenitors. Cell Stem Cell 13:102–116. https://doi.org/10.1016/j.stem.2013.05.014

Chapter 3

Generation of Antigen-Specific T Cells from Human Induced Pluripotent Stem Cells

Toshinobu Nishimura and Hiromitsu Nakauchi

Abstract

Human induced pluripotent stem cells (iPSCs) are a potential source of blood cells for transfusion therapies and a promising tool for studying the ontogeny of hematopoiesis. The development of widely varying reprogramming methods has enabled us nowadays to obtain iPSCs even from a small number of antigen-specific T cells from patients. As these T-cell-derived iPSCs (T-iPSCs) carry TCR gene rearrangements in their genomic DNA, they are likely useful for producing antigen-specific T cells and for studying T-cell development. T-cell immunotherapy is potentially an effective therapeutic strategy against many types of cancers and viral infections. If antigen-specific T cells tailored against diseases and for patients can be easily obtained, T-cell immunotherapy should become a popular choice of therapy. Here, we show the in vitro way to guide T-iPSCs sequentially to yield hematopoietic stem/progenitor cells (HSPCs), T-lineage cells, and mature CD8 single-positive T cells. These in vitro-generated $CD8^+$ T cells display antigen-specific cytotoxity and perform general T-cell functions. This novel protocol thus provides means to generate antigen-specific T cells as well as chances to study normal human lymphopoiesis. It may help identify, and then clear away, barriers to T-cell immunotherapy such as immunological tolerance and cell exhaustion. T-iPSCs can confer their juvenile status upon their descendant T cells during pluripotency reprogramming and redifferentiation. This phenomenon should help to eliminate T-cell exhaustion.

Key words Hematopoietic stem/progenitor cell, Human iPSCs, Immunotherapy, Rejuvenation, T cell

1 Introduction

Within human hematopoiesis, T-cell differentiation occurs at two locations. Hematopoietic stem/progenitor cells (HSPCs) differentiate into lymphoid progenitor cells and early T-cell progenitors (ETPs) in the bone marrow. After that, they move to the thymus and begin commitment and specification as T-lineage cells. Maturing T-lineage cells remain inside the thymus, which they leave after they have become CD4- or CD8-single positive cells. In vitro T-cell differentiation methods in essence mimic these processes by employing C3H10T1/2 stromal cells for HSPC generation [1, 2], OP9-DL1 stromal cells for T-lineage commitment [3, 4],

Ashleigh S. Boyd (ed.), *Immunological Tolerance: Methods and Protocols*, Methods in Molecular Biology, vol. 1899,
https://doi.org/10.1007/978-1-4939-8938-6_3, © Springer Science+Business Media, LLC, part of Springer Nature 2019

and peripheral blood mononuclear cells (PBMCs) for CD8-single positive maturation [5, 6]. In brief, C3H10T1/2 provides the environment for efficient hematopoietic differentiation, OP9-DL1 ignite Notch signaling via expression of delta-like 1 (DL1), one of the Notch ligands, and PBMCs assist in proliferation of stimulated maturing T cells. In this chapter, we describe detailed methods to yield T cells from T-iPSCs in vitro.

2 Materials

2.1 Culturing T-iPSCs

1. Phosphate-buffered saline (PBS): PBS used in the chapter is free from both Ca^{2+} and Mg^{2+}.
2. Essential 8 medium (Life Technologies, Carlsbad, CA) [7].
3. 5 μg/ml recombinant human vitronectin (VTN; Life Technologies) (*see* **Note 1**).
4. 5 mM EDTA (Sigma-Aldrich, St Louis, MO), dissolved in PBS and sterilized by 0.22-μm filtration.
5. 10 mM Rock inhibitor (Wako, Osaka, Japan): 1000× stock solution in water, stored at −20 °C. Avoid repeated freeze-thaw cycles.
6. Dimethyl sulfoxide (DMSO; Wako).
7. Freezing solution: Essential 8 medium containing 10% DMSO.
8. 6-Well culture dishes (TPP, Techno Plastics Products, Trasadingen, Switzerland).

2.2 Culturing C3H10T1/2 Feeder Cells

1. C3H10T1/2 cell line (RIKEN Bio-Resource Center, Tsukuba, Japan).
2. PBS.
3. Eagle's basal medium (BME; Invitrogen, Carlsbad, CA).
4. Fetal bovine serum (FBS) for C3H10T1/2 cells (Biological Industries, Kibbutz Beit-Haemek, Israel).
5. 10T1/2 medium: BME supplemented with 10% FBS for C3H10T1/2 cells and 2 mM L-glutamine.
6. 0.05% trypsin-EDTA (Sigma-Aldrich).
7. 0.1% gelatin from porcine skin (Sigma-Aldrich), dissolved in PBS and autoclaved (*see* **Note 2**).
8. 0.1% trypan blue (Sigma-Aldrich), dissolved in PBS.
9. 15 ml centrifuge tubes and 10 cm culture dishes (TPP®, Techno Plastics Products AG).

2.3 Culturing OP9-DL1 Feeder Cells

1. OP9-DL1 cell line (RIKEN Bio-Resource Center).
2. PBS.

3. Modified Eagle medium alpha (α-MEM) (Gibco, Carlsbad, CA).
4. FBS for OP9 cells (Biological Industries; *see* **Note 3**).
5. OP9 medium: α-MEM supplemented with 20% FBS for OP9 cells and 2 mM L-glutamine.
6. 0.05% trypsin-EDTA (Sigma-Aldrich).
7. 0.1% gelatin from porcine skin (Sigma-Aldrich), dissolved in PBS and autoclaved (*see* **Note 2**).
8. 0.1% trypan blue (Sigma-Aldrich), dissolved in PBS.
9. 15 ml centrifuge tubes and 10 cm culture dishes (TPP, Techno Plastics Products).

2.4 Differentiation of T-iPSCs into Multipotent Hematopoietic Stem/Progenitor Cells Via iPS-Sacs

1. PBS.
2. Iscove's modified Dulbecco's medium (IMDM; Sigma-Aldrich).
3. FBS for embryonic body (EB) formation (Gibco; *see* **Note 4**).
4. 100× insulin/transferrin/selenite (ITS) solution (Gibco): A cocktail of 10 μg/ml human insulin, 5.5 μg/ml human transferrin, and 5 ng/ml sodium selenite.
5. 50 mg/ml ascorbic acid (Sigma-Aldrich): 1000× stock solution in water, sterilized by 0.22 μm filtration. Store at 4 °C no longer than 1 month.
6. 450 μM α-monothioglycerol (MTG; Sigma-Aldrich): 1000× stock solution in PBS, sterilized by 0.22 μm filtration, and stored at −20 °C.
7. EB medium: IMDM supplemented with 15% FBS for EB formation, 1× ITS, 50 μg/ml ascorbic acid, 450 nM MTG, and 2 mM L-glutamine.
8. 20 μg/ml recombinant human vascular endothelial growth factor (hVEGF; R&D Systems, Minneapolis, MN): Dissolved in PBS containing 0.1% bovine serum albumin and stored at −20 °C. Avoid repeated freeze-thaw cycles.
9. 10 μg/ml recombinant human stem cell factor (hSCF; R&D Systems): Dissolved in PBS containing 0.1% bovine serum albumin and stored at −20 °C. Avoid repeated freeze-thaw cycles.
10. 10 μg/ml recombinant human thrombopoietin (hTPO; R&D Systems): Dissolved in PBS containing 0.1% bovine serum albumin and stored at −20 °C. Avoid repeated freeze-thaw cycles.
11. 10 μg/ml recombinant human FLT-3 ligand (hFLT-3L; Peprotech, Rocky Hill, NJ): Dissolved in PBS containing

0.1% bovine serum albumin and stored at −20 °C. Avoid repeated freeze-thaw cycles.

12. 10 μg/ml recombinant human interleukin-7 (hIL-7; Peprotech): Dissolved in PBS containing 0.1% bovine serum albumin and stored at −20 °C. Avoid repeated freeze-thaw cycles.
13. 2.5% trypsin (Invitrogen).
14. Knockout serum replacement (KSR; Gibco).
15. 100 mM $CaCl_2$ (Wako): 100× stock solution, dissolved in water and autoclaved. Stored at 4 °C no longer than 12 months.
16. hiPS dissociation solution: 0.25% trypsin, 1 mM $CaCl_2$, and 20% KSR in PBS. Stored at −20 °C no longer than 12 months.
17. 100 U/ml collagenase IV solution (Gibco): Dissolved in PBS and sterilized by 0.22 μm filtration. Stored at 4 °C no longer than 2 weeks.
18. 40 μm nylon cell strainer (BD Bioscience, San Jose, CA).
19. 0.1% gelatin from porcine skin (Sigma-Aldrich): dissolved in PBS and autoclaved.
20. 50 ml centrifuge tubes and 10 cm culture dishes (TPP, Techno Plastics Products).

2.5 Differentiation of Hematopoietic Stem/Progenitor Cells to T-Lineage Cells

1. OP9 medium; *see* above, Subheading 2.3.
2. 10 μg/ml hSCF (R&D Systems); *see* above, Subheading 2.3.
3. 10 μg/ml hTPO (R&D Systems); *see* above, Subheading 2.3.
4. 10 μg/ml hFLT-3L (Peprotech); *see* above, Subheading 2.3.
5. 10 μg/ml hIL-7 (Peprotech); *see* above, Subheading 2.3.
6. Antibody against (α)-CD34-FITC (BD Pharmingen, San Diego, CA).
7. α-CD38-PerCP/Cy5.5 (BioLegend, San Diego, CA).
8. α-CD45-V500 (BD Bioscience).
9. α-CD7-APC (BioLegend).
10. α-CD1a-PE (BioLegend).
11. α-CD45RA-APC/Cy7 (BioLegend).
12. α-CD56-PE/Cy7 (BD Bioscience).
13. α-CD3-eFluor450 (eBioscience, San Diego, CA).
14. α-TCRαβ-FITC (eBioscience).
15. α-CD5-Alexa Fluor 700 (BD Pharmingen).
16. α-CD4-APC/H7 (BD Bioscience).
17. α-CD8-PerCP/Cy5.5 (BioLegend).

18. 1 mg/ml propidium iodide (PI; Sigma-Aldrich): 1000× stock solution in PBS, stored in the dark at 4 °C. (Extremely toxic substance; follow local guidelines for safe use and disposal.)

2.6 Differentiation of T-Lineage Cells into CD8-Single Positive T Cells

1. RPMI-1640 (Sigma-Aldrich).
2. FBS for T cells (Gibco).
3. 10 μg/ml hIL-7 (Peprotech); *see* above, Subheading 2.3.
4. 10 μg/ml recombinant human interleukin-15 (hIL-15; Peprotech): dissolved in PBS containing 0.1% bovine serum albumin and stored at −20 °C. Avoid repeated freeze-thaw cycles.
5. R10 medium: RPMI-1640 medium supplemented with 10% FBS for T cells and 2 mM L-glutamine.
6. Lymphosepar (Takara Bio, Otsu, Japan).
7. 5 mg/ml phytohemagglutinin (PHA-L; Sigma-Aldrich): 1000× stock solution in water, sterilized by 0.22 μm filtration. Stored at 4 °C no longer than a year.
8. Multimer-PE (MBL, Aichi, Japan).
9. α-CD3-eFluor450 (eBioscience).
10. α-CD45-V500 (BD Bioscience).
11. α-CD4-APC/H7 (BD Bioscience).
12. α-CD8-APC (BioLegend).
13. α-CD7-FITC (BioLegend).
14. α-CD5-Alexa Fluor 700 (BD Pharmingen).
15. α-CD1a-PE (BioLegend).
16. α-CD56-PE/Cy7 (BD Bioscience).
17. 1 mg/ml PI (Sigma-Aldrich): *see* above, Subheading 2.5.
18. T25 flask (TPP, Techno Plastics Products).

3 Methods

3.1 Culturing T-iPSCs

T-iPSCs should be passaged when the cells are at 85% confluence (*see* **Note 5**).

3.1.1 Thawing T-iPSCs

1. Thaw T-iPSCs quickly in a 37 °C water bath.
2. Pipette the cell suspension slowly and gently from the cryovial tube into a 15 ml centrifuge tube.
3. Add 10 ml essential 8 medium drop by drop while shaking the 15 ml tube.
4. Centrifuge the cells at 200 × *g* min at RT for 5 min.
5. Aspirate the supernatant and resuspend the cells in 3 ml Essential 8 medium containing 10 μM Rock inhibitor.

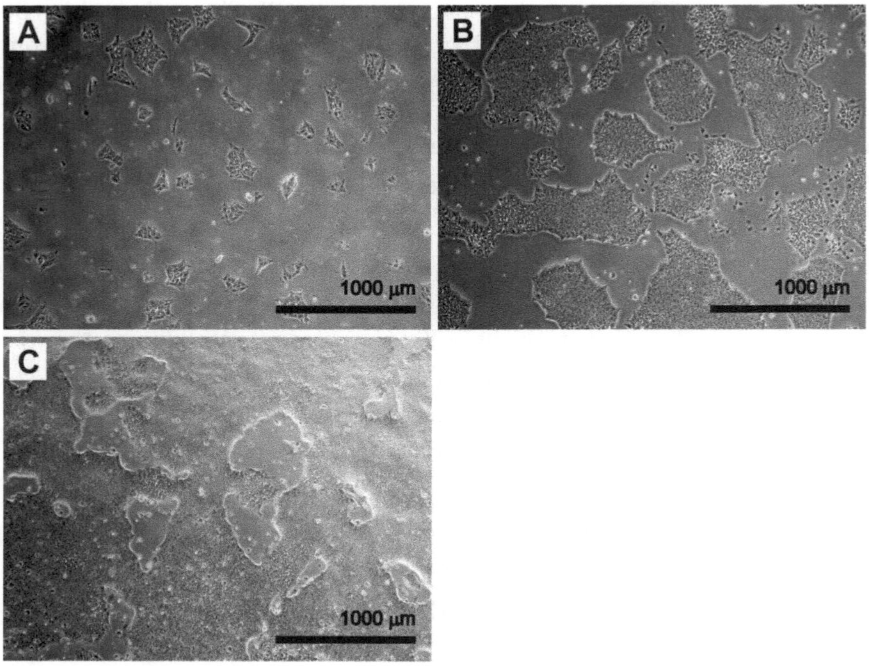

Fig. 1 Representative image of T-iPSCs. (**a**) Picture of T-iPSCs 1 day after passage. (**b**) Picture of T-iPSCs 3 days after passage. (**c**) Picture of T-iPSCs 5 days after passage. At this time point, they are at about 90% confluence

6. Transfer the resuspended cells into one well of a VTN-coated 6-well plate and place the dish in an incubator.
7. Incubate at 37 °C, 5% CO_2.

3.1.2 Maintaining T-iPSCs

1. Replace culture medium every day with 3–4 ml Essential 8 medium (Fig. 1b).
2. To passage the cells, remove the culture medium (Fig. 1c).
3. Wash the well twice (3 ml PBS in each wash).
4. Add 1 ml 5 mM EDTA solution and incubate the cells at 37 °C for 3–7 min until the cells start to separate everywhere in the colonies.
5. Aspirate away the EDTA solution and add to the cells 3 ml Essential 8 medium.
6. Pipette the cells 3–10 times, until colonies become clumps of 10–20 cells each.
7. Transfer 200–300 µl of cell suspension into each well of a VTN-coated 6-well plate containing 3 ml Essential 8 medium (no need to add Rock inhibitor).
8. Shake the plate to scatter the cell clumps evenly within the wells and place it in an incubator. Do not dawdle, because cell clumps begin to attach in as little as 3 min (Fig. 1a).

3.1.3 Freezing T-iPSCs

1. Prepare 5.5 ml freezing solution for T-iPSCs per well. Precool the solution on ice.
2. Passage the cells as described in **steps 2–4** of the previous subsection, and add 5 ml freezing solution to each well.
3. Disaggregate the T-iPSC colonies by pipetting 3–10 times, until colonies become clumps of 10–20 cells.
4. Aliquot 1 ml cell suspension per cryovial.
5. Freeze the cells at −80 °C. Transfer them to liquid nitrogen for storage.

3.2 Culturing C3H10T1/2 Stromal Cells

The C3H10T1/2 cells are spindle-shaped cells established from mesenchymal cells derived from C3H mouse embryo. C3H10T1/2 cells should be passaged when the cells are at 80% confluence (*see* **Notes 6** and 7).

3.2.1 Thawing C3H10T1/2 Cells

1. Thaw C3H10T1/2 cells quickly in a 37 °C water bath.
2. Pipette the cell suspension slowly and gently from the cryovial tube into a 15 ml centrifuge tube.
3. Add 10 ml 10T1/2 medium drop by drop while shaking the 15 ml tube.
4. Centrifuge the cells at 400 × *g* at RT for 5 min.
5. Aspirate the supernatant and resuspend the cells in 10 ml 10T1/2 medium.
6. Transfer the resuspended cells into a 10 cm dish and place the dish in an incubator.
7. Incubate at 37 °C, 5% CO_2.

3.2.2 Maintaining C3H10T1/2 Cells

1. For routine culture, change the culture medium every 2 days.
2. To passage the cells, remove the culture medium and wash the cells twice with 10 ml PBS in each wash.
3. Add 1 ml 0.05% trypsin-EDTA to each 10 cm dish and incubate at 37 °C for 5 min.
4. Add 10 ml 10T1/2 medium to each 10 cm dish and pipette well to disperse the cells into single cells.
5. Centrifuge the cells at 400 × *g* at RT for 5 min.
6. Aspirate away the supernatant and resuspend the cells in 8 ml 10T1/2 medium.
7. Transfer 1/8 volume (1 ml) of cell suspension into a 10 cm dish with 9 ml 10T1/2 medium (total 10 ml).
8. Place the dish in an incubator and incubate at 37 °C, 5% CO_2.

3.2.3 Preparation of C3H10T1/2 Feeder Cells for Hematopoietic Differentiation

1. Irradiate the C3H10T1/2 cells (in 10 cm dishes) at 50 Gy to stop cell growth.
2. Passage the cells as described in **steps 2–6** of the previous subsection.
3. Seed 1.0×10^6 C3H10T1/2 cells into each 10 cm dish coated with 0.1% gelatin.
4. Confirm that the cells are uniformly spread.

3.3 Culturing OP9-DL1 Stromal Cells

OP9-DL1 cells should be passaged when the cells are at 80% confluence (*see* **Note 8**).

3.3.1 Thawing OP9-DL1 Cells

1. Thaw OP9-DL1 cells quickly in a 37 °C water bath.
2. Pipette the cell suspension slowly and gently from the cryovial tube into a 15 ml centrifuge tube.
3. Add 10 ml OP9 medium drop by drop while shaking the 15 ml tube.
4. Centrifuge the cells at 400 × *g* at RT for 5 min.
5. Aspirate away the supernatant and resuspend the cells in 10 ml OP9 medium.
6. Transfer the resuspended cells into a 10 cm dish and place the dish in an incubator.
7. Incubate at 37 °C, 5% CO_2.

3.3.2 Maintaining OP9-DL1 Cells

1. For routine culture, change the culture medium every 2 days.
2. To passage the cells, remove the culture medium and wash the cells twice with 10 ml PBS in each wash.
3. Add 1 ml 0.05% trypsin-EDTA to each 10 cm dish and incubate at 37 °C for 5 min.
4. Add 10 ml OP9 medium and pipet well to disperse into single cells.
5. Centrifuge the cells at 400 × *g* at RT for 5 min.
6. Aspirate away the supernatant and resuspend the cells in 6 ml OP9 medium.
7. Transfer 1/6 volume of cell suspension (1 ml) into a 10 cm dish with 9 ml OP9 medium (total 10 ml).
8. Place the dish in an incubator and incubate at 37 °C, 5% CO_2.

3.3.3 Preparation of OP9-DL1 Feeder Cells for T-Lineage Differentiation

1. Irradiate the OP9-DL1 cells (in 10 cm dishes) at 50 Gy to stop cell growth.
2. Passage the cells as described in **steps 2–6** of the previous subsection.

3. Seed 1.0×10^6 OP9-DL1 cells into each 10 cm dish coated with 0.1% gelatin.
4. Confirm that the cells are uniformly spread.

3.4 Differentiation of Hematopoietic Progenitors Via an iPS-Sac on C3H10T1/2 Feeder Cells

For efficient induction of hematopoietic progenitors, to culture T-iPSCs at the appropriate density is important. Note that T-iPSCs grow less well when they are disaggregated into single cells.

3.4.1 Induction of iPS-Sacs

1. Prepare one well (6-well plate) of T-iPSCs 4–5 days before differentiation experiments for 8 dishes (10 cm dishes) of C3H10T1/2 feeder cells.
2. When T-iPSCs grow at 90% confluence, remove the culture medium and wash twice with 3 ml PBS in each wash.
3. Add 1 ml hiPS dissociation solution and incubate at 37 °C for 5–7 min.
4. When the rims of T-iPSC colonies roll up, aspirate away the hiPS dissociation solution.
5. Add 3 ml EB medium and disaggregate the T-iPSC colonies into 50-cell clumps by gentle pipetting (*see* **Note 9**).
6. Seed 200–300 μl of cell suspension into each 10 cm dish of C3H10T1/2 feeder cells in 10 ml EB medium containing 20 ng/ml hVEGF. About 100 clumps per 10 cm dish is appropriate for hematopoietic differentiation (Fig. 2a).
7. Incubate at 5% O_2 (hypoxia) for 6 days initially and at 20% O_2 (normoxia) for 6 days thereafter. Change the culture medium every 3 days.
8. At about 8 days of culture iPS-Sacs, including floating roundish cells, emerge (Fig. 2b).

3.4.2 Disruption of iPS-Sacs and Collection of Hematopoietic Stem/Progenitor Cells

1. Remove the culture medium and wash the cells twice with 10 ml PBS in each wash.
2. Add 10 ml collagenase IV solution (100 U/ml) to each dish and incubate at 37 °C for 45 min.
3. Collect and filtrate the collagenase IV solution through 40 μm cell strainers into 50 ml centrifuge tubes. Do not discard cell strainers, as it is reused in a later step.
4. Add 5 ml 0.05% trypsin/EDTA to each dish and incubate at 37 °C for 15–20 min.
5. Pipette the iPS-Sacs vigorously to dissociate the cells into single cells.
6. Filtrate cells/trypsin mixture through 40 μm cell strainers into the tubes that contain collagenase IV solution.

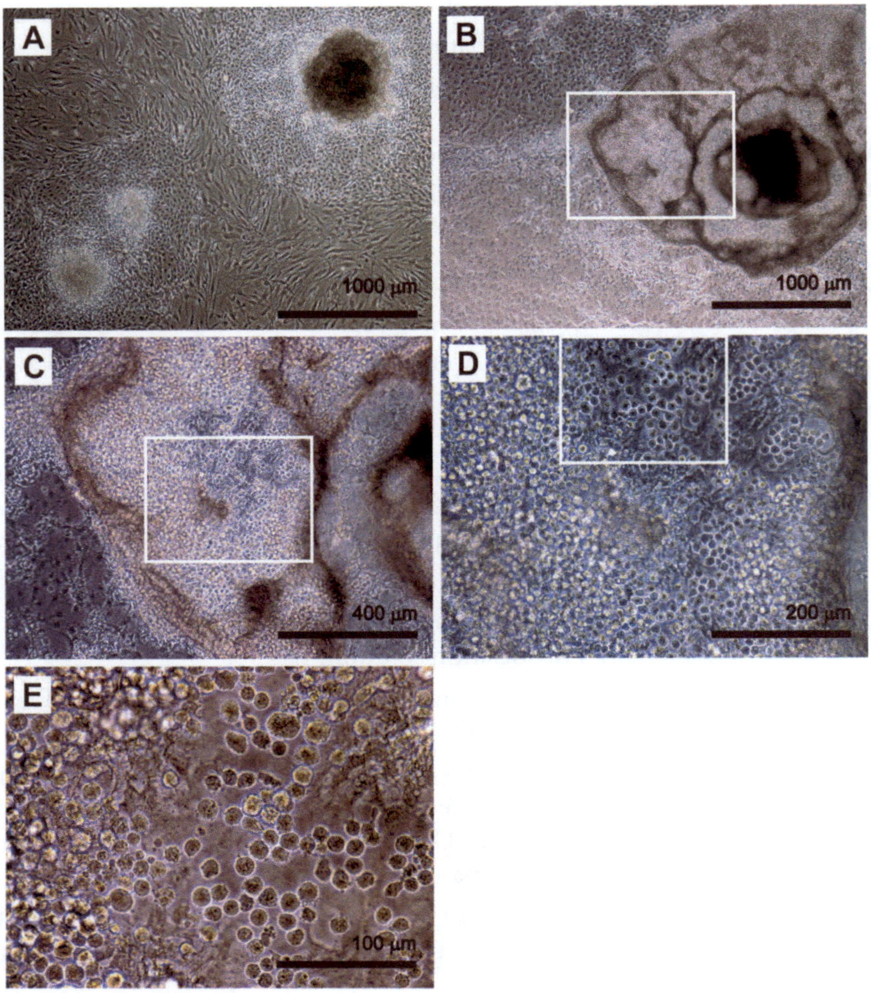

Fig. 2 Hematopoietic differentiation via T-iPS-Sacs. (**a**) Picture of T-iPS-Sacs on C3H10T1/2 feeder cells 3 days after seeding. (**b–e**) Picture of a T-iPSC-Sac on C3H10T1/2 feeder cells 14 days after seeding. (**c**), (**d**), and (**e**) are magnified images of the regions enclosed by white boxes in (**b**), (**c**), and (**d**), respectively

7. Rinse each 10 cm dish with 5 ml OP9 medium and combine the rinsings with the collagenase IV/cells/trypsin mixture (likewise, filtrating them through 40 μm cell strainers).
8. Centrifuge the cells at 300 × *g* at RT for 10 min.
9. Seed the cells onto 4 0.1% gelatin-coated 10 cm dishes in 10 ml per dish OP9 medium containing 10 ng/ml hSCF, 10 ng/ml hTPO, 10 ng/ml hFLT-3L, and 10 ng/ml hIL-7.
10. Incubate at 37 °C for 2–4 h and harvest the floating cells.

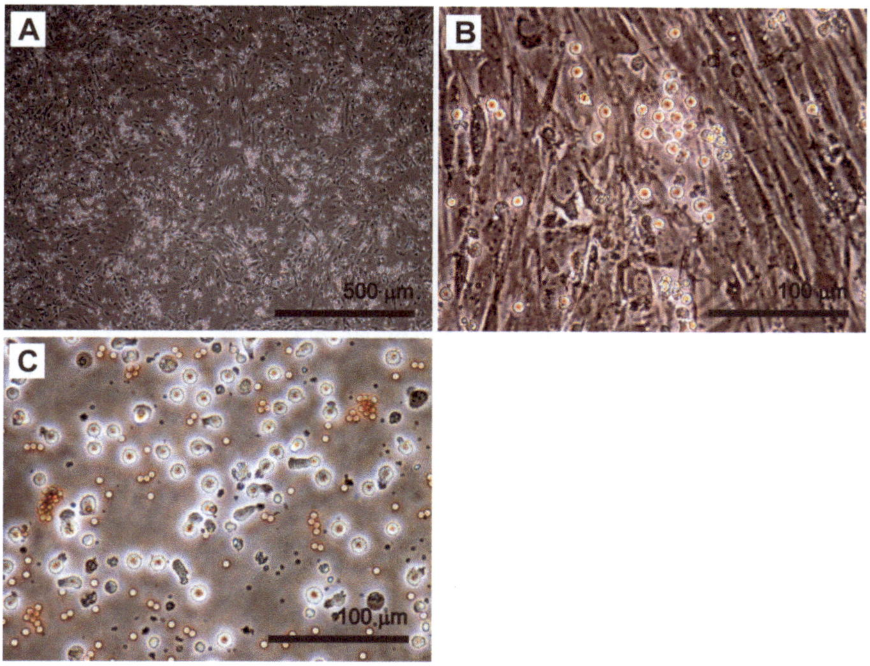

Fig. 3 T-lineage differentiating cells on OP9-DL1 feeder cells and CD8-single positive-maturing T cells. (**a**) Expanding HSPCs and/or lymphoid progenitor cells on OP9-DL1 feeder cells in the presence of hSCF and hTPO 6 days after seeding onto OP9-DL1 feeder cells. (**b**) T-lineage cells 24 days after differentiation on OP9-DL1 feeder cells. (**c**) CD8-single positive T cells 2 weeks after stimulation

3.5 Differentiation of Hematopoietic Progenitors into T-Lineage Cells on OP9-DL1 Feeder Cells

To cause the hematopoietic progenitors harvested from Subheading 3.4. to differentiate into T-lineage cells that express the hematopoietic cell marker (CD45), lymphoid cell markers (CD7, CD5, and CD1a), and T-lineage cell markers (CD3, CD4, CD8, and TCRαβ), coculture with OP9-DL1 is employed.

1. Seed the harvested floating cells into 10 cm dishes of OP9-DL1 feeder cells in 10 ml OP9 medium containing 10 ng/ml hSCF, 10 ng/ml hTPO, 10 ng/ml hFLT-3L, and 10 ng/ml hIL-7 (Fig. 3a) (*see* **Note 10**).
2. Coculture the cells on OP9-DL1 feeder cells for 6 days. Change half the culture medium every 3 days (*see* **Note 11**).
3. Harvest the floating cells and combine them into one container. Transfer the harvested, combined cells into a new 10 cm dish of OP9-DL1 feeder cells in 10 ml OP9 medium containing 5 ng/ml hFLT-3L and 1 ng/ml hIL-7 (Fig. 3b).
4. Coculture the cells on OP9-DL1 cells for 6 days. Change half the culture medium every 3 days (*see* **Note 11**).
5. Repeat **steps 3** and **4** twice more; i.e., total coculture time on OP9-DL1 cells is 24 days.

6. Harvest the floating cells. An aliquot is analyzed by FACS (Subheading 3.8.). The others are used for CD8-single positive maturation (see below).

3.6 Induction of CD8-Single Positive Maturation by TCR Stimulation and Coculture with PBMCs

3.6.1 Preparation of Freshly Isolated PBMCs

1. Mix 10 ml freshly isolated peripheral blood with 10 ml PBS (total 20 ml).
2. Pipette 20 ml Lymphosepar into a 50 ml centrifuge tube.
3. Add diluted peripheral blood to Lymphosepar gently, taking care not to disturb the boundary interface between peripheral blood and Lymphosepar.
4. Centrifuge the tube at 1500 rpm (240 × *g*) at RT for 30 min, braking as gently as possible (or allowing rotation to cease without braking).
5. PBMCs are concentrated at the phase boundary. Harvest them by gentle pipetting and transfer them into a new 50 ml centrifuge tube.
6. Add PBS to an end volume of 50 ml.
7. Centrifuge the cells at 300 × *g* at RT for 10 min.
8. Aspirate the supernatant and resuspend the cells in 20 ml PBS.
9. Wrap the tube cap with parafilm and irradiate the cells at 40 Gy to stop cell growth.
10. Centrifuge the cells at 300 × *g* at RT for 10 min.
11. Aspirate the supernatant and resuspend the cells in 10 ml R10 medium.

3.6.2 TCR Stimulation and Coculture with PBMCs

1. Combine the T-lineage cells and irradiated PBMCs in a T25 flask (total volume 10 ml).
2. Stimulate the cells with 5 μg/ml PHA-L in the presence of 10 ng/ml IL-7 and 10 ng/ml hIL-15.
3. Incubate at 37 °C for 2 weeks (*see* **Note 12**). Half the volume of culture medium is removed and replaced with fresh culture medium 5, 8, and 11 days after stimulation (*see* **Note 13**).
4. Harvest the cells (Fig. 3c), with an aliquot to be analyzed and/or sorted by FACS (Subheading 3.8).

3.7 FACS

3.7.1 FACS for T-Lineage Cells

1. Resuspend about 1×10^5 cells (corresponding to 0.1 test) in 50–100 μl PBS in a 15 ml centrifuge tube.
2. Add a quantity sufficient for 0.1 test of cells of antibody panel 1 (α-CD34-FITC, α-CD38-PerCP/Cy5.5, α-CD45-V500, α-CD7-APC, α-CD5-Alexa Fluor 700, α-CD1a-PE, and α-CD45RA-APC/Cy7) or antibody panel 2 (α-CD56-PE/Cy7, α-CD45-V500, α-CD3-eFluor450, α-TCRαβ-FITC, α-CD5-Alexa Fluor 700, α-CD1a-PE, α-CD4-APC/H7, and α-CD8-PerCP/Cy5.5).

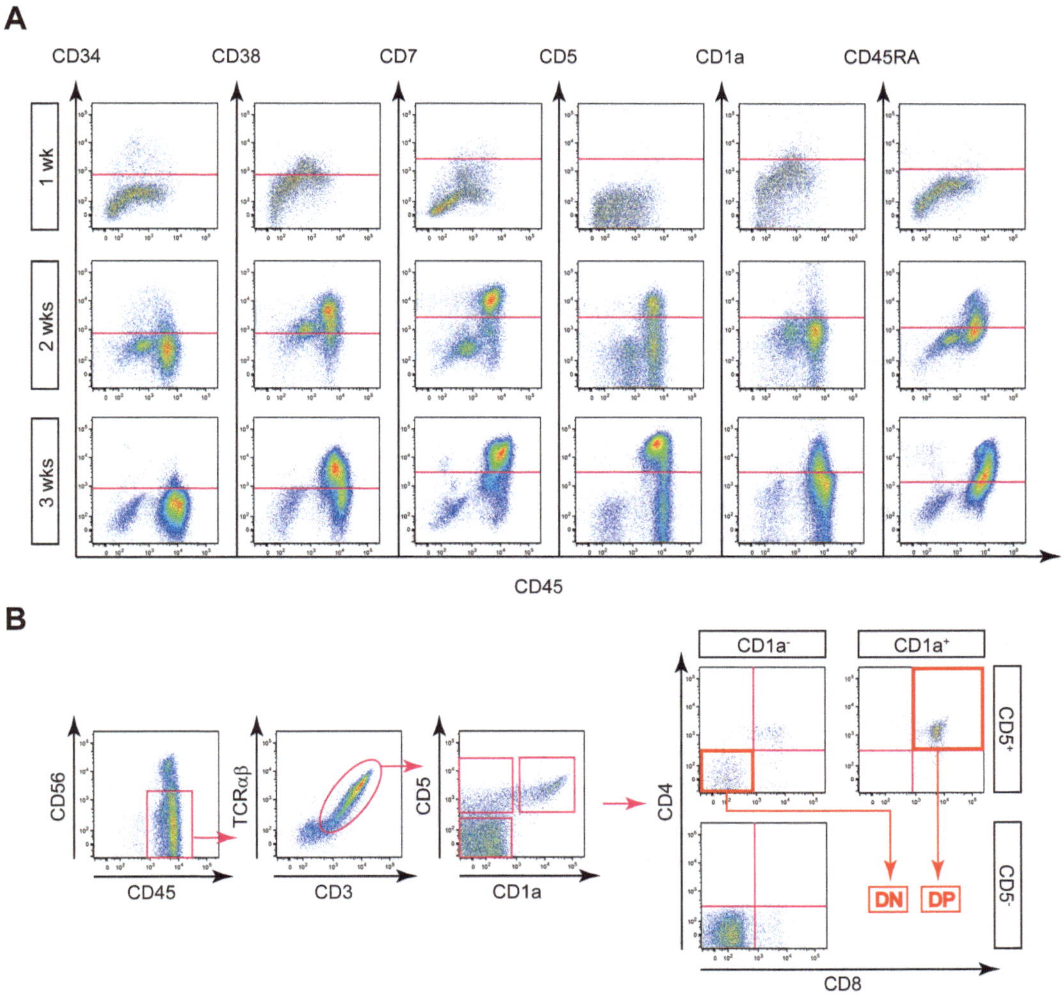

Fig. 4 FACS analyses for T-lineage cells on OP9-DL1 feeder cells. (**a**) Developmental progression from HSPCs in T-iPS-Sacs into T-lineage cells are shown in cell surface expression of CD34, CD38, CD7, CD5, CD1a, and CD45RA. (**b**) Cells floating on OP9-DL1 feeder cells were collected and analyzed 24 days after starting T-lineage differentiation

3. Incubate on ice for 30 min in the dark.
4. Wash the cells with 10 ml PBS.
5. Aspirate the supernatant and resuspend the cells in 200 μl PI/PBS.
6. Analyze the cells by FACS Aria II (Panel 1: Fig. 4a and panel 2: Fig. 4b).

3.7.2 FACS Analysis and/or Sorting for CD8-Single Positive T Cells Using Multimer

1. Resuspend 1×10^6 cells (corresponding to 1 test) in 100 μl PBS in a 15 ml centrifuge tube.
2. Add enough Multimer-PE for 1 test of cells.
3. Incubate on ice for 30 min in the dark.

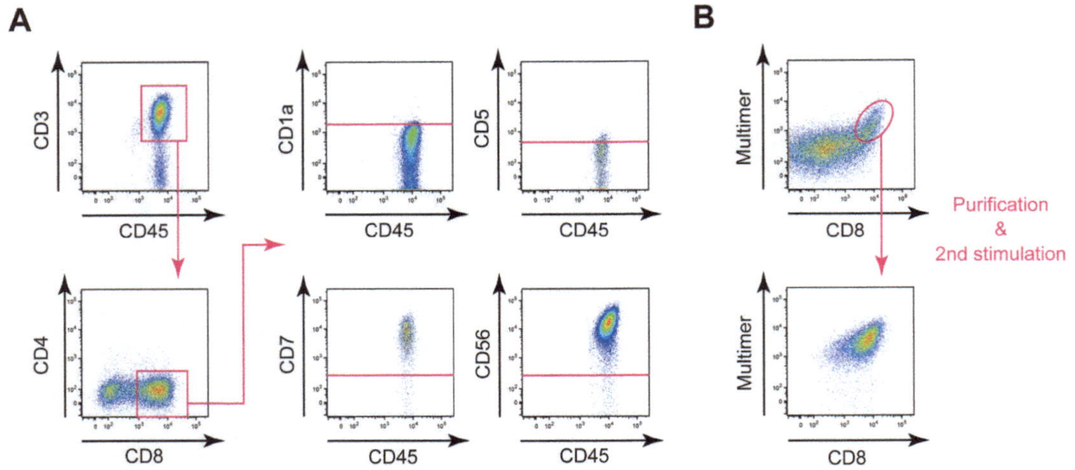

Fig. 5 FACS analyses for CD8-single positive mature T cells. (**a**) Flow cytometric analysis of the phenotypes of T cells 2 weeks after the stimulation of T-lineage cells. (**b**) Recognition of Multimer-PE 2 weeks after the stimulation of T-lineage cells (upper panel). Multimer-positive cells were sorted by FACS, then stimulated and cultured for an additional 14 days, after which the expanded T cells were re-analyzed for Multimer (lower panel)

4. Wash the cells with 10 ml PBS.
5. Resuspend the cells in 100 μl PBS.
6. Add enough α-CD3-eFluor450, α-CD45-V500, α-CD4-APC/H7, α-CD8-APC, α-CD1a-PE, α-CD7-FITC, α-CD5-Alexa Fluor 700, and α-CD56-PE/Cy7 for 1 test of cells.
7. Incubate on ice for 30 min in the dark.
8. Wash the cells with 10 ml PBS.
9. Aspirate the supernatant and resuspend the cells in 200 μl PI/PBS.
10. Analyze and/or sort the cells by FACS Aria II (Fig. 5).

3.8 Restimulation of CD8-Single Positive T Cells for Further Expansion

1. Sort $CD8^+$/$Multimer^+$ cells.
2. Prepare 10× as many freshly isolated and irradiated PBMCs (40 Gy) as sorted $CD8^+$/$Multimer^+$ cells.
3. Resuspend sorted $CD8^+$/$Multimer^+$ cells and irradiated PBMCs together in R10 medium at appropriate cell concentration ($<1.0 \times 10^6$ cells/ml).
4. Add PHA-L (5 μg/ml), hIL-7 (10 ng/ml), and hIL-15 (10 ng/ml).
5. Incubate at 37 °C for 2 weeks (*see* **Note 12**). Half the volume of culture medium is removed and replaced with fresh culture medium 5, 8, and 11 days after stimulation (*see* **Note 13**).

4 Notes

1. Add 1 ml 5 μg/ml VTN solution to each well of a 6-well plate. Incubate the plates at RT for 1 h, alternatively at 4 °C overnight. Aspirate the VTN solution and discard. It is not necessary to rinse the wells after the removal of VTN solution.
2. Add 1 ml 0.1% gelatin solution to each 10 cm dish. Incubate the plates at RT for 15 min. Aspirate the gelatin solution and discard. It is not necessary to rinse the wells after the removal of gelatin solution.
3. T-lineage induction efficiency is affected by FBS batch variation. Batch screening is recommended to obtain best results.
4. HSPC induction efficiency is affected by FBS batch variation. Batch screening is recommended to obtain best results.
5. Be careful not to allow T-iPSCs to become overgrown (>90% confluence) as they may lose their capacity for hematopoietic differentiation.
6. Be careful not to allow C3H10T1/2 cells to become overgrown (>90% confluence) as they may lose the ability to support hematopoietic differentiation of T-iPSCs.
7. For generating hematopoietic progenitors from hESCs or hiPSCs, coculture with OP9 cells is broadly used. We compared the ability of C3H10T1/2 cells and OP9 cells to support hematopoietic differentiation from hESCs and hiPSCs and found no significant difference in ability to support hematopoiesis between these two types of feeder cells.
8. Be careful not to allow OP9-DL1 cells to be overgrown (>90% confluence) as they may lose the ability to support T-lineage differentiation of HSPCs.
9. Be careful not to allow T-iPSCs to be triturated <20-cell clamps. Small T-iPSC clumps form iPS-Sacs poorly, reducing the yield of HSPCs. Minimize the time of trypsinization.
10. Differentiating cells float just above or loosely attach to the OP9-DL1 cells, so leave the culture dish undisturbed for a couple of minutes to allow the floating cells to settle onto the OP9-DL1 cells. Aspirate the culture medium slowly with the tip of the pipet continually touching the surface of the culture medium, never tilting the culture dish.
11. Measure the cell number of floating cells and seed them at the concentration of 1.0×10^6 cells per 10 cm dish of OP9-DL1 feeder cells.
12. If the cell concentration becomes $>1.5 \times 10^6$ cells/ml, reduce the cell concentration by increasing the culture medium volume and/or split the cells into more bottles.

13. Maturing cells float just above the bottom surface, so leave the culture flask undisturbed for a couple of minutes to allow the floating cells to settle onto the bottom of the culture flask. Aspirate the culture medium slowly with the tip of the pipet continually touching the surface of the culture medium, never tilting the culture flask.

References

1. Vodyanik MA, Bork JA, Thomson JA, Slukvin II (2005) Human embryonic stem cell-derived CD34+ cells: efficient production in the coculture with OP9 stromal cells and analysis of lymphohematopoietic potential. Blood 105:617–626
2. Takayama N, Nishikii H, Usui J, Tsukui H, Sawaguchi A, Hiroyama T, Eto K, Nakauchi H (2008) Generation of functional platelets from human embryonic stem cells in vitro via ES-sacs, VEGF-promoted structures that concentrate hematopoietic progenitors. Blood 111:5298–5306
3. Schmitt TM, Zuniga-Pflucker JC (2002) Induction of T cell development from hematopoietic progenitor cells by delta-like-1 in vitro. Immunity 17:749–756
4. La Motte-Mohs RN, Herer E, Zuniga-Pflucker JC (2005) Induction of T-cell development from human cord blood hematopoietic stem cells by Delta-like 1 in vitro. Blood 105:1431–1439
5. Nishimura T, Kaneko S, Kawana-Tachikawa A, Tajima Y, Goto H, Zhu D, Nakayama-Hosoya K, Iriguchi S, Uemura Y, Shimizu T et al (2013) Generation of rejuvenated antigen-specific T cells by reprogramming to pluripotency and redifferentiation. Cell Stem Cell 12:114–126
6. Vizcardo R, Masuda K, Yamada D, Ikawa T, Shimizu K, Fujii S, Koseki H, Kawamoto H (2013) Regeneration of human tumor antigen-specific T cells from iPSCs derived from mature CD8(+) T cells. Cell Stem Cell 12:31–36
7. Chen G, Gulbranson DR, Hou Z, Bolin JM, Ruotti V, Probasco MD, Smuga-Otto K, Howden SE, Diol NR, Propson NE et al (2011) Chemically defined conditions for human iPSC derivation and culture. Nat Methods 8:424–429

Part II

Isolation of Regulatory Lymphocyte Populations

Chapter 4

Isolation of Human Regulatory T Lymphocytes by Fluorescence-Activated Cell Sorting

Kate Milward, Joanna Hester, and Kathryn J. Wood

Abstract

Regulatory T cells (Tregs) are a population of lymphocytes that exerts suppressive effects upon the immune system. In human peripheral blood, the major population of T lymphocytes with suppressive capacity are defined by expression of the T cell co-receptor CD4 and the interleukin-2 receptor α-chain (CD25), combined with minimal expression of the interleukin-7 receptor α subunit (CD127). We begin by outlining the method for isolating peripheral blood mononuclear cells (PBMCs) from human blood by centrifugation of whole blood overlayed on a hydrophilic polysaccharide, with an additional erythrocyte lysis step. The protocol that follows utilizes Fluorescence-Activated Cell Sorting (FACS) for the isolation of this $CD4^{+}CD25^{+}CD127^{lo}$ population of regulatory T cells, with high yield and purity, from immunostained PBMCs. Prior to FACS isolation, this protocol exploits magnetic immunoselection for pre-enrichment of $CD25^{+}$ PBMC, which reduces the duration of the subsequent FACS isolation.

Key words Regulatory T cells, Treg, FACS, Fluorescence-activated cell sorting, Cell isolation

Abbreviations

cGMP	Current good manufacturing practice
FACS	Fluorescence-activated cell sorting
PBMC	Peripheral blood mononuclear cell
Treg	Regulatory T cell

1 Introduction

Regulatory T cells (Tregs) are a population of T lymphocytes that are capable of suppressing immune responses by modulating the proliferation, survival, or function of immune effector cells. The physiological role of Tregs in suppressing autoreactive effector populations that escape negative selection in the thymus serves to enforce peripheral tolerance to auto-antigen. Treg-mediated suppression is also implicated in homeostatic control of physiological

Ashleigh S. Boyd (ed.), *Immunological Tolerance: Methods and Protocols*, Methods in Molecular Biology, vol. 1899, https://doi.org/10.1007/978-1-4939-8938-6_4, © Springer Science+Business Media, LLC, part of Springer Nature 2019 immune responses, in order to minimize immunopathological tissue damage [1–4].

Unfortunately, no definitive pattern of cell surface antigen expression uniquely and universally marks human T cells with regulatory capacity. Indeed, regulatory function has been attributed to a plethora of T-cell subsets, each with its own characteristic set of molecular markers [5]: $CD8^+$ Tregs [6]; $CD4^-CD8^-$ Treg [7]; NKT cells [8]; $CD4^+CD25^+CD127^{lo}$ and γδ T cells [9]. Even $CD4^+$ Tregs can be subdivided into naïve (resting) versus activated (antigen-experienced) [10]; thymus-derived versus peripherally-induced [11]; Th-like Treg subsets [12]. The most reliable molecular correlate of Treg function is high expression of the transcription factor FoxP3, whose role in Treg development and function has been illuminated by genetic defects in FoxP3 deficient scurfy mice and IPEX (Immunodysregulation Polyendocrinopathy Enteropathy X-linked syndrome) patients and demonstrated in numerous experimental studies [1]. As such, CD4 and FoxP3 co-expression has come to define a widely-acknowledged "classical Treg" population. However, FoxP3 is also expressed by activated human effector T cells and, crucially, as this protein is absent from the cells surface, it cannot be tagged with antibody without disrupting the plasma membrane and killing the cells. As the most predominant, and best characterized, population of Tregs identified in human peripheral blood, this protocol focuses upon the isolation of $CD4^+CD25^+CD127^{lo}$ population of naturally-occurring Tregs. This population of Treg cells constitutes approximately 6% of $CD4^+$ T Cells in adult human peripheral blood [13]. There is strong consensus that the latter phenotype corresponds most closely to the $CD4^+FoxP3^+$ population [13, 14] and that sorting strategies incorporating depletion of $CD127^+$ cells yield the most suppressive Treg cells [13, 15, 16].

For research applications, there are two common methods for isolation of Tregs: magnetic immunoselection [17] and FACS [18]. Both methods rely upon labeling cell surface antigens with selectable particles. In the former method, these particles are antibodies against the antigenic marker, conjugated to magnetized metal particles or microbeads. When the labeled cell suspension is applied to a magnet, the magnetic particles or beads are captured, along with any cells expressing the antigen to which these particles are bound. Isolation based upon expression of multiple cell surface markers can be achieved by performing a limited number of positive and negative selection steps. Since only a single species of marker (the magnetized conjugate) is available and it is not possible to reverse the labeling of a cell sample, positive selection is restricted to a single antigen for a given isolation protocol. Despite this limitation, the majority of contaminating cell populations usually can be excluded in a single negative selection step, prior to positive selection, using an appropriate negative selection "cocktail" of bead-conjugated antibodies. Using a MACS Treg Isolation Kit for the selection of $CD4^{+}CD25^{+}CD127^{lo}$ from adult peripheral blood, we have isolated $CD4^{+}$ cells that were more than 80 per cent $FOXP3^{+}CD127^{lo}$ [19]. A further limitation of the magnetic isolation method is that it is inherently binary. Thus, this method can be used to separate cells that express the antigen from those that do not but cannot discriminate intermediate antigen expression levels, which may identify distinct cellular subpopulations. With respect to adaptation and refinement of the technology for the manufacture of cell products at a clinical grade and clinical scale, magnetic immunoselection technology is more advanced than the equivalent FACS technology, as exemplified my Miltenyi's CliniMACS system [20].

For FACS, cells are labeled using fluorochrome-conjugated antibodies with specificity for the antigenic marker. A cytometer detects the fluorescence emitted from these fluorochromes, upon laser excitation, as the cells are passed between fluorescence detectors in a stream of fluid droplets, each containing a single cell. The cytometer applies an electric charge to fluid droplets containing cells expressing surface markers matching the chosen selection parameters. The electric charge enables cell-containing droplets to be deflected into separate receptacles. Depending upon the model, a FACS cytometer can detect up to 18 colors, each marking a different antigen, simultaneously. In practise, it would be unwise to sort upon more than ten fluorochromes due to technical limitations in overcoming spectral overlap between a larger number of fluorochromes. Nonetheless, this allows the discrimination of cellular subsets with greater specificity, by incorporating more selection parameters. Moreover, the readout from these fluorochromes is analogue, reflecting the entire spectrum of antigen densities expressed by cells in the sample, which permits discrimination of cell populations defined by intermediate antigen expression. An additional advantage of FACS over magnetic selection is the ability to sort multiple cell populations simultaneously from the same sample. In this protocol, for example, it is recommended that effector T cells are sorted alongside regulatory T cells, to use as controls for research applications to which the sorted Tregs are destined.

For most applications, yield and purity are key criteria for cell isolation procedure. The challenge of generating large yields of Tregs can be overcome, independently of the cell isolation method, by expansion of naturally-occurring Tregs or by induction of adaptive Tregs from conventional T cells in vitro. The criterion of purity depends largely upon the efficiency of the cell isolation method, despite methods for removing contaminating cell populations from an impure population of Tregs after isolation, such as culturing a Treg-enriched population of T cells with Rapamycin to selectively eliminate $CD4^{+}$ effector T cells [21].

In addition to research applications, there is considerable interest in the isolation of Tregs for application as a cellular therapy to alleviate a spectrum of immunopathological conditions [22, 23]. Any protocol for the isolation of cells destined for adoptive cellular therapy must not only meet particularly stringent criteria for yield and purity but also must comply with cGMP legislation [24]. Until recently, Tregs utilized in clinical trials have been isolated by magnetic beads-based separation methods, by necessity, as clinical grade reagents and equipment for FACS were not available. However, with the development of clinical grade cytometers and reagents, FACs-isolated cells will become a viable source of cellular therapeutics. For example, promising data have been published from a trial in which Tregs sorted using a BD Influx cytometer were administered to type I diabetes patients, with no detectable toxicity or infection associated with the infusion [25].

The following protocol exploits FACS as the method of cell isolation but includes a pre-enrichment of $CD25^+$ cells by magnetic selection in order to reduce the duration of time required for the flow sort. Moreover, the $CD25^+$ cell fraction is depleted of monocytes, which can retard the flow sort by physically impeding the cytometer fluidics, due to their large size and adherence.

2 Materials

2.1 Isolation of Peripheral Blood Mononuclear Cells from Human Blood

1. Human blood, e.g., buffy coat, leukocyte cone, or heparinized blood sample.
2. Lymphocyte Separation Medium (LSM) (PAA, Pashing, Austria). Store at room temperature, protected from light.
3. PharmLyse solution (BD Pharmingen, Franklin Lakes, NJ, USA): dilute 2.5 mL of 10× concentrated stock solution with 22.5 mL sterile deionized water.
4. Hemocytometer.
5. Trypan blue 0.05% solution, sterile.
6. *Optional* RPMI 10%HS: 450 mL RPMI, 50 mL heat-inactivated (15 min at 55 °C) human AB serum (Lonza, Basel, Switzerland).

2.2 Magnetic Beads-Based Enrichment of $CD25^+$ Cells

1. Human CD25 microbeads (Miltenyi Biotech, Bergisch Gladbach, Germany).
2. MACS separator (Miltenyi Biotech, Bergisch Gladbach, Germany).
3. MACS magnet (Miltenyi Biotech, Bergisch Gladbach, Germany).
4. MACS LS (large) or MS (small) columns for MACS separator (Miltenyi Biotech, Bergisch Gladbach, Germany).

5. MACS buffer: 500 mL sterile PBS, 2 mL EDTA 0.5 M pH 8, 2.5 mL heat-inactivated foetal calf serum. Store on ice before and during procedure.
6. 50 μM cup filcon, sterile.

2.3 Immunostaining Reagent

1. Anti-CD4—ECD antibody, clone SFCI12T4D1 (Beckman Coulter, Brea, CA, USA).
2. Anti-human CD25—PE Cy7 antibody, clone M-A251 (BD Biosciences, Franklin Lakes, NJ, USA).
3. Anti-human CD127—PE antibody, clone hIL-7R-M21 (BD Biosciences, Franklin Lakes, NJ, USA).
4. FACS buffer: dissolve 0.1 g sodium azide in 480 mL sterile PBS and add 20 mL foetal calf serum.

2.4 Fluorescence-Activated Cell Sorting

1. Flow cytometer with cell sorting capacity, e.g., BD FACSAria cell sorter (BD Biosciences, Franklin Lakes, NJ, USA).
2. Sterile 5 mL polystyrene tube, with cap (BD Biosciences, Franklin Lakes, NJ, USA).
3. RMPI 10%HS (as above).
4. *Optional.* Freezing medium: 45% RPMI, 45%FCS (heat-inactivated), 10% DMSO.
5. *Optional* 1.5 mL cryovials.

3 Methods

Unless otherwise stated, all steps should be performed in a (class II) tissue culture hood, using sterile apparatus, consumables, and reagents.

3.1 Isolation of Peripheral Blood Mononuclear Cells (PBMCs) from a Human Blood

1. Dilute blood with an equal volume of PBS.
2. Take one 50 mL conical centrifuge tube per 25 mL of diluted blood and transfer 15 mL of lymphocyte separation medium to each tube.
3. For each tube, very gradually overlay 25 mL of diluted blood onto the lymphocyte separation medium, using a serological pipette or pasteur pipette to trickle the blood down the inside of the centrifuge tube (*see* **Note 1**).
4. Once all tubes are filled, transfer tubes to a centrifuge carefully, to avoid mixing the blood and LSM, and spin for 30 min at 800 rcf, 20 °C with the centrifuge break off (*see* **Note 1**).
5. Return the tubes to the tissue culture hood, again taking care to avoid mixing the layers. The blood should have separated into fractions, with the red cells pelleted below the LSM, the

plasma (yellow) retained above the LSM, and the leukocytes forming a thin white disk at the interface between the LSM and the plasma. Using a pasteur pipette, aspirate the buffy coat and transfer to a fresh tube. Avoid transferring any of the lower (LSM) phase and minimize the amount of the upper (plasma) phase (*see* **Note 2**). Collect buffy coats from all tubes into a single tube and disperse the buffy coats by pipetting up and down. Top of the volume of the tube to a total of 45 mL with PBS.

6. Spin the buffy coats for 10 min at 540 rcf and discard the resulting supernatant.
7. Prepare 25 mL of lysing buffer by adding 2.5 mL PharmLyse solution to 22.5 mL diH_2O.
8. Gradually resuspend the cell pellet in the lysing buffer. And mix well. Incubate at RT for 5 min (*see* **Note 3**). Add 20 mL PBS.
9. Spin the cell suspension for 10 min at 200 rcf, 4 °C and discard the resulting supernatant. This step should remove platelets. Resuspend the cell pellet in PBS (as a guide, a volume about equal to the initial blood volume usually gives a reasonable concentration for counting). Alternatively, at this stage, cells can be resuspended in complete culture medium (at least 20 mL) and stored overnight at 4 °C (*see* **Note 4**).
10. Take a 10 μL aliquot of the PBMC suspension, dilute with trypan blue, and count live cells using a hemocytometer. If platelets are still abundant, **step 9** can be repeated.

3.2 Enrichment of CD25$^+$ Cells from PBMCs (Adapted from Manufacturer's Protocol)

Throughout the procedure, the manufacturer recommends keeping all reagents on ice and working swiftly for optimal efficiency. After each addition, allow the column to run dry before proceeding to the next step.

1. Resuspend cell pellet in 30 μL MACS buffer per 10^7 cells.
2. Vortex CD25 Microbeads II thoroughly and add 6 μL beads per 10^7 cells (*see* **Note 5**). Incubate for 15 min in the fridge (not on ice).
3. In the meantime, prepare selection column(s) (*see* **Note 6**). First fix the selection column into the appropriate MACS magnet. Place a filter in the top if the column. Position an open 50 mL centrifuge tube below the outlet of the column, to collect the effluent. Wash the column by adding 3 mL MACS buffer into each LS column, or 0.5 mL buffer into each MS column, allowing the column reservoir to run dry.
4. Following the 15 min incubation, wash cells by adding at least 10 mL MACS buffer and centrifuging the cells for 7 min at 300 rcf, 4 °C. Aspirate the supernatant entirely and resuspend the pellet in 500 μL MACS buffer per 10^8 cells.

5. Transfer cell suspension into the filter placed on the top of the column. If the number of cells in the suspension exceeds the recommended capacity of the column (refer to the manufacturer's guidelines) then use multiple columns. Allow the column to run dry.
6. Wash column by adding 3 mL MACS buffer into each LS column, or 0.5 mL into each MS column, and allowing column to run dry. Repeat this wash step a further 2 times. The effluent, consisting of $CD25^+$-cell-depleted PBMC, can be discarded or utilized for other applications.
7. Remove the column from the magnet and place the column in a 15 mL centrifuge tube. Add 5 mL MACS buffer to each LS column and apply the plunger provided, depressing the plunger slowly but firmly, to expunge the buffer through the column. The resulting cell fraction should be highly enriched for CD25-expressing cells.

3.3 Immunostaining of $CD25^+$ Cells for FACS

The following quantities of reagents are appropriate for the normal range of $CD25^+$ cell yields from 50 mL of human blood (*see* **Note 7**).

1. Spin the cells for 7 min at 240 rcf and resuspend the cells in 60 μL FACS buffer.
2. Add 6 μL αCD4-ECD, 6 μL αCD127-PE, and 8 μL αCD25-PE-Cy7 antibodies. Incubate in the fridge for 30 min.
3. Wash the cells by adding at least 2 mL FACS buffer. Spin the cells for 7 min at 240 rcf at 4 °C.
4. Resuspend the cells in complete medium (approximately 50–150 × 10^6 cells/mL) (*see* **Note 8**).

3.4 FACS Isolation of Treg Cells

1. Prepare the cytometer for an aseptic sort, according to the manufacturer's protocol. It is recommended that BD FACS-Flow solution (*see* **Note 9**) or autoclaved PBS is used as sheath fluid during the sort. If a sample cooling system is available, set the sample temperature to 4 °C.
2. Using PBMC stained as above, or with the relevant isotype controls, set up a gating strategy for the sort as follows (*see* Fig. 1 for guidance), deriving each gate as a daughter of the gate set up the previous step:
   (a) Plot FSC vs. SSC and gate live lymphocytes. Take particular care to exclude monocytes from this gate, as these cells express CD4 and may exert pro-inflammatory effects that modulate Treg function or expansion [26].
   (b) Plot SSC-W vs. SSC-H and, using a gate descended from that constructed in (2a), gate on singlets (the bulk of the population with lower SSC-W).

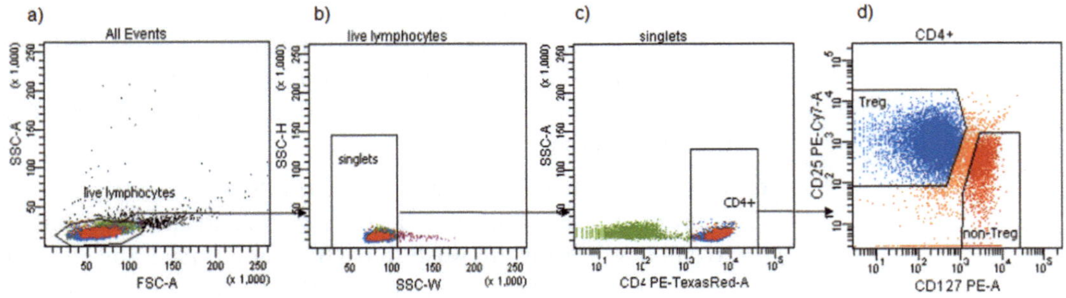

e)
Tube: sort

Population	#Events	%Parent	%Total
All Events	20,000	####	100.0
live lymphocytes	19,736	98.7	98.7
singlets	19,697	99.8	98.5
CD4+	14,986	76.1	74.9
Treg	10,487	70.0	52.4
non-Treg	2,912	19.4	14.6

Fig. 1 Gating hierarchy for sorting Treg from human PBMC pre-enriched for CD25$^+$ cells (**a**) First gate upon live lymphocytes on a FSC-A vs SSC-A plot. (**b**) From the lymphocytes gate, plot SSC-W vs SSC-H and gate upon the SSC-W^{lo} population of singlets, excluding doublets with higher SSC-W. (**c**) From the singlets, gate upon CD4$^+$ cells. (**d**) Plotting CD4$^+$ cells on a CD127 vs CD25 graph, two distinct populations should be visible: the CD25$^+$CD127^{lo} population (gated as "Treg" in plot (**d**)) and the CD127$^+$ population (gated as "non-Treg" in plot (**d**)) (**e**) population hierarchy for sorting human Treg

(c) Plot CD4 vs. SSC and gate on CD4$^+$ cells.

(d) Plot CD25 vs. CD127 and gate on the CD25$^+$CD127^{lo} subpopulation, which usually constitutes approximately 35–45% of CD4$^+$ cells after CD25$^+$ enrichment. As a control, gate separately the CD127$^+$ population.

3. Prepare two 15 mL centrifuge tubes, adding 2 mL complete medium to each, as collection tubes. Install the collection tubes into the collection chamber of the cytometer.
4. Pass the cell suspension from step 6.3.4 through a 70 μm filter into a sterile 5 mL FACS tube. Wash the filter with an equal volume of complete medium.
5. Load this tube into the cytometer and record ~20,000 events the sample and from each staining control sample. Adjust the gates, if necessary, based upon the staining controls. Once the gates are satisfactory, load the sample and begin the sort. After CD25$^+$ enrichment, usually 30–45% of cells are CD4$^+$CD25$^+$CD127^{lo}.
6. At the end of the sort, resuspend the sorted cells in complete medium. Take a small aliquot to run on the cytometer, under the same template as was used for the sort, to assess the purity of the sorted populations (*see* **Note 10**).
7. The sorted Tregs may be used immediately or cryopreserved (*see* **Note 11**). To cryopreserve Tregs, suspend the cells at a

density of 10–50 × 10^6 Tregs per mL of freezing medium, transfer to 1.5 mL cryovial(s). A freezing box should be used to store cryovials at −80 °C for 16–72 h before transferring the vials to −160 °C for long-term storage.

4 Notes

1. By maintaining a slow, steady trickle of blood down the side of the tube, the blood should spread across the surface of the lymphocyte separation medium without disturbing the meniscus and mixing with the medium below. Mixing of the blood with the LSM can be detrimental to the purity of the isolated PBMC, with greater contamination with erythrocytes. For this reason, also take care when transferring tubes of blood overlayed on LSM between the hood and the centrifuge, to avoid disturbing the layers. Likewise, disengaging the break of the centrifuge during this step prevents mixing of blood with LSM during centrifugation. At a cost, some labor-saving devices are available to aid PBMC isolation. For example, one may choose to use specialized conical centrifuge tubes containing a porous insert that forms a physical barrier between the buffy coat and the LSM. The insert allows blood to be added more rapidly and buffy coats removed more easily.
2. The lower (LSM) phase contains erythrocytes and granulocytes. The majority of these cells should pellet as the bottom of the tube but some may deposit just below the buffy coat so take care to avoid collecting anything red. Again, tubes containing a porous insert can facilitate collection of the buffy coat. The upper (plasma) phase contains platelets, so should be avoided if contamination with platelets is likely to impact upon the application of your PBMC after isolation. Subsequent centrifugation steps are designed to exclude platelets and can be repeated if there is evidence of excessive platelet contamination. Should these phases fail to separate properly, or become mixed slightly, they can be recovered by repeating the 30-min spin. If this fails, collect all of the layers into which the lymphocytes might have been mixed, wash the cells twice in PBS, spinning them for 5 min at 380 rcf. Resuspend the cell pellet in RPMI, overlay the resulting cell suspension of LSM, and proceed from step 6.1.4.
3. Continuing the red cell lysis reaction for longer than 5 min is not recommended, due to adverse effects on PBMC viability. If the pellet looks red after centrifuging the cells following the lysis step, this step can be repeated.
4. We have found no difference in the phenotype of Tregs isolated on the day after blood collection and PBMC isolation,

compared with Treg isolated from blood on the day of collection; however, it may be advisable to conduct a comparison of those parameters that are particularly relevant to your application.

5. These volumes differ from those recommended by the manufacturer and were chosen to maximize yield, economically.
6. Refer to the manufacturer's guidelines to select the correct size and number of MACS columns, depending upon the total number of cells in your sample and the expected number of labeled cells. As a guideline, you can expect less than 3% of unstimulated human PBMC to be labeled by the CD25 microbeads. Therefore, total cell number will be the limiting factor for column capacity: Load no more than 2×10^8 cells onto a MS column and no more than 2×10^9 cells onto an LS column. Exceeding the recommended capacity of the column can result in the column becoming blocked or saturated, which will impair the purity or yield of the selection.
7. As we routinely perform Treg isolation from blood products of a standardized volume (approximately 50 mL), we have not titrated antibody concentrations across a range of cell yields and would recommend performing this procedure if you plan to stain PBMC from volumes of blood much smaller or larger than 50 mL.
8. The cell densities recommended here are based upon the use of a BD FACSAria instrument and upon our preferred sorting flow rate and event rate and are, as such, only a guideline.
9. If using FACSFlow solution as sheath fluid, to minimize potential cytotoxic effects of prolonged exposure to preservative compounds, it is recommended to replace the collection tubes every 30 min during the sort and resuspend the cells collected in fresh medium.
10. If the purity of the sorted sample is inadequate for your application, the purity may be enhanced by repeating the sort. Resuspend the impure sorted cells at a suitable cell density in complete medium and proceed from step 6.4.5.
11. There is some controversy regarding the cryopreservation of Treg cells. In our experience, isolated Treg cells frozen as described above can be retrieved with a loss of fewer than 30% of cells and no substantial or permanent alteration of phenotype or suppressive potency [16]. However, several studies report altered phenotype or viability of Treg cells following cryopreservation [27–29] and so we recommend conducting a side-by-side comparison of cryopreserved and freshly-isolated Tregs, from the same donor and isolation batch, in your standard assays. Alternatively, a short period of stimulation in culture may restore Treg phenotype and function after cryopreservation [20].

Acknowledgements

KM holds a British Heart Foundation Research Studentship. The work from the authors' own laboratory was supported by grants from The Wellcome Trust and European Union FP7 project The ONE Study.

References

1. Rudensky AY (2011) Regulatory T cells and Foxp3. Immunol Rev 241:260–268
2. Benoist C, Mathis D (2012) Treg cells, life history, and diversity. Cold Spring Harb Perspect Biol 4:a007021
3. Miyara M, Sakaguchi S (2011) Human FoxP3 (+)CD4(+) regulatory T cells: their knowns and unknowns. Immunol Cell Biol 89:346–351
4. Vignali D a a, Collison LW, Workman CJ (2008) How regulatory T cells work. Nat Rev Immunol 8:523–532
5. Wood KJ, Bushell A, Hester J (2012) Regulatory immune cells in transplantation. Nat Rev Immunol 12:417–430
6. Reibke R, Garbi N, Ganss R et al (2006) CD8+ regulatory T cells generated by neonatal recognition of peripheral self-antigen. Proc Natl Acad Sci U S A 103:15142–15147
7. Juvet SC, Zhang L (2012) Double negative regulatory T cells in transplantation and autoimmunity: recent progress and future directions. J Mol Cell Biol 4:48–58
8. Monteiro M, Almeida CF, Caridade M et al (2010) Identification of regulatory Foxp3+ invariant NKT cells induced by TGF-beta. J Immunol 185:2157–2163
9. Hayday A, Tigelaar R (2003) Immunoregulation in the tissues by gammadelta T cells. Nat Rev Immunol 3:233–242
10. Miyara M, Yoshioka Y, Kitoh A et al (2009) Functional delineation and differentiation dynamics of human CD4+ T cells expressing the FoxP3 transcription factor. Immunity 30:899–911
11. Bluestone J a, Abbas AK (2003) Natural versus adaptive regulatory T cells. Nat Rev Immunol 3:253–257
12. Duhen T, Duhen R, Lanzavecchia A et al (2012) Functionally distinct subsets of human FOXP3+ Treg cells that phenotypically mirror effector Th cells. Blood 119:4430–4440
13. Seddiki N, Santner-Nanan B, Martinson J et al (2006) Expression of interleukin (IL)-2 and IL-7 receptors discriminates between human regulatory and activated T cells. J Exp Med 203:1693–1700
14. Liu W, Putnam AL, Xu-Yu Z et al (2006) CD127 expression inversely correlates with FoxP3 and suppressive function of human CD4+ T reg cells. J Exp Med 203:1701–1711
15. Ukena SN, Höpting M, Velaga S et al (2011) Isolation strategies of regulatory T cells for clinical trials: phenotype, function, stability, and expansion capacity. Exp Hematol 39:1152–1160
16. Nadig SN, Wieckiewicz J, Wu DC et al (2010) In vivo prevention of transplant arteriosclerosis by ex vivo-expanded human regulatory T cells. Nat Med 16:809–813
17. Miltenyi S, Müller W, Weichel W et al (1990) High gradient magnetic cell separation with MACS. Cytometry 11:231–238
18. a Herzenberg L, Parks D, Sahaf B et al (2002) The history and future of the fluorescence activated cell sorter and flow cytometry: a view from Stanford. Clin Chem 48:1819–1827
19. Milward K, Issa F, Hester J et al (2013) Multiple unit pooled umbilical cord blood is a viable source of therapeutic regulatory T cells. Transp J 95:85–93
20. Peters JH, Preijers FW, Woestenenk R et al (2008) Clinical grade Treg: GMP isolation, improvement of purity by CD127 depletion, Treg expansion, and Treg cryopreservation. PLoS One 3:e3161
21. Battaglia M, Stabilini A, Roncarolo M-G (2005) Rapamycin selectively expands CD4 +CD25+FoxP3+ regulatory T cells. Blood 105:4743–4748
22. Wieckiewicz J, Goto R, Wood KJ (2010) T regulatory cells and the control of alloimmunity: from characterisation to clinical application. Curr Opin Immunol 22:662–668
23. Safinia N, Leech J, Hernandez-Fuentes M et al (2013) Promoting transplantation tolerance; adoptive regulatory T cell therapy. Clin Exp Immunol 172:158–168
24. Mcintyre CA, Flyg BT, Fong TC (2010) Fluorescence-activated cell sorting for CGMP processing of therapeutic cells

25. Rzonkowska NAMA (2012) Regulatory T cells preserves b -cell function in type 1 diabetes in children. 35:3–6
26. Walter GJ, Evans HG, Menon B et al (2013) Interaction with activated monocytes enhances cytokine expression and suppressive activity of human CD4+CD45ro+CD25+CD127(low) regulatory T cells. Arthritis Rheum 65:627–638
27. Golab K, Leveson-Gower D, Wang X-J et al (2013) Challenges in cryopreservation of regulatory T cells (Tregs) for clinical therapeutic applications. Int Immunopharmacol 16:371–375
28. Sattui S, de la Flor C, Sanchez C et al (2012) Cryopreservation modulates the detection of regulatory T cell markers. Cytometry B Clin Cytom 82:54–58
29. Elkord E (2009) Frequency of human T regulatory cells in peripheral blood is significantly reduced by cryopreservation. J Immunol Methods 347:87–90

Chapter 5

Identification and Isolation of Regulatory B Cells in Mouse and Human

Madhvi Menon, Elizabeth C. Rosser, and Claudia Mauri

Abstract

Regulatory B cells (Bregs) suppress immune response via the provision of IL-10. Due to the phenotypic heterogeneity of described Bregs, it is important to have standardized protocols for their isolation and identification. Previous work by our laboratory has shown that the immature B-cell populations in the murine spleen and human peripheral blood produce the highest levels of IL-10 on engagement of CD40, and can suppress pro-inflammatory T-cell differentiation. In this chapter, we describe the methods necessary for the isolation of this subset of Bregs and their activation via CD40 in vitro.

Key words Regulatory B cells, Inflammation, IL-10, T2-MZP B cells, Immature B cells, CD40

1 Introduction

B cells are classically viewed as positive effectors of immune responses due to their ability to produce antibody and present antigen. However, in recent years, it has become evident that certain subsets of B cells negatively regulate immune responses by skewing lymphocyte differentiation in favor of a regulatory phenotype. Immunosuppressive subsets of B cells are collectively known as regulatory B cells (Bregs) [1].

Multiple subsets of Bregs have been described in both mice and humans [2]. For example, in different mouse models of inflammation, Bregs have been identified as $CD19^{+}CD21^{hi}CD23^{+}CD24^{hi}$ transitional-2 marginal zone precursor (T2-MZP) B cells [3], $CD19^{+}CD21^{hi}CD23^{-}CD24^{hi}$ marginal zone B cells [4], Tim-1+ B cells [5], and $CD5^{+}CD1d^{hi}$ B (B10) cells [6]. Similarly in humans, Bregs have been identified as both $CD19^{+}CD24^{hi}CD38^{hi}$ immature B cells [7] and $CD19^{+}CD24^{hi}CD27^{+}$ B cells [8]. Despite this phenotypic heterogeneity, most Breg subsets produce IL-10 in

Madhvi Menon and Elizabeth C. Rosser contributed equally to this work.

Ashleigh S. Boyd (ed.), *Immunological Tolerance: Methods and Protocols*, Methods in Molecular Biology, vol. 1899,
https://doi.org/10.1007/978-1-4939-8938-6_5,

response to engagement of CD40, toll-like receptor agonists and the B cell receptor (BCR) [1]. Thus, it is important to have reliable protocols that allow for the identification of IL-10-producing B cell subsets (Bregs) in both mouse and human.

Previous research by our laboratory has shown that in the context of autoimmunity, Bregs are contained within the immature population of B cells found in the murine spleen or human peripheral blood, and that engagement of CD40 is fundamental for their survival and function. In the murine spleen, T2-MZP B cells isolated from mice in remission from arthritis are the highest producers of IL-10 following stimulation with agonistic anti-CD40 in vitro, and are the only B-cell subset that can suppress arthritis on adoptive transfer [3]. Within human peripheral blood mononuclear cells (PBMCs), $CD19^{+}CD24^{hi}CD38^{hi}$ B cells produce the highest amount of IL-10 among the different B-cell subsets on activation of CD40 in vitro, and most importantly suppress effector T-cell responses [7, 9]. Of note, $CD19^{+}CD24^{hi}CD38^{hi}$ B cells are both functionally and numerically defective when isolated from patients with autoimmune disease [7, 9].

In this chapter, we describe the detailed methods needed for the isolation of $CD19^{+}CD21^{hi}CD23^{+}CD24^{hi}$ T2-MZP B cells from mice, and $CD19^{+}CD24^{hi}CD38^{hi}$ immature B cells from human peripheral blood. We also describe how to identify IL-10-producing B cells in these subsets by flow cytometry following CD40 activation in vitro.

2 Materials

Prepare all solutions in a sterile hood. Store all reagents at 4 °C (unless otherwise stated).

2.1 Materials Needed for the Identification and Isolation of Regulatory B Cells in Mice

1. C57BL/6 8–12 week old mice (*see* **Note 1**).
2. 5 mL syringes.
3. 70 μM Cell Strainers.
4. 15 mL and 50 mL Falcon Tubes.
5. Polypropelene FACS tubes.
6. Supplemented RPMI 1640 (with L-Glutamine and $NaHCO_3$): RPMI, 10% fetal calf serum (FCS), 0.01% penicillin-streptomycin, and 50 μM 2-mercaptoethanol.
7. MACS Buffer: 0.5% FCS, 2 mM EDTA in 1× PBS.
8. Trypan Blue for cell counts.
9. OPTIONAL STEP: CD43 (Ly-48) microbeads and LD columns for B cell isolation (Milteyi: Used according to the manufacturer's instructions).

10. Flourochrome conjugated anti-mouse CD19 (1D3), CD21 (7G6), CD23 (B3B4), and CD24 (M1/69) (*see* **Note 2**).
11. DAPI (0.05 μg/mL–0.1 μg/mL).
12. Sort collection media: 1:1 mixture of MACS Buffer and FCS.
13. Cell sorter.
14. Agonistic anti-CD40 (10 μg/mL).
15. PMA (50 ng/mL) and Ionomycin (500 ng/mL).
16. Golgi-stop containing Monensin (BD Biosciences, used according to the manufacturer's instructions).
17. Flourochrome conjugated anti-mouse IL-10 (JES5-16E3) (*see* **Note 2**).
18. Intracellular fixation buffer (eBiosciences).
19. Permeabilization buffer (eBiosciences).
20. Live/Dead fixable Dead Cell stain kit.
21. FACS Buffer: 0.5% FCS, 2 mM EDTA in 1× PBS, 0.01% NaN_3.
22. Flow cytometer.
23. Flowjo Software, or similar flow cytometry platform.

2.2 Materials Needed for the Identification and Isolation of Regulatory B Cells in Humans

1. Peripheral blood in heparin (*see* **Note 3**).
2. Ficoll-Paque.
3. 25 mL stripettes.
4. 15 mL and 50 mL Falcon Tubes.
5. 3 mL Pasteur pipettes.
6. Polypropelene FACS tubes.
7. Supplemented RPMI 1640 (with L-Glutamine and $NaHCO_3$): RPMI, 10% fetal calf serum (FCS) and 0.01% penicillin-streptomycin.
8. Freezing media: 90% FCS and 10% DMSO.
9. Mr. Frosty® Freezing container.
10. Cryovials.
11. MACS Buffer: 1% FCS, 2 mM EDTA in 1× PBS.
12. Trypan blue for cell counts.
13. Hemocytometer.
14. OPTIONAL STEP: EasySep magnet and Human B cell enrichment kit for B cell isolation (StemCell: Used according to the manufacturer's instructions) (*see* **Note 4**).
15. Fluorochrome conjugated anti-human CD19 (HIB19), CD24 (SN3), and CD38 (HB7) (*see* **Note 5**).
16. Live/Dead fixable Dead Cell stain kit.

17. DAPI (0.05 μg/mL–0.1 μg/mL).
18. Sort collection media: 1:1 mixture of MACS Buffer and FCS.
19. Cell sorter.
20. Chinese hamster ovary (CHO) cells expressing CD154 and untransfected control.
21. Supplemented DMEM containing 4500 μg/mL glucose, 110 μg/mL sodium pyruvate, and 2 mM L-glutamine: 5% FCS and 0.01% penicillin-streptomycin.
22. Tissue culture flasks: T25 or T75 flasks.
23. Irradiator.
24. PMA (50 ng/mL) and Ionomycin (250 ng/mL).
25. Brefaldin A (5 μg/mL).
26. Intracellular fixation buffer (eBiosciences).
27. Permeabilization buffer (eBiosciences).
28. IL-10 (JES3-19F1) (*see* **Note 5**).
29. FACS Buffer: 0.5% FCS in 1× PBS, 0.01% NaN_3.
30. Flow cytometer.
31. FlowJo Software or similar flow cytometry platform.

3 Methods

3.1 Identification and Isolation of Bregs in Mice

In this section, we describe the basic protocols needed to identify regulatory B cells isolated from spleens dissected from mice.

3.1.1 Isolation of Mouse Splenocytes

1. Euthanize mice by CO_2 inhalation, cervical dislocation, or any other approved method.
2. Dissect spleens from mice and put in 15 mL falcon tubes containing ice cold RPMI containing 0.1% Penicillin/Streptomycin, and place directly on ice.
3. In a sterile hood, gently mash spleens through a 70 μM cell strainer into a 50 mL Falcon tube using the flat end of the plunger from a 5 mL syringe. Wash filter with 15 mL of RPMI. Centrifuge for 10 min, 4 °C, 500 × *g* (*see* **Note 6**).
4. Discard the supernatant, and resuspend in 1 mL/spleen of red cell lysis buffer, leave for 2 min on ice. Following incubation with red cell lysis buffer, fill tube to the top with supplemented RPMI. Centrifuge for 10 min, 4 °C, 500 × *g*.
5. Resuspend cells in 5–10 mL of MACs buffer/spleen and count. Centrifuge for 10 min, 4 °C, 500 × *g*.

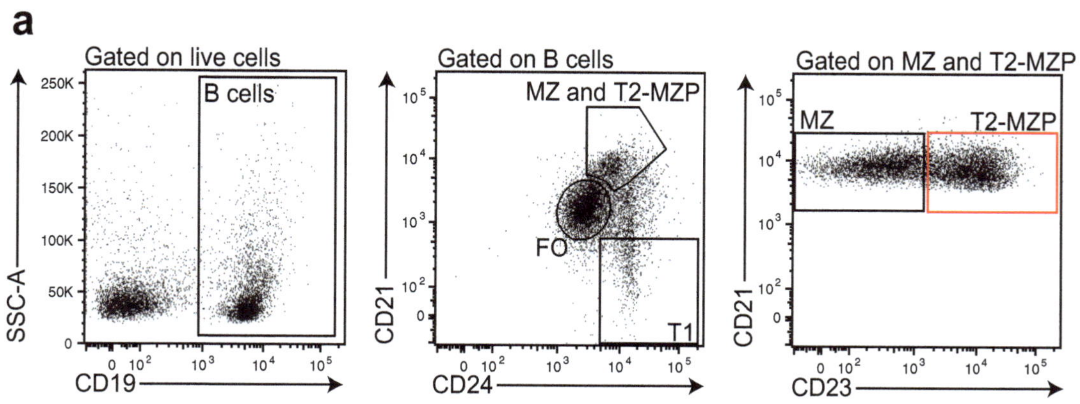

Fig. 1 Gating strategy Breg isolation from mouse splenocytes. Isolated splenic B Cells from mice were stained with monoclonal antibodies against CD19, CD21, CD23, and CD24 for FACS sorting. (**a**) Representative flow cytometry dot plots showing gating strategy for purification of B-cell subsets. Highlighted gate in red shows population of interest, in this case T2-MZP

3.1.2 Sorting and Activation of B-Cell Subsets

1. OPTIONAL STEP: Negatively isolate resting B cells using CD43 (ly-48) microbeads and LD columns according to the manufacturer's instructions. Count cells. Centrifuge for 10 min, 4 °C, 500 × *g* (*see* **Note 7**).
2. Resuspend cells at a concentration of 50 × 10^6 cells/mL. To identify T2-MZP B cells stain cells with suggested monoclonal antibodies against CD19, CD21, CD23, and CD24 (staining concentrations in **Note 2**, *see* Fig. 1a for representative FACS plots). Concurrently, prepare single stain controls for compensation. Incubate cells with antibodies for a minimum of 20 min on ice.
3. Wash twice by filling tube with ice-cold MACS buffer and centrifuging for 10 min, 4 °C, 500 × *g*. Resuspend at 30–50 × 10^6 for cell sorter.
4. To prevent blockage of the cell sorter, remove clumps of cells by straining sample through a 40 μM filter. Transfer cells to 5 mL polystyrene FACS tubes for sorting.
5. Add DAPI (final concentration of 0.05 μg/mL–0.1 μg/mL) to samples and DAPI single stained control.
6. Take sample to cell sort into B-cell subsets. Use polypropelene tubes containing 1–2 mLs of sort collection medium to collect sorted B-cell subsets.
7. Collect sorted T2-MZP Bregs, and other subsets of interest, and centrifuge for 500 × *g*, 4 °C for 10 min.
8. Count cells, and prepare cells for downstream analysis (*see* **Note 8**).

3.1.3 Detecting IL-10⁺ Bregs by Flow Cytometry Using C57BL/6 Mice

1. For activation of B-cell subsets in vitro with agonistic anti-CD40, plate out the appropriate number of B cells for subsequent assays (~250,000 cells/well is adequate for detection of IL-10) in a final volume of 200 μL and stimulate with agonistic anti-CD40 (10 μg/mL) in a sterile 96-well cell culture plate.
2. Sorted B-cell subsets are left in culture for 48 h.
3. Collect cell culture supernatants after 43 h and store at −80 °C for subsequent use.
4. Add 50 ng/mL PMA, 500 ng/mL ionomycin and Monensin in supplemented RPMI to cells for the last 5 h of culture to a final volume of 200 μL.
5. Centrifuge plate at 500 × *g*, 4 °C for 5 min, discard the supernatant, and wash cells twice by adding 200 μL/well of 1× PBS and centrifuging at 500 × *g*, 4 °C for 5 min.
6. Discard the supernatant and resuspend cell pellets by gently vortexing plate.
7. Stain the cells with a fixable live/dead cell staining fluorescent dye for 20 min at 4 °C. Include a well for a single stain control for the dead cell stain. Centrifuge plate at 500 × *g*, 4 °C for 5 min, discard the supernatant, and wash cells twice by adding 200 μL/well of FACS buffer and centrifuging at 500 × *g*, 4 °C for 5 min. Discard the supernatant.
8. Add 50 μL/well of FACS buffer containing monoclonal antibodies against CD19 diluted to appropriate concentration (*see* **Note 2**) and incubate for 20 min at 4 °C in the dark. Prepare single stain controls.
9. Centrifuge plate at 500 × *g*, 4 °C for 5 min, discard the supernatant, and wash cells twice by adding 200 μL/well of FACS buffer and centrifuging at 500 × *g*, 4 °C for 5 min.
10. Add 100 μL/well intracellular fixation buffer (for detecting cytokines) to each well for 15 min at 4 °C in the dark.
11. Permeabilize cells by washing twice with 200 μL of 1× permeabilization buffer and centrifuging at 500 × *g*, 4 °C for 5 min.
12. Incubate cells with 200 μL of 1× permeabilization buffer for 20 min at RT, then centrifuge at 500 × *g*, 4 °C for 5 min.
13. Incubate the cells with 50 μL of permeabilization buffer containing monoclonal antibodies against IL-10 diluted to appropriate concentration for 45 min at 4 °C in the dark.
14. Wash cells twice with permeabilization buffer and once with FACs buffer, before resuspending in 200 μL FACs buffer.
15. Transfer the cells to polystyrene FACS tubes, acquire data, and analyze using FlowJo or similar analysis platform.
16. Identify IL-10 producing B cells.

3.2 Identification and Isolation of Bregs in Humans

In this section, we describe the basic protocols needed to identify regulatory B cells isolated from the human peripheral blood mononuclear cells (PBMCs).

3.2.1 Isolation of PBMCs by Density Gradient Centrifugation

1. In a sterile hood, transfer whole venous blood into 50 mL falcon tubes, diluted 1:1 in serum-free RPMI 1640 media.
2. Layer 33 mL of diluted blood on 15 mL Ficoll without mixing, and centrifuge the tubes at a speed of 800 × *g* at 21 °C for 30 min with minimum acceleration and brake.
3. Carefully extract the PBMCs from the interface using a 2 mL Pasteur pipette and dilute 1:1 with RPMI.
4. Wash the extracted PBMCs twice by topping up the 50 mL tube with supplemented RPMI 1640 and centrifuging at 500 × *g*, 4 °C for 10 min. Discard the supernatant.
5. Resuspend cells in 0.5 mL supplemented RPMI/mL blood and count the cells using a hemocytometer.
6. Centrifuge cells at 500 × *g*, 4 °C for 10 min, discard the supernatant, and resuspend in freezing media to a concentration of 10^7 cells/mL. Quickly transfer cells to cryogenic vials.
7. Freeze cryovials at −80 °C in a Nalgene® Mr. Frosty® Freezing container containing isopropyl alcohol (*see* **Note 9**), followed by storage in liquid nitrogen at −196 °C until subsequent use.

3.2.2 Sorting and Activation of B-Cell Subsets

1. For isolation of B-cell subsets, thaw frozen PBMCs in supplemented RPMI media and wash twice by filling tube with MACS buffer and centrifuging at 500 × *g*, 4 °C for 5 min.
2. OPTIONAL STEP: Negatively isolate B cells using Human B-cell enrichment kit and EasySep Magnet according to the manufacturer's instructions. Count cells. Centrifuge at 500 × *g*, 4 °C for 10 min (*see* **Note 4**).
3. Resuspend cells at a concentration of 5×10^7 cells/mL in MACS buffer. To identify immature B cells, incubate the cells with monoclonal antibodies against CD19, CD24, and CD38 (used at 10 μL per 5×10^7 cells) (staining concentrations in **Note 5**, *see* Fig. 2a for representative FACS plots). Concurrently, prepare single stain controls for compensation. Incubate cells with antibodies for a minimum of 20 min on ice.
4. Wash cells twice by filling tube with MACS buffer and centrifuging at 500 × *g*, 4 °C for 5 min. Resuspend at a concentration of 30–50 × 10^6 cells/mL for cell sorter.
5. To prevent blockage of the cell sorter, remove clumps of cells by straining sample through a 40 μM filter. Transfer cells to 5 mL polystyrene FACS tubes for sorting.

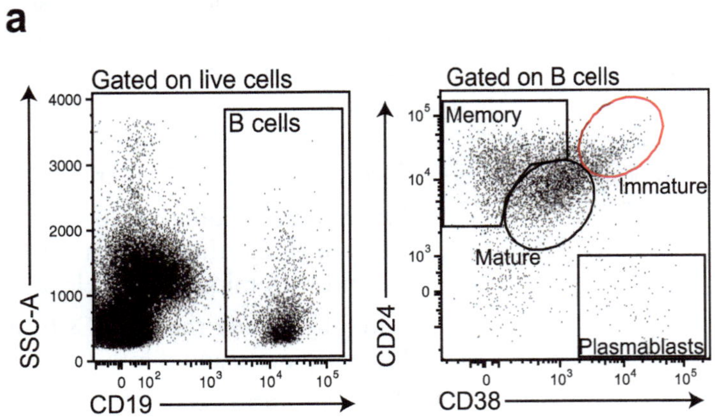

Fig. 2 Gating strategy Breg isolation from human PBMCs. Isolated human PBMCs were stained with monoclonal antibodies against CD19, CD24, and CD38 for FACS sorting. (**a**) Representative flow cytometry dot plots showing gating strategy for purification of B-cell subsets. Highlighted gate in red shows population of interest, in this case immature B cells

6. Add DAPI (final concentration of 0.05 μg/mL–0.1 μg/mL) to samples and prepare a single stained control.
7. Sort the PBMCs on a FACs sorter based on the expression of CD19, CD24, and CD38. B-cell subsets are identified as immature ($CD19^{+}CD24^{hi}CD38^{hi}$), mature ($CD19^{+}CD24^{int}CD38^{int}$), and memory ($CD19^{+}CD24^{hi}CD38^{-}$) B cells.
8. Collect the sorted B-cell subsets in polypropylene tubes containing 1–2 mL sort collection medium.
9. Prepare 96-well U-bottomed cell culture plates with CD154 (CD40L) transfected CHO cells as described in Subheading 3.2.3. Estimate the number of B cells to be plated and plate out sufficient CHO cells for a 1:10 ratio of CHO:B cells. Leave CHO cells for at least 2 h in an incubator at 37 °C to allow the cells to adhere to the plate.
10. Wash sorted B cell subsets twice by filling collection tubes with supplemented RPMI and centrifuging at 500 × *g*, 4 °C for 10 min.
11. Count the number of B cells in each sorted subset and add cells to wells containing CD154 (CD40L) transfected CHO cells (or control CHO cells). 250,000 B cells/well is sufficient for detecting IL-10 by flow cytometry (*see* **Note 10**). The final volume in the wells should be 200 μL. Handling CHO cells is explained in Subheading 3.2.3.

3.2.3 Working with CHO Cells

1. Thaw aliquot of CD154-transfected and untransfected CHO cells in pre-warmed supplemented DMEM media in a 50 mL tube.
2. Wash twice by filling tube with DMEM and centrifuging at 500 × *g*, 4 °C for 5 min.
3. Resuspend cells in 20 mL of supplemented DMEM media and seed in a T25 or T75 flask for 3–4 days or until 90% confluent (*see* **Note 11**).
4. Irradiate CHO cells-dose of 70 Gray (*see* **Note 12**).
5. Remove media from the T25 flasks and wash twice with 1× sterile PBS. Rinse around the inside of the flask a few times each wash.
6. Add 1.5 mL Trypsin-EDTA to detach the adherent confluent CHO cells (*see* **Note 13**).
7. Incubate at 37 °C for 3–4 min. Tap the flask to check whether the cells have detached.
8. Once detached, add 10 mL of supplemented DMEM to inhibit enzymatic reaction. Transfer cells from flask to a 50 mL tube.
9. Wash twice by filling tube with supplemented RPMI and centrifuging at 500 × *g*, 4 °C for 5 min.
10. Count cells and plate for culture with B cells (**step 9** of Subheading 3.2.2).

3.2.4 Detecting Bregs by Flow Cytometry

1. The sorted B-cell subsets are in culture with CHO cells for 72 h (Subheading 3.2.2).
2. Collect cell culture supernatants after 67 h and store at −80 °C for subsequent use.
3. Add 50 ng/mL PMA, 250 ng/mL ionomycin and brefaldin A in supplemented RPMI to cells in culture for the last 5 h to a final volume of 200 μL.
4. Centrifuge plate at 500 × *g*, 4 °C for 5 min, and discard the supernatant, and wash cells twice by adding 200 μL/well 1× PBS and centrifuging at 500 × *g*, 4 °C for 5 min.
5. Discard the supernatants and resuspend cell pellets by gently vortexing the plate.
6. Stain the cells with a fixable live/dead cell staining fluorescent dye for 20 min at 4 °C. Include a well for a single stain control for the dead cell stain. Centrifuge the plate at 500 × *g*, 4 °C for 5 min, discard the supernatant, and wash cells twice by adding 200 μL/well of 1× FACS buffer and centrifuging at 500 × *g*, 4 °C for 5 min. Discard the supernatant.
7. Add 50 μL/well of FACS buffer containing monoclonal antibodies against CD19 diluted to appropriate concentration and

incubate for 20 min at 4 °C in the dark. Prepare single stain controls.

8. Centrifuge plate at 500 × *g*, 4 °C for 5 min, discard the supernatant, and wash cells twice by adding 200 μL/well of FACS buffer and centrifuging at 500 × *g*, 4 °C for 5 min.
9. Add 100 μL/well intracellular fixation buffer (for detecting cytokines) to each well for 15 min at 4 °C in the dark.
10. Wash once with FACs buffer by adding 200 μL/well of FACS buffer and centrifuging at 500 × *g*, 4 °C for 5 min.
11. Permeabilize cells by washing twice with 200 μL of 1× permeabilization buffer and centrifuging at 500 × *g*, 4 °C for 5 min.
12. Incubate the cells with 50 μL of permeabilization buffer containing monoclonal antibodies against IL-10 diluted to appropriate concentration for 45 min at 4 °C in the dark.
13. Wash cells twice with permeabilization buffer and once with FACs buffer, before resuspending in 200 μL FACs buffer.
14. Transfer the cells to polystyrene FACs tubes, acquire data and analyze using FlowJo or similar analysis platform.
15. Identify regulatory B cells as IL-10$^+$CD19$^+$ B cells within the immature B cells (*see* **Note 14**). In addition to IL-10 production, regulatory function of B cell subsets can also be assessed by suppression assay [7, 9].

4 Notes

1. You can use mice of any strain, sex, or age for these experiments. However, the number of Bregs changes over age, and varies between strains, and the representative gating we have provided is for C57BL/6 8–12 week-old female mice. It is also important to note that Bregs are rare in naïve mice, and expanded following remission from autoimmune disease. Given these factors, we recommend using 8–12 week old mice that are in remission from autoimmune disease for the isolation of murine Bregs. For experiments where cells will be collected to assess the ability of Bregs to suppress pro-inflammatory responses in vivo or in vitro, samples can be pooled to achieve sufficient numbers of Bregs for assays. Furthermore, the use of IL-10eGFP reporter mice allows ex vivo identification of IL-10 by flow cytometry without the need for in vitro stimulation.
2. These suggested clones of anti-CD19, anti-CD21, anti-CD23, and anti-CD24 antibodies are used at staining concentrations of 0.8 μg/mL, and anti-IL-10 is used at a staining

concentration of 4 μg/mL. Other clones can be used but they would need to be optimized.

3. Whole venous blood must be collected in sodium heparin-coated tubes or sterile 50 mL centrifuge tubes containing 2 IU/mL heparin.
4. This enrichment of B cells using a negative selection kit is to shorten the time it takes to sort the B-cell subsets by flow cytometry.
5. These clones of anti-CD19, anti-CD24, and anti-CD38 antibodies are used at a staining concentration of 2 μg/mL, and the noted clone of anti-IL-10 is used at 4 μg/mL. Other clones would need to be optimized prior to use.
6. Other techniques to isolate splenocytes can be used. However as we usually work with large numbers of mice, we find this technique the most convenient and the least variable.
7. As the purpose of this step is to enrich for B cells in order to make the cell sort run faster than if B cells were sorted directly from splenocytes, several different B cell enrichment kits can be used, and as 100% purity is not necessary, reagents can be diluted further than recommended. However, we would recommend using kits that negatively select for B cells.
8. At this point, cells can also be used to assess their ability to suppress pro-inflammatory response both in vivo and in vitro. Assessment of disease suppression by Bregs in vivo remains the gold standard for their identification and analysis of their function in mice, as IL-10 production does not correlate with the suppressive capacity of B cells in all models of inflammation. In the context of arthritis, we have described the protocols necessary to assess Breg suppression in vivo in a previous edition of molecular methods in molecular biology [10].
9. This is to ensure freezing at a controlled rate of −1 °C/min, resulting in improved viability of PBMCs.
10. 1 μg/mL *Mega*CD40L from Enzo LifeSciences can be used as an alternative to CHO-CD40L cells to stimulate B cells. Although the induction of Bregs is not equivalent, it is comparable.
11. The CHO cells must be cultured 3–4 days prior to setting up culture with isolated B-cell subsets.
12. In order to expand and aliquot CHO cells for future use, do not irradiate the cells (skip to **step 4**). The cells should not have more than 3 passages as they lose the expression of CD40L. Once cells have been detached, wash twice with supplemented DMEM media and freeze cells in 2–5 million cells/mL aliquots in freezing media.

13. The trypsin-EDTA solution must be pre-warmed in a water bath at 37 °C for detachment of adherent CHO cells.
14. The presence of CHO cells does not affect the detection of IL-10-producing Bregs. Majority of the CHO cells will be attached to the well, and those detached can be discriminated from lymphocytes on the FSC-SSC plot.

Acknowledgments

We would like to thank Dr. Paul Blair for his constructive criticism of the manuscript. Madhvi Menon is funded by a Wellcome Trust PhD studentship (090406/Z/09/Z). Elizabeth C. Rosser was funded by an Arthritis Research UK PhD studentship (MP/19314).

References

1. Mauri C, Bosma A (2012) Immune regulatory function of B cells. Annu Rev Immunol 30:221–241. https://doi.org/10.1146/annurev-immunol-020711-074934
2. Mauri C and Menon M 2015. The expanding family of regulatory B cells. Int Immunol, Vol. 27, No. 10, pp. 479–486
3. Evans JG, Chavez-Rueda KA, Eddaoudi A, Meyer-Bahlburg A, Rawlings DJ, Ehrenstein MR, Mauri C (2007) Novel suppressive function of transitional 2 B cells in experimental arthritis. J Immunol 178(12):7868–7878
4. Miles K, Heaney J, Sibinska Z, Salter D, Savill J, Gray D, Gray M (2012) A tolerogenic role for toll-like receptor 9 is revealed by B-cell interaction with DNA complexes expressed on apoptotic cells. Proc Natl Acad Sci U S A 109 (3):887–892. https://doi.org/10.1073/pnas.1109173109
5. Ding Q, Yeung M, Camirand G, Zeng Q, Akiba H, Yagita H, Chalasani G, Sayegh MH, Najafian N, Rothstein DM (2011) Regulatory B cells are identified by expression of TIM-1 and can be induced through TIM-1 ligation to promote tolerance in mice. J Clin Invest 121 (9):3645–3656. https://doi.org/10.1172/JCI46274
6. Yanaba K, Bouaziz JD, Haas KM, Poe JC, Fujimoto M, Tedder TF (2008) A regulatory B cell subset with a unique CD1dhiCD5+ phenotype controls T cell-dependent inflammatory responses. Immunity 28(5):639–650. https://doi.org/10.1016/j.immuni.2008.03.017
7. Blair PA, Norena LY, Flores-Borja F, Rawlings DJ, Isenberg DA, Ehrenstein MR, Mauri C (2010) CD19(+)CD24(hi)CD38(hi) B cells exhibit regulatory capacity in healthy individuals but are functionally impaired in systemic lupus Erythematosus patients. Immunity 32 (1):129–140. https://doi.org/10.1016/j.immuni.2009.11.009
8. Iwata Y, Matsushita T, Horikawa M, Dilillo DJ, Yanaba K, Venturi GM, Szabolcs PM, Bernstein SH, Magro CM, Williams AD, Hall RP, St Clair EW, Tedder TF (2011) Characterization of a rare IL-10-competent B-cell subset in humans that parallels mouse regulatory B10 cells. Blood 117(2):530–541. https://doi.org/10.1182/blood-2010-07-294249
9. Flores-Borja F, Bosma A, Ng D, Reddy V, Ehrenstein MR, Isenberg DA, Mauri C (2013) CD19+CD24hiCD38hi B cells maintain regulatory T cells while limiting TH1 and TH17 differentiation. Sci Transl Med 5 (173):173ra123. https://doi.org/10.1126/scitranslmed.3005407
10. Rosser EC, Mauri C (2014) Regulatory B cells in experimental mouse models of arthritis. Methods Mol Biol 1190:183–194. https://doi.org/10.1007/978-1-4939-1161-5_13

Chapter 6

An Innovative Standard Operation Procedure for Isolating GMP-Grade $CD4^+CD25^+$ T Cells from Non-Mobilized Leukapheresis

Wei Zhang, Suzanne M. Watt, and David J. Roberts

Abstract

This SOP describes a closed system for isolating GMP-grade $CD4^+CD25^+$ T cells from non-mobilized leukapheresis collections (nMLCs), independent of a clean room in a certified GMP premises, by using CliniMACS format GMP grade reagents (CD25-labeled magnetic beads with/without pre-depletion of $CD8^+$ T cells and $CD19^+$ B cells), a GMP grade-A laminar hood and CliniMACS cell processing system.

Key words GMP, CD25, Leukapheresis collection, CliniMACS, Magnetic beads

1 Introduction

Good manufacturing practice (GMP) is a production and testing practice which helps to ensure a quality product [1]. In many countries pharmaceutical industry and other healthcare providers follow mandatory legislation and guidelines. The SOP described here was developed and validated by the National Health Service Blood and Transplant, Oxford Centre. It complies with the guidelines of the Human Tissue Authority in the UK for the procurement and subsequent cell selection to GMP without further manipulation [2], which is achieved by processing cells within a closed system, usage of GMP-grade reagents, demonstration of reproducibility, product safety and traceability during cell processing.

Apheresis is a medical procedure in which the blood of a donor or patient is passed through an apparatus that separates out one particular constituent and returns the remainder to the circulation [3]. Leukapheresis is one type of apheresis which selectively harvests mononuclear leucocytes from a donor's circulation using apheresis machines [4]. Cell type specific gravity, as shown in Table 1, governs specificity in cell selection. It is worth noting

Ashleigh S. Boyd (ed.), *Immunological Tolerance: Methods and Protocols*, Methods in Molecular Biology, vol. 1899,
https://doi.org/10.1007/978-1-4939-8938-6_6,

Table 1
Specific gravity of different blood components

Blood component	Specific gravity
Plasma	1.025
Platelets	1.040
Lymphocytes	1.050–1.061
Monocytes	1.065–1.070
Granulocytes	1.087–1.092
Red blood cells (RBC)	1.093–1.096

that performance of different apheresis machines can vary in terms of their selectivity. We found when using the setting of Donor Lymphocyte Collection Program for harvesting nMLCs, Cobe Spectra collected significantly higher number of lymphocytes and platelets than Spectra Optia [5]. The setting of apheresis machines targets for hematopoietic stem cells may therefore need to be optimized for lymphocytes [6, 7] and subsequently validated as needed for future works.

Allo-Bone Marrow Transplanation (BMT) or hematpoietic stem cell transplantation (HSCT) is a well-established treatment for a range of malignant and other hematological diseases [8, 9]. Its success depends on graft-versus-leukemia (GvL) or graft-versus-tumor (GvT) effects of donor lymphocytes [10]. However, these lymphocytes may induce graft-versus-host disease (GvHD), a multi-organ acute and chronic disease leading to serious morbidity and mortality in allogeneic HSCT recipients. GvHD contributes to 40% of the immediate transpant related mortality. Furthermore, over half of the patients who survive suffer from chronic GvHD requiring long periods of immunosuppression and reducing their quality of life [8–10]. Elegant studies in mouse models of HSCT have shown that $CD4^+CD25^+$ (Tregs) can suppress GvHD while sparing the beneficial effect of GvL [11]. Encouraging results from several clinical trials using Tregs with or without expansion, as prophylaxis or treatment option for acute GvHD have been published [12–17]. A study in Oxford Cancer Centre of 100^+ patients received non manipulated HSCT has shown patients received grafts which contained higher than median Tregs (as percentage of $CD4^+$ T cells) had a significantly higher 5 years overall survivor [18]. Further clinical trials are required to refine the trial protocols and unravel the mechanisms underline the observed beneficial effect of Tregs in HSCT.

We found that multiple factors, which are likely to be shared by several other published methods, affected the yield of $CD4^+CD25^+$ cells [5]. There were no positive correlations between the numbers of $CD4^+$ T cells in the $CD25^+$ products and the total white blood cells (WBC) in the nMLCs. There was a substantial variation in the number of $CD4^+$ T cells in the nMLCs from different donors despite the fact that these nMLCs have a similar total number of WBC. However, positive correlations between the yield of $CD4^+CD25^+$ cells and lymphocyte numbers in the nMLCs and the $CD8^-CD19^-$ fractions were observed. In addition, we found complete depletion of $CD8^+$ T cell and $CD19^+$ B cell was achieved using the stringent *depletion program 2.1*. However, this CliniMACS negative depletion step was associated with substantial bystander cell loss. For patients receiving non-manipulated grafts, which contained a large number of leukocytes, selection for $CD25^+$ cells without $CD8^+$ T cells and $CD19^+$ B cells depletion maybe a possible option in the future as not only would cell loss be minimized during cell isolation but also a substantial financial saving would be possible.

We have made an assumption that all fluid used in this protocol is 1 mL volume equals 1 g weight. This allows us to calculate the volume from a known weight and vice versa. While $CD4^+CD25^+$ T cells are selected from nMLCs by following this SOP, the same principles and methods described here are also applicable for other cellular products, which can be enriched from peripheral blood by leukapheresis and express a specific cell surface marker allows for magnetic bead labeling, e.g. magnetic bead labeled with anti-CD34, CD14, CD56 and HLA-tetramer-antigen-complex for hematopoietic stem cells, monocytes, NK cells and pathogen-specific T cells, respectively. Post isolation manipulation is beyond the scope of this SOP. It is worth bearing in mind that complicated post isolation manipulation increases the cost, risk of contamination and complicity in legislation requirement. In vitro suppression assays have been used to demonstrate the suppressive function of $CD4^+CD25^+$ T cells. They are likely to be applied during validation procedures and as a retrospective measure of in vitro efficacy rather than as a product release criterion, due to the long processing time for these assays and lack of any evidence for a close relationship between these laboratory assays and what happens in the recipient. Much more work is needed to establish the efficacious dose, the timing of administration, the potential side-effects of cellular therapy products to patients and negative impact of GvHD prophylaxis drugs on cellular therapy products such as Tregs.

2 Materials

2.1 Material for Cell Processing

1. nMLC (*see* **Note 1**), collected by a qualified Apheresis unit using an Apheresis machine (*see* **Note 2**). Once the donor is identified and the date of donation is set, sticky labels with a donor/patient-specific barcode are generated for labeling the nMLCs and cellular product along each step of cell processing.

2. Peripheral blood samples collected into 4 mL Vacutainer (BD, 367844) pre- and post- leukapheresis collection.
3. A certified GMP premises (*see* **Note 3**), nMLCs for cell isolation must stay in the defined cell processing space within the premises once received and signed in.
4. A Grade A laminar Hood, Labcaire, Fisher Scientific, Loughborough, UK.
5. A Hematology analyzer, Sysmex XE-2100, Sysmex Corp, Kobe, Japan.
6. Centrifuge, Heraeus Megafuge 2.0RS, Rotor 2708, Thermo Scientific, Loughborough, UK.
7. CliniMACS, Miltenyi Biotec, Surrey, UK.
8. Tuber sealer, SEBRA, Haemonetics, Coventry, UK.
9. Sterile docking device, Terumo SCD II, Surrey, UK.
10. Balance, Excell, UKAS, Middlesex, UK.
11. −20 °C freezer, Fisher Scientific, Loughborough, UK.
12. Fridge, Fisher Scientific, Loughborough, UK.
13. Flat-bed rocker, Grant-Bio, Cambridgeshire, UK.
14. Plastic Spencer Wells, Fisher Scientific, Loughborough, UK.
15. Plasma press, Fenwal Europe sprl, Mont Saint Guibert, Belgium.
16. Cold packs, 216-0196, VWR, Jencons Whitworth, UK.
17. Timer.
18. One bottle each of CliniMACS format GMP-grade CD8, CD19 and CD25 microbeads for CliniMACS, Miltenyi Biotec, Surrey, UK.
19. 600 mL standard transfer bags, TerumoBCT, Surrey, UK.
20. CliniMACS tubing sets, 162-01 and 161-01, Miltenyi Biotech, Surrey, UK.
21. Pre-system filters, 130-018-101, Miltenyi Biotech, Surrey, UK.
22. Zenalb® 20, a 200 g/L of human albumin solution for infusion (20% Solution), BPL, Herts, UK.
23. CliniMACS buffer (Cat no. 700-25) 4 × 1 L supplemented with 0.5% Zenalb. It must be used at room temperature or 4 °C for different parts of the protocol—remove from cold room and allow to come to room temperature (RT) before use for all but the specified 4 °C step.
24. 2.85 mL of Gammaguard (Gammagard, Baxter, Thetford, UK) at 5%. Reconstitute Gammaguard following the manufacturer's instruction.

25. 5 mL, 10 mL, 20 mL, and 50 mL Syringes and needles, TerumoBCT, Surrey, UK.
26. Forms and bottles for aerobic and anaerobic blood cultures, BD BacTec, Oxford, UK.
27. Female sample side couplers, OriGen Biomedical, West Midlands, UK.
28. Klerwipe 70/30, Shield Medicare, Farnham, UK.
29. Processing recording sheet (Fig. 1).

2.2 Materials for Immuno-Fluorescent Staining and Flow Cytometer Analysis

1. Centrifuge, Heraeus Megafuge 1.0R, Rotor 2704, Thermo Scientific, Loughborough, UK.
2. Tube-Segment-Opener, D-51588, SARSTEDT, Leicester, UK.
3. PBS, Sigma-Aldrich, Dorset, UK.
4. 1.5 mL Eppendorfs, Eppendorf UK Limited, Stevenage, UK.
5. P20, P200, P1000 Gilson Pipettes, Gilson Scientific Ltd., Bedfordshire, UK.
6. Filter Tips, Renin, Mettler Toledo Ltd., Leicester, UK.
7. Truecount tubes, Oxford, Becton Dickenson (BD), UK.
8. 4 mL FACS tubes, Oxford, BD, UK.
9. Red cell lyses buffer, Oxford, BD, UK.
10. Antibodies: mouse anti-human CD3-FICT, CD4-PerCPCy5.5, CD8-APC-Cy7, CD20-PE, CD25-PE, BD.
11. Pan CD45-APC, R&DSystem, Abingdon, UK.
12. Live/Dead Fixable dye-blue, Invitrogen, L23105. Optional.
13. FcR blocker, Miltenyi Biotec, Surrey, UK.
14. Anti-FOXP3-APC, Miltenyi Biotec, Surrey, UK.
15. FOXP3 staining kit, Miltenyi Biotec, Surrey, UK.
16. Set of Compbeads, BD.
17. Flow cytometer with UV, blue and red lasers and appropriate long pass and band pass filters (example shown in Table 2).

3 Methods

3.1 Preparation for Cell Isolation

1. On the day of leukapheresis collection take a pigtail sample (*see* **Note 4**) from the leukapheresis bag.
2. Transfer nMLCs from the leukapheresis bag to a transfer bag by sterile docking of the leukapheresis bag with cells to a transfer bag (*see* **Note 5**). Release the Spencer Wells forceps to allow the contents of the leukapheresis bag to be completely transferred

Donor			
Donor/Patient Name	DOB:	Date of Process:	
Gender:	Hospital Number:	Weight (Kg):	Volume:
Leukapheresis Sample Analysis by Sysmex			
WBC concentration:	Total WBC	Lymph concentration:	Total lymph
Leukapheresis Sample Analysis by FACS			
$CD8^+$ T cells:		$CD19^+$ B Cells:	
CliniMACS Procedure			
CD8 Lot No.	Expiry Date:	CD19 Lot No.	Expiry Date:
Tubing Set Lot No.	Expiry Date:	Power Filter No.	Expiry Date:
Process Code:		Process Length:	
Final Volume (ml)			
$CD8^+CD19^+$:		$CD8^-CD19^-$:	Waste:
CD25 Lot No.		Expiry Date:	
Tubing Set Lot No.	Expiry Date:	Power Filter NO.	Expiry Date:
Process Code:		Process Length:	
Final Volume (ml)			
$CD25^+$:		$CD25^-$:	Waste:

Total Cell Counts (by Sysmex) $\times 10^6$ cells	WBC	Mono.	Lymph	Gran.	Platelets
Leukapheresis*					
$CD8^+CD19^+$					
$CD8^-CD19^-$					
$CD25^+$					
$CD25^-$*					

Total Cell Counts (by FACS) $\times 10^6$ cells	$CD45^+$	$CD3^-CD20^+$	$CD3^+CD8^+$	$CD3^+CD4^+$	$CD4^+CD25^+$	$CD25^+FOXP3^+$
Leukapheresis*						
$CD8^+CD19^+$						
$CD8^-CD19^-$						
$CD25^+$						
$CD25^-$*						

$CD4^+CD25^+$ cell product Storage/Issue in Cryobags				
Bags	Vol (ml)	$CD4^+CD25^+$ Stored	Date Issued	Fresh/Frozen
1				
2				

Operator's signature:____

*1 in 10 dilutions of these samples is used for Sysmex and FACS analysis.

Fig. 1 Processing recording sheet for CliniMACS selection of $CD4^+CD25^+$ cells from non-mobilized leukapheresis

Table 2
Cytometer set ups

Laser	Antigen	Conjugate	Filter setting
UV (355 nm, 20 mW)	Viability	Live/dead fixable dye	Non, 450/50
Blue (488 nm, 100 mW)	CD3 CD20 or CD25 CD4	FITC PE PerCP-Cy5.5	505LP, 530/30 550LP, 575/26 685LP, 695/40
Red (633 nm, 40 mW)	CD8 CD45 or FOXP3	APC-Cy7 APC	755LP, 780/60 Non, 660/20

to the transfer bag (*see* **Note 6**). Seal the tube with a tube sealer. Detach both bags.

3. Weigh the bag. Record the net volume of nMLC onto recording sheet. Store the bag at 4 °C overnight.
4. Label a 1.5 mL Eppendorf as NEAT nMLC. Transfer the contents of the pigtail sample to this vial (*see* **Note 7**).
5. Make a master dilution of nMCL for Sysmex and FACS cell quantitation. Label a 1.5 mL Eppendorf as 1:10 nMLC. Transfer 450 μL of PBS and 50 μL of NEAT nMLC to this vial (*see* **Note 8**).
6. Perform cell count by Sysmex (*see* **Note 9**) and FACS analysis (*see* Subheading 3.3, **step 7**) to determine the absolute number of cells of interest in the nMLC.
7. Record cell number onto the recording sheet after Sysmex and FACS analysis. The total number of WBC and the total percentage of $CD8^+$ T cells and $CD19^+$ B cells should be entered into the CliniMACS for the depletion step.

3.2 Reagent Preparation

Perform the following preparations in a grade A GMP tissue culture hood.

1. Draw the thawed Gammaguard into a 5 mL syringe.
2. Draw the contents of CD25 bead bottle into a 10 mL syringe.
3. Draw the contents of CD8 and CD19 bead into a 20 mL syringe.
4. Each time replace the needles with female sample side couplers. Store these syringes in individual sealed bags in a GMP-grade fridge.
5. Prepare 4 × 1 L CliniMACS buffer supplemented with 0.5% Zenalb (*see* **Note 10**).
6. Record the Lot number and expiry date onto the recording sheet at the end of reagent preparation.

3.3 Immuno-Fluorescent Staining for Lymphocyte Phenotyping

Sample preparation:

1. Label Eppendorfs correspondent to each pigtail sample. Transfer samples from pigtail tubes to Eppendorfs following **Note 7**.
2. A one in ten master dilution is made from nMLC and $CD25^{-}$ fractions due to high cell concentration follow **Note 8**.
3. Label one set of Trucount tubes according to the name and number (n) of samples for lymphocyte phenotyping.

   Antibody preparation:
   See Table 3 for details.
   Staining procedure:

4. Transfer 100 μL of each sample to the correspondent Trucount tubes. Accurate sample volume is important for calculation. Apply the two steps pipetting method or use an electronic pipette for obtaining accurate sample volume.
5. Transfer 40 μL of the antibody mix from panel one to each Trucount tube; mix well; and leave the tubes to incubate in the dark for 15 min at room temperature.
6. At the end of incubation, add 1 mL of red cell lyses buffer to each tube; check the tubes frequently. Once the solution turned from cloudy to clear (take about 4–6 min at RT), the samples are ready for analysis on FAC machine.
7. CST beads must be run on the day of experiment for instrument set up. Compbeads staining with single color is used for setup compensation. Instrument setup by CST beads is recommended for achieving maximal detection sensitivity.

Lymphocyte concentration (#/μL) = # of $CD45^{+}$ events/ # of events in absolute count beads region × # of beads per test* /test volume (100 μL).

* This number is Trucount tube batch specific; it is on the bag of Trucount tube. Make sure to use correct number.

Absolute number of lymphocyte in the sample = Lymphocyte concentration (#/μL) × volume of the sample × dilution factor.

Table 3
Antibody mix for lymphocyte typing

	CD45	CD3	CD4	CD8	CD20
	APC	FITC	PERCPCy5.5	APC-Cy7	PE
SAMPLE × n	5 μL	10 μL	10 μL	5 μL	10 μL
	× n	× n	× n	× n	× n

N = number of samples to be stained

Total number of lymphocyte subsets (e.g. $CD3^{+}CD4^{+}$ T cells) = Total number of lymphocyte in the sample × % of $CD3^{+}CD4^{+}$ cells in the lymphocyte gate.

Collect Sysmex and FACS report, Bead CE certificate and the recording sheet ready for the next day process.

3.4 Leukapheresis Preparation

Wash to reduce the number of platelets and the volume of the nMLC for the bead labeling.

1. Sterile dock the bag with cells to the MACS buffer bag. Increase the volume of nMLC to 550 mL (*see* **Note 11**). Seal the tube with a tube sealer and detach the MACS buffer bag.
2. Sterile dock the bag with cells to a new empty transfer bag (*see* **Note 12**).
3. Place the bags and a balance bag (*see* **Note 13**) in the buckets of a centrifuge (*see* **Note 14**). Centrifuge at 200 × *g* for 10 min with brake off. Total time required for this step is about 20 min.
4. At the end of centrifugation, carefully remove the bag with cells from the bucket. To remove the supernatant, hang the bag onto the plasma presser or extruder, push the hook forward. Release the presser from the stationary or fixed position to allow it to come into contact with the bag. Release the Spencer Wells to allow supernatant to flow from the nMLC bag to the empty transfer bag. Try to remove as much supernatant as possible without disturbing the pellet. Avoid moving the position of the bag during releasing supernatant.
5. Clamp the tube with two Spencer Wells when the cell pellet starts to be disturbed. Seal the tube with a tube sealer. Detach the bags.
6. Resuspend the pellet (*see* **Note 15**).
7. Sterile dock the syringe containing Gammaguard to the bag containing cells. Release Spencer Wells and push the plunge to transfer Gammaguard to the cell bag. Seal the tube and detach the bags. Mix Gammaguard and cells by inverting the bag a few times.
8. Increase the volume of nMLC for bead labeling. Sterile dock MACS buffer bag to the bag with cells. Transfer buffer to nMLC bag as described in **Note 11**. The volume of cell suspension for the negative depletion is 90 mL.

3.5 CD8 and CD19 Depletion

1. Transfer CD8 and CD19 beads to the nMLCs bag. Connect the syringe containing CD8 and CD19 beads and the bag containing cells by sterile docking. Seal the tube with tube sealer after the contents of the syringe has been completely transferred to the bag. Detach the syringe. Mix well and

incubate for 30 min at controlled RT, no higher than 25 °C. Rotate gently on the flat bed rocker mixer.

2. Wash cells to remove excessive beads. At the end of incubation, sterile dock the bag with MACS buffer bag. Transfer buffer to the bag with cells (*see* **Note 11**). Clamp and seal the tube then sterile dock the cell bag to a new transfer bag (*see* **Note 12**) before centrifugation.
3. Repeat **steps 4–6** under Subheading 3.3. At the end of centrifugation, change the temperature setting of the centrifuge to 4 °C for all the rest of centrifugation steps.
4. Increase the volume of nMLCs to 100 mL for CliniMACS run. Sterile dock the cell bag and MACS buffer. Transfer MACS buffer to the now completely resuspended cells (*see* **Note 11**). Seal and detach the bags.
5. To connect a 162-01 tubing set with cell bag, buffer bag and cell collection bag. In a GMP grade A hood, check to make sure that all connections in the tubing set are properly sealed; connect a bag of **cold** MACS buffer and a pre-system filter to the tubing set. **Clamp** tubes connecting CliniMACS tubing set to the MACS buffer bag and the pre-system filter with Spencer Wells (*see* **Note 16**). Sterile dock a new transfer bag to the output tube of the 162-01 tubing set for collecting cells.
6. Hook up the MACS buffer bag, cell bag and the waste wash bag onto the CliniMACS. Install the tubing set following CliniMACS instructions. Select *depletion program 2.1* from the manual. Input the total number of WBC and the total percentage of CD8 and CD19 labeled cells. Set machine to RUN and release Spencer Wells. Once the cell suspension starts to fill the power filter, gently tap the filter till there are no air bubbles going up; this minimizes air bubbles trapped on the filter and increases efficiency. While the negative depletion is in progress, sandwich the bag for the negative fraction (containing $CD8^{-}CD19^{-}$ cells) between two cold blocks. The depletion takes about 80 min and uses $\leq$1 L of buffer for an average size of nMLC.
7. While the depletion is in progress record Lot number and expiry date of the 162-01 tubing set used and processing time (this will show on CliniMACS machine) onto the recording sheet. Label the bags using sticky labels.
8. At the end of CliniMACS depletion step, record the CliniMACS protocol number onto the recording sheet; clamp or seal all the tubes in and out of the CliniMACS tubing set and remove the bags from hooks.
9. Detach the bag containing $CD8^{-}CD19^{-}$ fraction and promptly proceed to the CD25 positive isolation.

10. Take a pigtail sample (*see* **Note 4**) from each of the bags containing $CD8^{+}CD19^{+}$ and $CD8^{-}CD19^{-}$ cells. Label the samples.
11. Weigh the bags and record the net volume onto the recording sheet.

3.6 CD25 Isolation

1. For the CD25 beads labeling, the incubation volume is 380 mL (± 10%). Increase or decrease the volume of the $CD8^{-}CD19^{-}$ fraction depending on its volume. If the weight of the cell bag is in the range of 380–440 g go straight into CD25 bead selection.
2. Transfer CD25 beads to the bag of cells via a sample side coupler using a sterile docking system. Mix well. Sandwich the bag in between one cold block stored in a fridge at 4 °C and one stored in a freezer at −20 °C. Wrap in cling film and place the bundle on a rocker and incubate for 15 min.
3. Wash the cells to remove excessive beads. At the end of incubation, sterile dock the bag with cells with a bag containing cold MACS buffer. Transfer MACS buffer to cell bag (*see* **Note 11**).
4. Seal the bag then sterile dock the bag with cells to a new transfer bag (*see* **Note 12**) before centrifugation.
5. Repeat **steps 4–6** under Subheading 3.3 above.
6. Resuspend cell pellet (*see* **Note 15**).
7. Increase the volume of $CD8^{-}CD19^{-}$ to 100 mL for CliniMACS run (*see* **Note 11**).
8. In a GMP grade A hood, connect the bag with cells, the pre-system filter and buffer bag to a CliniMACS tubing set 161-01 by repeating Subheading 3.4, **step 5** (*see* **Note 16**).
9. Hook up buffer bag, bag of cells, and waste collection bag. Install the tubing set to the CliniMACS. Select program *enrichment 3.1*. Press RUN and release the Spencer Wells.
10. While the positive selection is in progress, record Lot number and expiry date of the 161-01 tubing set used, and processing time onto the recording sheet. Label the bags using sticky labels generated earlier.
11. At the end of the enrichment program, record the CliniMACS protocol number onto the recording sheet; seal all the tubes in and out of the CliniMACS tubing set. Remove all bags and the tubing set and then shut down CliniMACS.
12. Weigh the bags containing $CD25^{+}$ and $CD25^{-}$ fractions and record the net volume of the content (*see* **Note 17**). Take a pigtail sample from both $CD25^{-}$ and $CD25^{+}$ fractions for Sysmex and FACS analysis (*see* **Note 4**). Label the pigtail samples.

Table 4
Antibody mix for Treg semi-quantification

	CD3	CD4	CD25		FOXP3 APC
	FITC	PERCPCy5.5	PE	Fix&Perm	
FMO FITC		10 μL	20 μL		20 μL
FMO PERCPCy5.5	10 μL		20 μL		20 μL
FMO PE	10 μL	10 μL			20 μL
FMO APC	10 μL	10 μL	20 μL		
SAMPLE × *n*	10 μL	10 μL	20 μL		20 μL
	× *n*	× *n*	× *n*		× *n*

13. In the GMP grade A hood, take a sample from the negative fraction (*see* **Note 18**); inoculate 3 mL of the negative fraction to each of the aerobic and anaerobic blood cultures. Fill in the form and send the bottles to local microbiology department.
14. Operators must complete and sign the production form.

3.7 Immuno-Fluorescent Staining for Semi-Quantification of Regulatory T Cells Number in the Donor Peripheral Blood and the nMLCs Before and Throughout Each Step of the GMP Cell Isolation Process

1. Label another set of FACS tubes according to the name and number (*n*) of samples and FMOs (Table 4) for Treg semi quantification.
2. Transfer 100 μL of each (diluted or neat) sample as used for the lymphocyte quantification to the correctly-labeled FACS tubes including FMO-1 controls for Treg quantification.
3. Add 40 μL of Treg antibody mix or FMO mixes to the cell suspension. **Mix well** and leave to incubate at RT for 20 min.
4. At the end of incubation, top up the tubes with 3 mL of PBS and centrifuge at 300 × *g* for 5 min.
5. Discard the supernatant. Vortex tubes to resuspend cells (*see* **Note 19**).
6. Lyse red cells as described in the lymphocyte staining protocol and wash cells once with 3 mL of PBS and centrifuge at 300 × *g* for 5 min.
7. Discard the supernatant and blot the tube on a piece of tissue paper. This will reduce the residual buffer to around 50 μL. Vortex tubes to resuspend cells.
8. Live/Dead stain is optional. Make the Live/Dead stain working solution by diluting the stock of Live/Dead solution 1/1000 in PBS (*see* **Note 20**). Add 1 mL of this **Live/Dead stain** working solution to each FACS tube. Leave the sample to incubate at RT for 10 min.

9. At the end of incubation, top up the tubes with 3 mL of PBS and centrifuge at 300 × *g* for 5 min.
10. Discard the supernatant. Vortex tubes to resuspend cells.
11. Add 0.5 mL of freshly prepared diluted **fix buffer** from the FOXP3 staining buffer kit to each tube; incubate the tubes in a fridge @ 4 °C for at least 30 min.
12. At the end of incubation, top up the tubes with 3 mL of PBS and centrifuge at 300 × *g* 4 °C for 5 min.
13. Discard the supernatant. Vortex tubes to resuspend cells.
14. Wash the cell one more time in 1 mL of **perm buffer** per sample.
15. Discard the supernatant and blot the tube on tissue paper. Vortex tubes to resuspend cells.
16. Add 5 μL of FcR blocker to the cell suspension and incubate for 5–10 min at RT.
17. Add 20 μL of anti-FOXP3 to each tube and incubate the tubes at 4 °C in the dark for 30 min.
18. At the end of incubation, top up the tubes with 1 mL of perm buffer, leave it to stand for 2 min before centrifuge at 300 × *g* 4 °C for 5 min.
19. Discard the supernatant and resuspend the pellet in PBS.
20. Repeat **steps 18** and **19**. Cells are ready for FACS analysis.

(Assume cells lost to different subsets in the sample occurred in equal proportion.)

Number of Treg = Absolute number of $CD3^{+}CD4^{+}$ T cell in a sample × % of $CD25^{+}FOXP3^{+}$ cells in the $CD3^{+}CD4^{+}$ T cell gate of the sample.

4 Notes

1. Use of nMLCs for research and development requires ethical permission from local Ethics Committee.
2. Spectra Optia (TerumoBCT, Surrey, UK) is the one currently provided on contract to NHS National Blood and Transplant in the UK.
3. Certified GMP premises is regulated, maintained, and inspected according to national guidelines. For details of guidelines in UK consult the MHRA at http://www.mhra.gov.uk/Howweregulate/Medicines/Inspectionandstandards/GoodManufacturingPractice/index.htm

4. To take a pigtail line sample, the line is stripped back six times while mixing the bag, before being sealed off and removed using the RF tube sealer. The length of the line to be taken is dependent on the cell concentration of the solution. Samples such as nMLCs, and $CD25^-$ fraction have a high cell concentration. 1 cm of line containing cell solution is sufficient. Master dilutions must be prepared from the neat solutions for cell quantitation by Sysmex counter (takes about 200 μL per run) and FACS (take 100 μL per FACS panel). 1.5 cm of line or approximately 500 μL of cell solution to be taken for other samples ($CD8^+CD19^+$, $CD8^-CD19^-$ and $CD25^+$).
5. Sterile dock the bags (or sample side coupler). Make sure there is sufficient length of tube to allow for the sterile docking. First, clamp the tubes from both the bags with Spencer Wells, then perform the sterile docking using the sterile docking device. Check the sterile docking is intact. The Spencer Wells provide an additional guarantee of an enclosed system, but can still allow for liquid transfer to take place when they are released at the time indicated in the protocol.
6. The size of a leukapheresis bag is too big for the height of hanger of the CliniMACS. The weight of a leukapheresis and a 600 mL transfer bag is 40 g and 30 g, respectively.
7. To empty the contents of a pigtail line, cut one end of the tube and insert the open end to a vial or Eppendorf tube. Insert a Tube-Segment-Opener to the other end of the tube. The contents of the pigtail line will drain freely into the vial. Check the vial labeling is correct and discard the pigtail line and the Tube-Segment-Opener.
8. Apply the two-step pipetting technique or use an electronic pipette to minimize pipetting error. Use a master dilution to avoid inconsistency.
9. Operate the Sysmex counter following the instrument manual.
10. Wipe the detachable metal lid with an alcohol wipe before lifting it from a Zenalb bottle. Draw 2.5 mL of Zenalb® 20 from the bottle. Replace the needle with a sample side coupler. Connect the syringe to the tube of a buffer bag using a sterile docking device. Inject the contents of the syringe into the buffer bag. Seal the tube using a tube sealer and detach the syringe from the bag. Repeat this for the remaining three bags of buffer.
11. Once the sterile docking is completed, place the bag with nMLC on a balance and top up the bag with MACS buffer by releasing the two Spencer Wells and monitor the weight. The volume for all washing steps and CliniMACS runs is 550 mL and 100 mL, so clamp the tube with Spencer Wells when the weight of the bag is 580 g or 130 g, respectively. The volume

for CD8 and CD19 beads incubation is 90 mL, so clamp the bag when the weight of bag reaches 120 g.

12. The empty bag is for discarded supernatant after centrifugation. Docking before centrifugation minimizes the risk of disturbing the cell pellet.
13. Wrap the empty bag and tube around the Spencer Wells so the empty bag and the Spencer Wells can be tucked down tightly and neatly in the centrifugation bucket in the next step. Have the non-covered side of the bag facing outside of the bucket. Tuck down with tissue and make sure the bag stands upright without folds and bends, so that a compact pellet will form at the end of centrifugation step.
14. A balance bag is prepared in advance by transferring 550 mL of distilled water into a transfer bag. The tube is sealed and clamped with a Spencer Well for balancing purposes.
15. To disperse the cell pellet, hold the two ends of the bag and roll it against the edge of a bench. Hold the bag against a light source to check for any visible cell clumps. Repeat this until no visible clumps remain before proceeding to the next step. It is important to completely resuspend the cell pellet to minimize cell loss in the pre-system filters. Make sure the cell pellet is well resuspended before increasing the volume as better cell resuspension is achieved in a smaller volume.
16. If the tubes leading to the pre-system filter are not clamped, cells and buffer will flood the CliniMACS set. These cells will be flushed to the waste bag during the subsequent CliniMACS tubing set preparation. It is therefore important to clamp all the tubes that lead to the pre-system filter before hanging up CliniMACS tubing set.
17. The content of CliniMACS positive isolation is 50 mL by default. We found the real volume is between 45 and 50 mL. We recommend recording the real volume to avoid overestimation of cell number.
18. Use the negative fraction to inoculate each of the aerobic and anaerobic blood cultures to minimize the waste of $CD25^+$ cells.
19. Make sure cell pellets are well resuspended after each centrifugation.
20. Make sure cells are washed in PBS to remove proteins before staining with Live/Dead dye as this dye is amine reactive.

Acknowledgments

We would like to acknowledge the support of NHS Blood and Transplant, the National Institute for Health Biomedical Research

Centre Program and the NHSBT and Department of Haematology Trust Funds. This report presents independent research commissioned by the National Institutes for Health Research (NIHR) under its Programme Grants for Applied Research Programme (Grant Reference Number RP-PG-0310-1003) (WZ, DJR, SMW). The views expressed in this publication are those of the authors and not necessarily those of the NHS, the NIHR, or the Department of Health.

The authors wish to thank all donors who participated in this study and the Therapeutic Apheresis Services Unit NHSBT Oxford for providing the leukapheresis collections.

References

1. http://www.who.int/medicines/areas/quality_safety/quality_assurance/about/en/index.html
2. http://www.hta.gov.uk/
3. Burgstaler EA (2006) Blood component collection by apheresis. J Clin Apher 21:142–151
4. Hester J (2000) Peripheral blood stem cell collection: the interaction of technology, procedure, and biological factors. Transfus Sci 23:125–132
5. Zhang W, Frith E, Belfield H, Smythe J, Clarke S, Watt SM, Danby R, Benjamin S, Peniket A, Roberts DJ (2015) An innovative method to generate a GMP-grade regulatory T cell product from non-mobilised leukapheresis donors independent of a clean room facility. Cytotheropy
6. Hester J, Bojko P, Rondon G, Champlin R (1996) Integration of biological, procedural, apheresis principles of peripheral blood stem cell transplantation programs. Transfus Sci 17:585–590
7. Steininger PA, Smith R, Geier C, Zimmermann R, Eckstein R, Strasser EF (2013) Leukapheresis in non-cytokine-stimulated donors with a new apheresis system: first-time collection results and evaluation of subsequent cryopreservation. Transfusion 53:747–756
8. Welniak LA, Blazar BR, Murphy WJ (2007) Immunobiology of allogeneic hematopoietic stem cell transplantation. Annu Rev Immunol 25:139–170
9. Gyurkocza B, Rezvani A, Storb RF (2010) Allogeneic hematopoietic cell transplantation: the state of the art. Expert Rev Hematol 3 (3):285–299
10. Ringden O, Karlsson H, Olsson R, Omazic B, Uhlin M (2009) The allogeneic graft-versus-cancer effect. Br J Haematol 147(5):614–633
11. M E, Hoffmann P, Ermann J, Drago K, Fathman CG, Strober S, Negrin RS (2003) CD4+CD25+ regulatory T cells preserve graft-versus-tumor activity while inhibiting graft-versus-host disease after bone marrow transplantation. Nat Med 9(9):1144–1150
12. Trzonkowski P, Bieniaszewska M, Juścińska J, Dobyszuk A, Krzystyniak A, Marek N, Myśliwska J, Hellmann A (2009) First-in-man clinical results of the treatment of patients with graft versus host disease with human ex vivo expanded CD4+CD25+CD127- T regulatory cells. Clin Immunol 133(1):22–26
13. Di Ianni M, Falzetti F, Carotti A, Terenzi A, Del Papa B, Perruccio K, Ruggeri L, Sportoletti P, Rosati E, Marconi P, Falini B, Reisner Y, Velardi A, Aversa F, Martelli MF (2011) Immunoselection and clinical use of T regulatory cells in HLA-haploidentical stem cell transplantation. Best Pract Res Clin Haematol 24(3):459–466
14. Edinger M, Hoffmann P (2011) Regulatory T cells in stem cell transplantation: strategies and first clinical experiences. Curr Opin Immunol 23(5):679–684
15. Brunstein CG, Miller JS, Cao Q, McKenna DH, Hippen KL, Curtsinger J, Defor T, Levine BL, June CH, Rubinstein P, McGlave PB, Blazar BR, Wagner JE (2011) Infusion of ex vivo expanded T regulatory cells in adults transplanted with umbilical cord blood: safety profile and detection kinetics. Blood 117 (3):1061–1070
16. A G, Landau DA, Martin GH, Bonduelle O, Grinberg-Bleyer Y, Matheoud D, Grégoire S, Baillou C, Combadière B, Piaggio E, Cohen JL (2011) Immune reconstitution is preserved in hematopoietic stem cell transplantation coadministered with regulatory T cells for GVHD prevention. Blood 117(10):2975–2983

17. Martelli MF, Di Ianni M, Ruggeri L, Falzetti F, Carotti A, Terenzi A, Pierini A, Massei MS, Amico L, Urbani E, Del Papa B, Zei T, Iacucci Ostini R, Cecchini D, Tognellini R, Reisner Y, Aversa F, Falini B, Velardi A (2014) HLA-haploidentical transplantation with regulatory and conventional T-cell adoptive immunotherapy prevents acute leukemia relapse. Blood 124(4):638–644

18. Danby RD, Zhang W, Medd P, Littlewood TJ, Peniket A, Rocha V, Roberts DJ (2016) High proportions of regulatory T cells in PBSC grafts predict improved survival after allogeneic haematopoietic SCT. Bone Marrow Transplantation 51:110–118

Part III

Mechanisms and Induction of Immunological Tolerance

Chapter 7

Measuring CTLA-4-Dependent Suppressive Function in Regulatory T Cells

Tie Zheng Hou, Omar S. Qureshi, and David M. Sansom

Abstract

Regulatory T cells (Treg) have a central role in controlling the activation of self-reactive T cells and maintaining peripheral tolerance in our body. Many effector mechanisms for Treg function have been described including a role for the protein CTLA-4 which is constitutively expressed by these cells. Despite its importance, there is currently little consensus in the methods and protocols for studying CTLA-4 function, which is partially due to debate over CTLA-4 function itself. In this chapter, we outline protocols used in our lab to study CTLA-4 function, which have been generated based on the observation that CTLA-4 acts to physically remove and degrade its ligands expressed by antigen presenting cells. Accordingly, we provide protocols for isolation of human monocytes and their differentiation into dendritic cells (DC), purification of conventional and regulatory T-cell populations, and the assembly of CTLA-4-dependent Treg suppression assays. We hope that this will offer a reliable platform for dissecting the biology of CTLA-4 on Treg and for testing reagents aimed at modulating CTLA-4 function. Such assays are increasingly vital for the study of immune function in both healthy individuals and patients with a variety of autoimmune and immune dysregulation syndromes.

Key words Conventional T cells, Regulatory T cells, CTLA-4, CD80, CD86, CD28, Transendocytosis, Dendritic cell, Costimulation, Suppression

1 Introduction

Regulatory T cells (Treg) are key regulators in the immune system and play an essential role in maintaining immune homeostasis and tolerance [1]. Loss of Treg due to mutation in the key transcription factor Foxp3 results in profound autoimmunity [2, 3]. This has focused attention on the effector mechanisms whereby Treg suppress self-reactivity and multiple mechanisms have been identified. These include cell-contact dependent molecules and soluble factors that are expressed on and secreted by Treg, respectively [4–8]. However, among these mechanisms, is a role for the protein CTLA-4 which is increasingly recognized as imparting a dominant suppressive function to Treg in vivo [9–12]. Accordingly, animals lacking CTLA-4 die from fatal autoimmune disease characterized

Ashleigh S. Boyd (ed.), *Immunological Tolerance: Methods and Protocols*, Methods in Molecular Biology, vol. 1899, https://doi.org/10.1007/978-1-4939-8938-6_7,

by multiple tissue infiltration and organ failure caused by self-reactive T cells [13–15]. Interestingly, it is also evident that autoimmunity due to the lack of CTLA-4 is dependent on the presence of the immune stimulatory protein CD28 and its ligands CD80 and CD86 for which CTLA-4 is a shared receptor. The importance of the CD28/CTLA-4 pathway has therefore led to the development of numerous therapeutic interventions in recent years including the generation of multiple soluble CTLA-4 variants [16], the use of Treg for adoptive therapies [17], and the use of anti-CTLA-4 for tumor therapy [18]. While CTLA-4 is accepted as a crucial negative regulator of T-cell responses, there is still controversy over its fundamental behavior at a molecular level [19]. This debate appears to have impeded the development of robust assays for CTLA-4 function and as a result, there are no widely accepted protocols available.

Accepting the on-going mechanistic controversies, it is nonetheless our view that there is compelling evidence that CTLA-4 works in a cell-extrinsic manner: that is CTLA-4 expressed on Treg works via influencing the antigen presenting cells (APC) [10]. A number of in vivo studies point to the fact that CTLA-4 expressing cells can control CTLA-4 deficient cells indicating a cell-extrinsic function. More importantly from an assay perspective we recently observed a novel-molecular mechanism (transendocytosis) where CTLA-4 acts to capture and destroy its ligands CD80/CD86 from cells in contact. This cell-extrinsic function deprives the APC of the capacity to costimulate T cells via CD28 [20]. The core of this new idea is that T cells expressing CTLA-4 control costimulatory signals derived from CD28 interactions with its ligands. It is well established that CD28 costimulation is generally required for full T-cell activation and CTLA-4 therefore acts to limit this function [21]. A more detailed consideration of this idea reveals that the function of CTLA-4 is likely not ubiquitous, but rather limited to specific contexts. Perhaps most germane to this argument, is the fact that CTLA-4 function cannot be measured if the T-cell response is not specifically dependent on the presence of CD28 ligands. Accordingly, widely used protocols using beads coated with CD3 and CD28 antibodies cannot be used to measure CTLA-4 functions. In addition, the balance between the total number of ligands (CD80/CD86) and the amount of CTLA-4 available will also determine the functional efficacy of CTLA-4 behavior. Accordingly, low amounts of ligand will generally be susceptible to CTLA-4 suppression. In contrast high levels of ligand and/or relatively low levels of CTLA-4 would permit CD28 costimulation. We have shown that such predictions hold true in experimental models and act to predict CTLA-4-dependent Treg function [22]. Based on this concept, we have developed quantitative assays to examine Treg suppressive function mediated by CTLA-4 which are capable of identifying defects in CTLA-4 expression [23]. Here, we describe the details of isolation and differentiation of relevant cells and the assembly of in vitro assays capable of measuring CTLA-4-dependent regulatory T-cell function in humans.

2 Materials

2.1 Reagents and Monoclonal Antibodies

1. For reagents *see* Table 1.
2. For monoclonal antibodies *see* Table 2.

2.2 Isolation Buffer and Culture Media

1. Isolation buffer: PBS supplemented with 2 mM EDTA and 0.5% bovine serum albumin.
2. Culture media: RPMI 1640 supplemented with 10% FBS, 1% Penicillin (10,000 U/ml), 1% streptomycin (10 mg/ml), and 1% L-glutamine (2 mM).
3. Culture conditions: cells are cultured at 37°C, 95% humidity and 5% CO_2 in an incubator.

2.3 Cellular Components

2.3.1 Isolation of Human Peripheral Blood Mononucleated Cells

1. 50 ml fresh blood from healthy individuals is diluted at 1:1 with PBS.
2. Peripheral blood mononucleated cells (PBMC) isolations are performed by density gradient centrifugation (1000 × *g* for 25 min) following overlay of 25–30 ml diluted blood onto 15 ml Ficoll-Paque PLUS.
3. Yield is approximately 50–100 × 10^6 depending on donors.
4. PBMC are resuspended at 100 × 10^6/ml in isolation buffer for further separation and phenotyping by flow cytometry.

2.3.2 Isolation of Human CD14⁺ Monocytes by Magnetic Particle Separation

1. Monocytes are purified from PBMC by negative selection using human monocyte enrichment kit as follows:
2. PBMC are incubated with bispecific tetrameric antibody complexes containing monoclonal antibodies against CD2, CD3, CD16, CD19, CD20, CD56, CD66b, CD123, glycophorin A and dextran at 50 μl/ml of PBMC at 4 °C for 10 min in a 5 ml tube.
3. Dextran-coated D magnetic particles are vortexed thoroughly and added to the cells at 50μl/ml and incubated at 4 °C for 5 min.
4. Isolation buffer is added to a total volume of 2.5 ml and the tube is placed into the magnet for 5 min.
5. While still attached to the magnet, cells (containing negative fraction-enriched $CD14^+$ monocytes) are poured into a new 5 ml tube.
6. The magnetized tube is left inverted for 2–3 s and magnetically labeled (positive fraction/$cocktail^+$ cells) cells remain.

Table 1
Reagents

Reagent name	Alternative name Or abbreviation	Source	Catalog no.
Phosphate buffered saline	PBS	OXOID	BR0014G
Ethylenediaminetetraacetic acid	EDTA	Fisher Scientific	BP2482-1
Bovine Serum Albumin	BSA	ACROS ORGANICS	268131000
Roswell Park Memorial Institute 1640 medium	RPMI 1640 medium	Invitrogen or Life Tech	21875-034
Fetal bovine serum	FBS	Biosera or Life Tech	FCS-SA500-30401
Penicillin and streptomycin	P/S	GIBCO or Life Tech	15140-122
L-glutamine	L-G	GIBCO or Life Tech	25030-024
Ficoll-Paque PLUS	NA	GE Healthcare	17-1440-03
Human monocyte enrichment kit	NA	StemCell Technologies	19059
Human granulocyte-macrophage colony-stimulating factor	hGM-CSF or LEUKINE liquid Sargramostim	BERLEX	NA
Human interleukin 4	hIL-4	Miltenyi Biotec	130-093-924
Human $CD4^+$ T cell enrichment kit	NA	StemCell Technologies	19052
Human naïve $CD4^+$ T cell enrichment kit	NA	StemCell Technologies	19155
CD25 TAC custom kit	NA	StemCell Technologies	19309
CellTrace violet stain	CTV	Molecular Probes or Invitrogen	C34557
Human $CD4^+CD127^{low}CD49d^-$ regulatory T cells enrichment kit	NA	StemCell Technologies	19232
CTLA-4-Ig	Abatacept or ORENCIA	Bristol-Myers Squibb	1218778A3
Anti-CD3 antibody	OKT3	Hybridoma from ATCC	NA

(continued)

Table 1
(continued)

Reagent name	Alternative name Or abbreviation	Source	Catalog no.
Anti-CTLA-4	Tremelimumab or Ticilimumab	Gifts or Pharmacy	NA
CD3/CD28 T cell expander Dynabeads	Dynabeads human T-activator CD3/CD28	Invitrogen	111.31D
AccuCheck counting bead	NA	Invitrogen	PCB100

Table 2
Anti-human monoclonal antibodies

Target specificity	Isotype	Clone	Format	Source	Catalog no.
CD3	Mouse IgG1, κ	SK7	FITC	BD Pharmingen	345764
CD4	Mouse IgG1, κ	RPA-T4	PE APC	BD Pharmingen	555346 555349
CD4	Mouse IgG2b, κ	OKT4	PB	eBioscience	57-0048-71
CD11c (αX integrin chain)	Mouse IgG1, κ	Bly6	APC	BD Pharmingen	559877
CD14	MouseIgG2b, κ	MϕP9	PerCP	BD Pharmingen	345786
CD25 (IL-2Rα)	Mouse IgG1, κ	M-A251	PE	BD Pharmingen	555432
CD45RA	Mouse IgG2b, κ	HI100	PE	BD Pharmingen	555489
CD45RO	Mouse IgG2a, κ	UCHL1	FITC	BD Pharmingen	555492
CD49d (α4 integrin chain)	Mouse IgG2b, κ	9F10	FITC	BD Pharmingen	560840
CD80 (B7-1)	Mouse IgG1, κ	L307.4	PE	BD Pharmingen	557,227
CD86 (B7-2)	Mouse IgG1, κ	2331 (FUN-1)	FITC	BD Pharmingen	555657
CD127 (IL-7Rα)	Mouse IgG1, κ	HIL-7R-M21	PE-Cy7	BD Pharmingen	560822
CD152 (CTLA-4)	Mouse IgG2a, κ	BN13	PE	BD Pharmingen	555853
FoxP3 (Scurfin)	Mouse IgG1, κ	236A/E7	APC	eBioscience	17-4777-42

7. The magnetic removal step is repeated to improve yield and negatively selected cells are collected into a 20 ml universal.
8. Yield is approximately 10–15% of PBMC depending on donors.

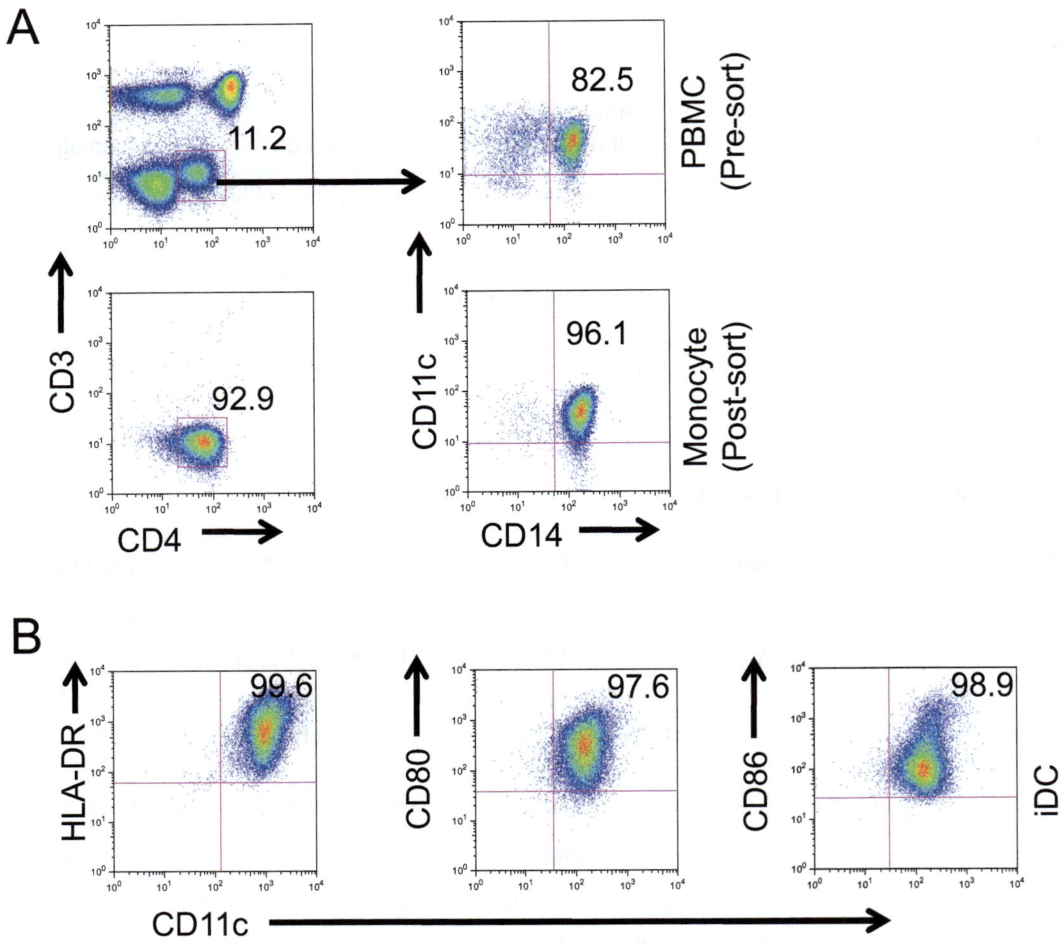

Fig. 1 Generation of human iDC (**a**) Purification of human monocytes. Monocytes are sorted from PBMC by negative selection using human monocyte enrichment kit. Pre-sort PBMC populations are FACS stained with CD3 and CD4 and gated to show the expression of CD11c and CD14 (upper panels) in CD3 and CD4 low compartments. Purified monocytes are re-analyzed to show the sorting efficacy (lower panels). (**b**) Phenotype of differentiated human iDC from sorted monocytes in A. Human monocytes were cultured with GM-CSF and IL-4 for 7 days and stained for CD11c, HLA-DR, CD80, and CD86 expression

9. Monocytes are resuspended in culture media at a density of 2×10^6/ml for further differentiation into DC in culture.
10. Monocytes are phenotyped by flow cytometry and are typically $CD3^-$ $CD4^{low}CD14^+CD11c^+$ cells (Fig. 1a).

2.3.3 Differentiation of Immature DC Derived from Human CD14⁺ Monocytes

1. Monocytes are cultured in flat-bottom 24-well plates in 0.5 ml (1×10^6 cells)/well in culture media supplemented with human GM-CSF at 20 ng/ml and human IL-4 at 100 ng/ml.
2. At day 2, cultures are further supplemented with 0.5 ml fresh culture media containing human GM-CSF and IL-4 at final volume of 1 ml.

3. At day 7, immature DC (iDC) are harvested for use in T-cell stimulations. When collecting DC, the culture plate is placed on ice for 20 min to reduce adherence. Wells are washed with ice-cold PBS and cells are suspended by gentle pipetting.
4. Yield is approximately 25–40% or 0.25–0.4 $\times$ 10^6/well depending on donors.
5. iDC are resuspended in culture media at a density of 0.36 $\times$ 10^6/ml and used as APC in T-cell proliferation and suppression assays.
6. iDC are phenotyped by flow cytometry and typically $CD11c^+HLA\text{-}DR^+CD80^+CD86^+$ cells (Fig. 1b).

2.3.4 Enrichment of Human Total $CD4^+$ T Cells by Magnetic Particle Separation

1. Total $CD4^+$ T cells are purified from PBMC by negative selection using human $CD4^+$ T cell enrichment kit as follows:
2. PBMC are incubated with bispecific tetrameric antibody complexes containing monoclonal antibodies against CD8, CD14, CD16, CD19, CD20, CD36, CD56, CD123, TCRγδ, glycophorin A and dextran at 25μl/ml at room temperature for 10 min in a 5 ml tube.
3. Dextran-coated D magnetic particles are vortexed thoroughly and added to the cells at 50μl/ml and incubated at room temperature for 5 min.
4. Isolation buffer is added to a total volume of 2.5 ml and the tube is placed into the magnet for 5 min.
5. While still attached to the magnet, cells (containing negative fraction-$CD4^+$ T cells) are poured into a new 5 ml tube.
6. The magnetized tube is left inverted for 2–3 s and magnetically labeled (positive fraction-linage/$cocktail^+$ cells) cells remain.
7. The magnetic removal step is repeated to improve yield and negatively selected cells are collected into a 20 ml universal.
8. Yield is approximately 20–30% of PBMC depending on donors.
9. $CD4^+$ T cells are resuspended in culture media at a density of 100 $\times$ 10^6/ml for further separations.

2.3.5 Isolation of Human $CD4^+CD25^-$ Naïve Conventional T Cells by Magnetic Particle Separation

1. $CD4^+CD25^-$ naïve conventional T cells (nTcon) are further purified from total $CD4^+$ T cells (following step Subheading 2.3.4) by negative selection using human naïve $CD4^+$ T cell enrichment kit as follows:
2. Cells are incubated with biotinylated anti-CD45RO antibody at 50 μl/ml at room temperature for 15 min in a 5 ml tube.
3. To obtain purified $CD25^-$ conventional T cells by depleting $CD25^+$ Treg, anti-CD25 tetrameric antibody complexes at 50 μl/ml are also added in combination with the above step.

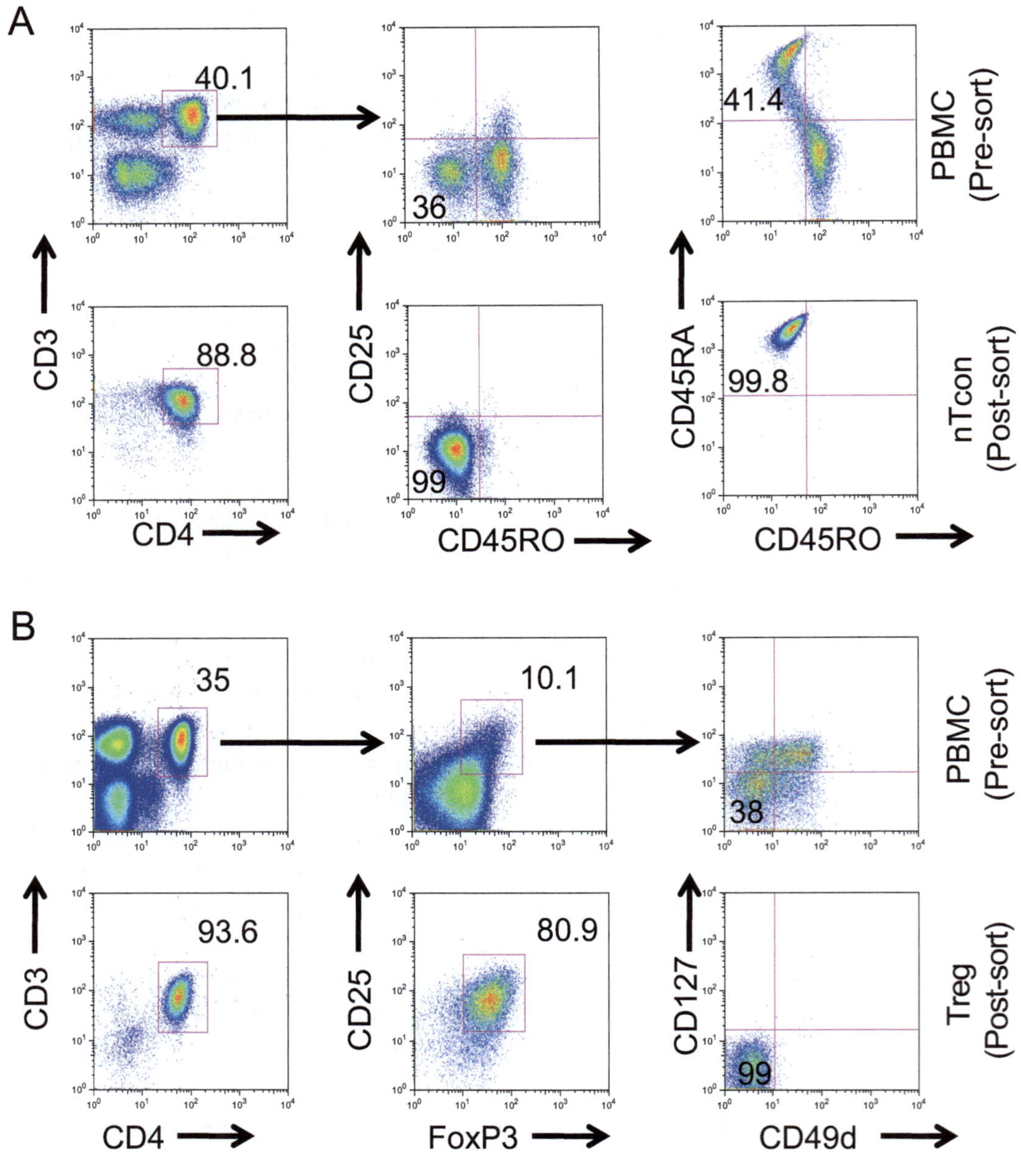

Fig. 2 Purification of human CD4$^+$ nTcon and Treg (**a**) Purity of human CD4$^+$CD25$^-$ nTcon. Purification of nTcon is performed in two successive steps: (1) total CD4$^+$ T-cell enrichment by negative selection using human CD4$^+$ T enrichment kit and (2) nTcon isolation by negative selection using human naïve CD4$^+$ T enrichment kit combined with Treg depletion by negative selection using anti-CD25. PBMC are stained and CD3$^+$CD4$^+$ T cells were gated to show the expression of CD25, CD45RA, and CD45RO (upper panels). Freshly purified nTcon were re-analyzed to show the sorting efficacy (lower panels). (**b**) Purity of human CD4$^+$ Treg. Purification of Treg is performed in two successive steps: (1) total CD4$^+$ T-cell enrichment by negative selection using human CD4$^+$ T enrichment kit and (2) Treg isolation by negative selection using human CD4$^+$CD127^{low}CD49d$^-$ Treg enrichment kit. PBMC are stained and CD3$^+$CD4$^+$ T cells are gated to show the expression of CD25, FoxP3, CD127, and CD49d (upper panels). Freshly sorted Treg are re-analyzed to show the sorting efficacy (lower panels)

4. Add the bispecific tetrameric antibody complexes containing monoclonal antibodies against CD8, CD14, CD16, CD19, CD20, CD36, CD56, CD66b, CD123, TCRγ/δ, glycophorin A and dextran at 50 μl/ml at room temperature for 10 min.
5. Dextran-coated magnetic nanoparticles are mixed thoroughly and added to the cells at 100 μl/ml and incubated at room temperature for 10 min.
6. Isolation buffer is added to a total volume of 2.5 ml and the tube is placed into the magnet for 10 min.
7. While still attached to the magnet, cells (containing negative fraction- nTcon) are poured into a new 5 ml tube.
8. The magnetized tube is left inverted for 2–3 s and magnetically labeled (positive fraction-linage/cocktail$^+$ cells) cells remain.
9. The magnetic removal step is repeated to improve yield and negatively selected cells are collected into a 20 ml universal.
10. Yield is approximately 10–50% of total CD4$^+$ T cells depending on donors.
11. nTcon are phenotyped by flow cytometry and are typically CD3$^+$CD4$^+$CD45RA$^+$CD45RO$^-$CD25$^-$ cells (Fig. 2a).
12. Cells are then labeled with 2.5 μM CellTrace Violet Stain reagent as follows:
13. Cells were washed twice with PBS and resuspended at a density of 5–10 × 10^6/ml in a 20 ml universal.
14. CellTrace Violet Stain is added at 2.5 μM and cells are incubated at 37 °C for 20 min.
15. To quench the labeling reaction, the universal is filled with 25 ml culture media and cell are incubated at 37 °C for a further 10 min followed by two washes with culture media.
16. CellTrace Violet labeled nTcon are resuspended in culture media at a density of 1.8 × 10^6/ml (or 90,000/50 μl) and used as responder cells in T-cell proliferation and suppression assays.

2.3.6 Isolation of Human CD4$^+$CD127^{low}CD49d$^-$ Treg by Magnetic Particle Separation

1. Treg are further purified from total CD4$^+$ T cells (following Subheading 2.3.4) by negative selection using human CD4$^+$CD127^{low}CD49d$^-$ Treg enrichment kit as follows:
2. Cells are incubated with human CD4$^+$CD127^{low}CD49d$^-$ Treg enrichment cocktail at 50 μl/ml at room temperature for 10 min in a 5 ml tube.
3. D2 magnetic particles are vortexed thoroughly and added to the cells at 100 μl/ml and incubated at room temperature for 5 min.

4. Isolation buffer is added to a total volume of 2.5 ml and the tube is placed into the magnet for 5 min.
5. The magnet holding the tube is picked up and desired fraction are poured into a new 5 ml tube. The tube is left inverted for 2–3 s.
6. The tube containing unwanted cells from the magnet is removed and discarded.
7. 50 μl of dextran selection cocktail is added to the cell suspension in the new tube and incubated at room temperature for 10 min.
8. 50 μl of D2 magnetic particles are added to the cells and incubated at room temperature for 5 min.
9. The magnet holding the tube is picked up and cells (Negative fraction-Treg) are poured into a new 5 ml tube. The tube is left inverted for 2–3 s.
10. The magnetic removal step is repeated to improve yield and negatively selected cells are collected into a 20 ml universal.
11. Yield is approximately 2–5% of total $CD4^+$ T cells depending on donors.
12. Treg are resuspended in culture media at a density of 1.8×10^6/ml (or 90,000/50 μl) and used as suppressors in T-cell suppression assays (*see* **Note 1**).
13. Treg are phenotyped by flow cytometry and typically $CD3^+CD4^+FoxP3^+$ $CD25^+CD127^{low}CD49d^-$ cells (Fig. 2b).

2.4 Flow Cytometric Analysis

1. FACS staining buffer: RPMI 1640 supplemented with 2% FBS.
2. PBMC, isolated monocytes and differentiated iDC, isolated nTcon and Treg are FACS stained using monoclonal Abs (*see* Table 2) at 4 °C for 30 min for flow cytometry (Figs. 1 and 2).
3. Single cell suspension is acquired by FACS-LSRII (Becton Dickinson) and analyzed by FlowJo (TreeStar).

3 Methods

3.1 CTLA-4 Dependent Treg Suppression Assay

1. To establish Treg suppression assay, iDC, nTcon, and Treg are cocultured in 250 μl culture media in the presence of anti-CD3. The ratio of iDC:Treg is the key variable for CTLA-4 function. Accordingly we routinely titrate the iDC:Treg ratio (*see* **Note 2**).
2. In a typical setting, 90,000 of CellTrace Violet labeled nTcon are added into culture as responder T cells, typically along with 9000 of iDC and 9000 of Treg (Fig. 3B).
3. To test the effect of CTLA-4 blockade on the proliferative response of nTcon, anti-CTLA-4 blocking Ab is added into

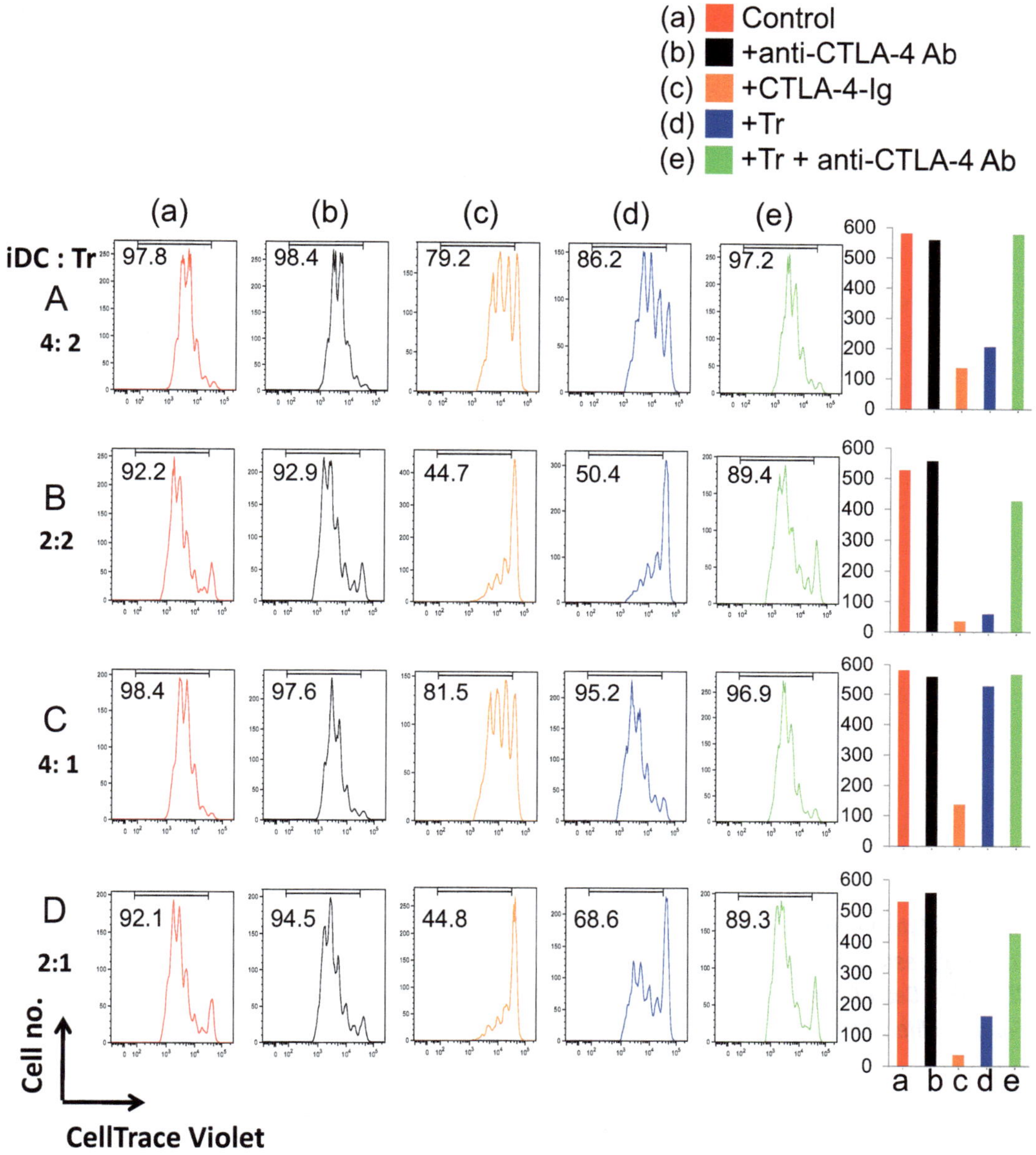

Fig. 3 CTLA-4-mediated Treg suppression is associated with low iDC and high Treg frequency. Violet labeled responder human $CD4^{+}CD^{25-}$ nTcon are activated with human monocyte-derived iDC and soluble anti-CD3 Ab. Culture was either untreated (**a**, red) or treated with anti-CTLA-4 Ab (**b**, black), CTLA-4-Ig (**c**, orange), Treg (**d**, blue), or Treg plus anti-CTLA-4 Ab (**e**, green). The proliferation of responder T cells is measured by the division of violet dye shown in histogram. The number of proliferating T cells ($\times 10^3$) is calculated using counting beads and are plotted in bar chart. In (**A** and **B**) Treg:nTcon ratio is 1:10 and (**C** and **D**) Treg:nTcon ratio is 1:20. Proliferation was measured at d5

culture condition without Treg. We routinely find blocking CTLA-4 alone has little or no effect on responder T-cell proliferation in the absence of Treg (Fig. 3B).

4. To test the CD80/CD86 dependency of T-cell responses, CTLA-4-Ig which blocks CD80/CD86 is added into culture at 10 μg/ml final concentration (Fig. 3C). The purpose of CTLA-4-Ig is to serve as a control to establish that the response is CD28-CD80/CD86 dependent. We routinely find high number of iDC is less CD80/CD86 dependent (Fig. 3A (c) and C(c)) (*see* **Note 3**).
5. To stimulate T-cell receptor (TCR), soluble agonistic anti-CD3 Ab is added into culture at typically at 0.5 μg/ml final concentration. This needs to be determined for each antibody. Soluble agonistic anti-CD3 Ab alone (i.e., without iDC) is included as negative control (*see* **Note 4**).
6. To test the effect of Treg numbers on responder T-cell proliferation, different numbers of Treg are added into culture (*see* **Note 5**). We find the suppressive effect of high number (relative to iDC) of Treg is more pronounced than that of low numbers (Fig. 3(d), A vs. B).
7. To test the CTLA-4 dependency of Treg suppression, anti-CTLA-4 blocking Ab is added together with Treg into cultured at 40 μg/ml final concentration (*see* **Note 6**). We find consistently that CTLA-4 blockade is able to largely if not completely reverse Treg suppression in CD80/CD86 dependent T-cell responses (Fig. 3B, (d) and (e)).
8. The proliferation of responder nTcon is measured by the dilution of CellTrace Violet. The absolute number of proliferating T cells is calculated using counting beads (*see* **Note 7**).

3.2 Nondetectable Treg Suppression in CD3/CD28 Bead Driven T-Cell Proliferation

1. To test the effect of Treg on nTcon proliferation in a non-CD80/CD86 dependent model, we include a control using T cells stimulated by CD3/CD28 beads in which T cells are still stimulated in TCR and CD28 driven signals but no ligand (CD80/CD86) exists in this system.
2. To test the impact of the number of CD3/CD28 beads on Treg suppression. The ratio between the number of CD3/CD28 bead and Treg is titrated.
3. The remaining settings are same as in Subheading 3.1, **steps 2–4** and **6–8**.
4. We find that Treg cannot suppress T-cell proliferation driven by CD3/CD28 beads regardless of the bead dose (Fig. 4(d), A vs. B). This is consistent with that CTLA-4-Ig has no impact on this type of T-cell proliferation (Fig. 4(c)). This suggests that the presence of ligand (CD80/CD86) is required for CTLA-4-mediated Treg suppression.

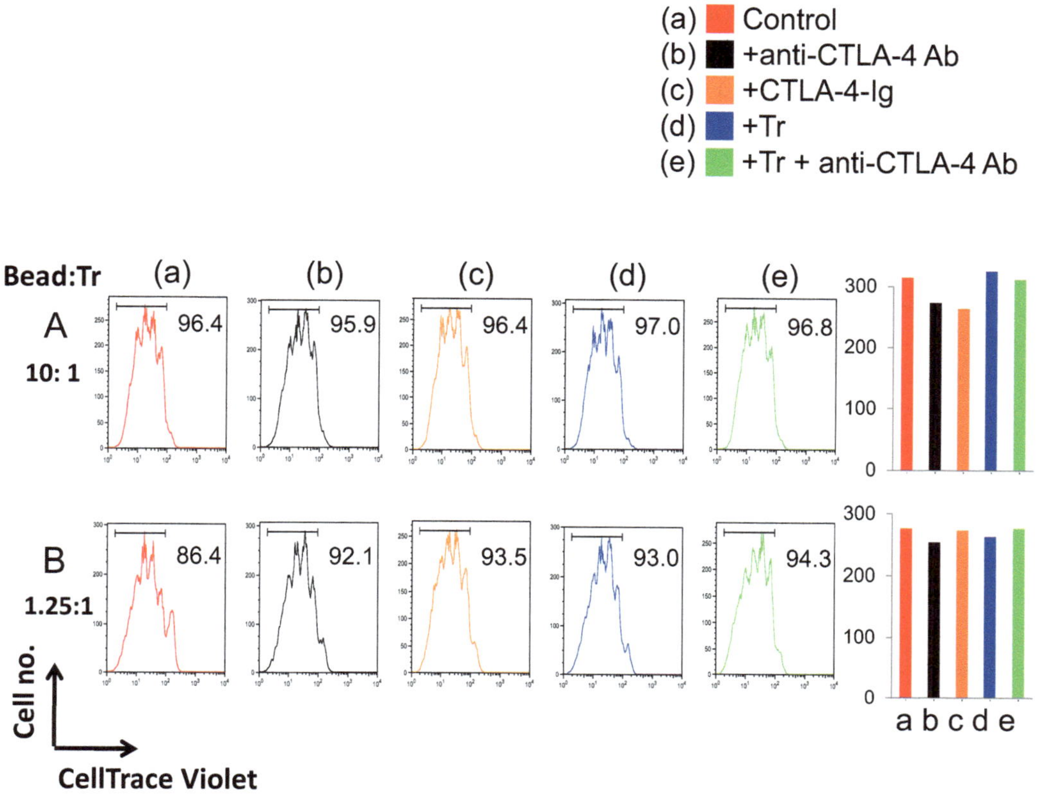

Fig. 4 Treg suppression is not observed in the absence of CD80 and CD86. Violet labeled responder human $CD4^{+}CD25^{-}$ nTcon are activated with CD3/CD28 beads. Culture is either untreated (**a**, red) or treated with anti-CTLA-4 Ab (**b**, black), CTLA-4-Ig (**c**, orange), Treg (**d**, blue), or Treg plus anti-CTLA-4 Ab (**e**, green). The proliferation of responder T cells is measured by the division of violet dye shown in histogram. The number of proliferating T cells is calculated using counting beads and are plotted in bar chat. (**A** and **B**) Treg:nTcon ratio is 1:5

4 Notes

1. A mixed leukocyte reaction is not detected even though nTcon and Treg are from the same donors whereas iDC are originated from different donors. This is because in the presence of soluble anti-CD3 Ab, responder nTcon proliferate more rapidly and in greater numbers, such that any alloresponse is not observed.
2. The number of responder nTcon cells and concentration of soluble anti-CD3 Ab are the same in all culture conditions, whereas the number of iDC and Treg are titrated to vary the ratio between iDC and Treg (or CD80/CD86 and CTLA-4).
3. We find a strong correlation between inhibitory effect of CTLA-4-Ig blockade and Treg suppression mediated by CTLA-4 (cell bound). This indicates that CTLA-4 on Treg

only suppress T-cell responses that are driven by CD80/CD86 costimulation.

4. The soluble form and low concentration of anti-CD3 used here provides a relatively weak TCR signal. This signal alone without costimulation provided by CD80/CD86 on iDC is insufficient to drive T-cell proliferation.
5. The proliferation of unlabeled Treg is not taken into account. The readout is determined by the proliferation of CellTrace Violet labeled responder nTcon as even after several (typically 1–6) rounds of division responder T cells can still be distinguished from unlabeled (violet negative) Treg by FACS analysis.
6. The reasons why we use relatively high concentration (40 μg/ml) of anti-CTLA-4 blocking antibody are as follows. First, although anti-CTLA-4 is very effective (almost 100%) at blocking, accessibility of the antibody to the intracellular and recycling CTLA-4 at immune synapses is likely limiting. Second, we only give one dose of anti-CTLA-4 at the beginning of the 5-day assays and the antibody bound to CTLA-4 is internalized and degraded. Blocking at 20 μg/ml is marginally less effective in our hands.
7. The quantitative nature of this assay is sufficient to reveal functional defects (i.e., impairment of Treg suppression) in patients with point mutations in their CTLA-4 [23].

Acknowledgments

TZH was funded by the Wellcome Trust.

References

1. Sakaguchi S, Yamaguchi T, Nomura T, Ono M (2008) Regulatory T cells and immune tolerance. Cell 133:775–787
2. Ziegler SF (2006) FOXP3: of mice and men. Annu Rev Immunol 24:209–226
3. Josefowicz SZ, Lu LF, Rudensky AY (2012) Regulatory T cells: mechanisms of differentiation and function. Annu Rev Immunol 30:531–564
4. Shevach EM (2009) Mechanisms of foxp3+ T regulatory cell-mediated suppression. Immunity 30:636–645
5. Tang Q, Bluestone JA (2008) The Foxp3+ regulatory T cell: a jack of all trades, master of regulation. Nat Immunol 9:239–244
6. Vignali DA, Collison LW, Workman CJ (2008) How regulatory T cells work. Nat Rev Immunol 8:523–532
7. Wing K, Yamaguchi T, Sakaguchi S (2011) Cell-autonomous and -non-autonomous roles of CTLA-4 in immune regulation. Trends Immunol 32:428–433
8. Yamaguchi T, Wing JB, Sakaguchi S (2011) Two modes of immune suppression by Foxp3 (+) regulatory T cells under inflammatory or non-inflammatory conditions. Semin Immunol 23:424–430
9. Read S, Malmstrom V, Powrie F (2000) Cytotoxic T lymphocyte-associated antigen 4 plays an essential role in the function of CD25(+) CD4(+) regulatory cells that control intestinal inflammation. J Exp Med 192:295–302

10. Walker LS, Sansom DM (2011) The emerging role of CTLA4 as a cell-extrinsic regulator of T cell responses. NatRevImmunol 11:852–863
11. Wing K, Onishi Y, Prieto-Martin P, Yamaguchi T, Miyara M, Fehervari Z, Nomura T, Sakaguchi S (2008) CTLA-4 control over Foxp3+ regulatory T cell function. Science 322:271–275
12. Yamaguchi T, Kishi A, Osaki M, Morikawa H, Prieto-Martin P, Wing K, Saito T, Sakaguchi S (2013) Construction of self-recognizing regulatory T cells from conventional T cells by controlling CTLA-4 and IL-2 expression. ProcNatlAcadSciUSA 110:E2116–E2125
13. Ise W, Kohyama M, Nutsch KM, Lee HM, Suri A, Unanue ER, Murphy TL, Murphy KM (2010) CTLA-4 suppresses the pathogenicity of self antigen-specific T cells by cell-intrinsic and cell-extrinsic mechanisms. Nat Immunol 11:129–135
14. Tivol EA, Borriello F, Schweitzer AN, Lynch WP, Bluestone JA, Sharpe AH (1995) Loss of CTLA-4 leads to massive lymphoproliferation and fatal multiorgan tissue destruction, revealing a critical negative regulatory role of CTLA-4. Immunity 3:541–547
15. Waterhouse P, Penninger JM, Timms E, Wakeham A, Shahinian A, Lee KP, Thompson CB, Griesser H, Mak TW (1995) Lymphoproliferative disorders with early lethality in mice deficient in Ctla-4. Science 270:985–988
16. Gardner D, Jeffery LE, Sansom DM (2014) Understanding the CD28/CTLA-4 (CD152) pathway and its implications for costimulatory blockade. Am J Transplant 14:1985–1991
17. Tang Q, Bluestone JA (2013) Regulatory T-cell therapy in transplantation: moving to the clinic. Cold Spring Harb Perspect Med 3
18. Pardoll DM (2012) The blockade of immune checkpoints in cancer immunotherapy. Nat Rev Cancer 12:252–264
19. Walker LS, Sansom DM (2015) Confusing signals: recent progress in CTLA-4 biology. Trends Immunol
20. Qureshi OS, Zheng Y, Nakamura K, Attridge K, Manzotti C, Schmidt EM, Baker J, Jeffery LE, Kaur S, Briggs Z, Hou TZ, Futter CE, Anderson G, Walker LS, Sansom DM (2011) Trans-endocytosis of CD80 and CD86: a molecular basis for the cell-extrinsic function of CTLA-4. Science 332:600–603
21. Soskic B, Qureshi OS, Hou T, Sansom DM (2014) A transendocytosis perspective on the CD28/CTLA-4 pathway. Adv Immunol 124:95–136
22. Hou TZ, Qureshi OS, Wang CJ, Baker J, Young SP, Walker LS, Sansom DM (2015) A transendocytosis model of ctla-4 function predicts its suppressive behavior on regulatory T cells. J Immunol 194:2148–2159
23. Schubert D, Bode C, Kenefeck R, Hou TZ, Wing JB, Kennedy A, Bulashevska A, Petersen BS, Schaffer AA, Gruning BA, Unger S, Frede N, Baumann U, Witte T, Schmidt RE, Dueckers G, Niehues T, Seneviratne S, Kanariou M, Speckmann C, Ehl S, Rensing-Ehl A, Warnatz K, Rakhmanov M, Thimme R, Hasselblatt P, Emmerich F, Cathomen T, Backofen R, Fisch P, Seidl M, May A, Schmitt-Graeff A, Ikemizu S, Salzer U, Franke A, Sakaguchi S, Walker LS, Sansom DM, Grimbacher B (2014) Autosomal dominant immune dysregulation syndrome in humans with CTLA4 mutations. Nat Med 20(12):1410–1416

Chapter 8

Alloanergization Method for Inducing Allospecific Hyporesponsiveness in PBMC Exposed to Allostimulation In Vitro in the Context of Costimulatory Molecule Blockade

Christine M. Barbon, Kenneth J. Janec, Rowan H. Kelner, James E. Norton, and Eva C. Guinan

Abstract

Alloantigen-specific hyporesponsiveness can be induced in alloreactive T cells contained within the whole peripheral blood mononuclear cell (PBMC) population by stimulating these responder cells ex vivo with HLA-mismatched stimulator PBMC as the antigen presenting cell (APC) source, in the presence of a CD28 costimulation blocking agent. As a result of this approach, specific alloreactivity is markedly decreased (by 1–2 logs), but third-party alloresponses and in vitro responses relying on the activation of pathogen- and tumor-associated antigen T-cell functional activities are not globally impinged upon (Guinan et al. N Engl J Med 340(22):1704–1714, 1999, Davies et al. Transplantation 86(6):854–864, 2008, Davies et al. Cell Transplant 21(9):2047–61, 2012). This method has been used clinically to alloanergize bone marrow and PBMC allografts, creating ex vivo cell therapies for adoptive transfer to blood cancer patients at high risk of disease relapse whose best option was to receive haploidentical hematopoietic cell transplants. These early phase trials consisting of, or containing, alloanergized T-cell infusions show promise in reducing graft-versus-host disease (GvHD), providing more rapid immune reconstitution, and decreasing severe post-transplant infectious complications and disease relapse. Herein, we describe this straightforward technique for generating alloanergized PBMC as it is performed in the research lab setting using belatacept for CD28-mediated costimulatory blockade (CSB) and PBMC isolated by Ficoll Hypaque gradient centrifugation as responders and APC. We also describe methods for evaluating subsequent alloproliferation to first and third party stimulation as well as assessment of cell division, pathogen-specific immunity, or allosuppression. The technique has successfully been transferred to collaborating labs, largely owing to the flexibility of using fresh or frozen PBMC, the lack of a requirement for specially isolated APC populations, and the ability to scale up or scale down the cell numbers that are to be anergized.

Key words Anergy, Alloanergy, Regulatory T cell (Treg), Alloantigen-specific response, alloreactivity, T-cell costimulation, Mixed lymphocyte reaction (MLR), Immune tolerance, Costimulatory molecule blockade

1 Introduction

Ex vivo alloanergization takes advantage of the principles of T-cell activation during which T-cell interactions with APC result in

Ashleigh S. Boyd (ed.), *Immunological Tolerance: Methods and Protocols*, Methods in Molecular Biology, vol. 1899,
https://doi.org/10.1007/978-1-4939-8938-6_8,

"signal 1" in which the T cell's antigen-specific T-cell receptor (TCR) binds cognate ligand on APC and "signal 2" consisting of costimulatory molecule engagement between the APC presenting the antigen and T-cell counterreceptors, most critically the B7-CD28 interaction. Without costimulatory reinforcement of TCR signaling by APC (i.e., absent signal 2), T cells can either be deleted, or display hyporesponsiveness upon subsequent repeat TCR signaling as a result of cell intrinsic factors [4, 5]. Belatacept, a second generation recombinant human Cytotoxic T Lymphocyte Antigen 4 (CTLA4)-Immunoglobulin (Ig) fusion protein combining the extracellular portion of CTLA4 with the Fc domain of human IgG1, competitively inhibits the binding of the T-cell costimulatory receptor CD28 to the APC ligands B7.1 and B7.2 [6].

2 Materials

1. RPMI-10% HuAB serum Complete Medium: 440 mL RPMI 1640 medium supplemented with phenol red and 1× L-glutamine or 1× L-glutamax (Gibco/Life Technologies or equivalent) to which is added 50 mL of human AB serum (Gemini Biomedical or equivalent) (*see* **Note 1**), 1× penicillin/streptomycin, 1× HEPES, and 1× gentamicin. Media should be made in a laminar flow biosafety cabinet and filter sterilized, 0.22 μM, stored in sterile bottles, and used within 30 days (*see* **Note 2**). Media should be pre-warmed to 37 °C prior to use.
2. Sterile Tissue Culture Labware: including 25 cm^2 tissue culture flasks, 96-well round-bottom plates, reagent reservoirs, 15- and 50 mL conical centrifuge tubes, 2.0 mL cryopreservation vials, serological pipettes, and filter barrier pipet tips.
3. Pipetman and single or multichannel pipetors.
4. Ficoll-Paque Plus lymphocyte separation medium (GE Healthcare Lifesciences).
5. Sterile Dulbeccos Phosphate-buffered Saline (DPBS).
6. Trypan Blue.
7. Cell Counter or Microscope and Hemocytometer.
8. Nulojix® (belatacept): (Bristol-Myers Squibb, Princeton, New Jersey (*see* **Note 3**)): Resuspend to 25 mg/mL in sterile deionized water using the syringe enclosed with the drug in its packaging. Follow the package insert instructions for avoiding excess foaming during reconstitution, then dilute the stock with DPBS to a final concentration of 10 mg/mL. Freeze in small single use aliquots at −20 °C for up to 1 year. Thaw on ice immediately prior to use and discard any remaining drug.
9. Lyophilized activating anti-human CD3 (Cat # IM0178) and anti-human CD28(Cat # IM1376) antibodies (Beckman

Coulter, Fullerton, CA): reconstituted to 200 μg/mL in sterile deionized water.

10. Tritiated Thymidine, [Methyl-3H]-, Specific Activity: 20 Ci (740 GBq)/mMole, >97%, 1 mCi (37 MBq), Perkin Elmer, Cat# NET027X001MC, or equivalent, diluted 1:25 in RPMI-10% HuAB serum Complete Medium, such that 25 μL = 1 μCi ^{3}H-thymidine (*see* **Note 4**).
11. 96-well plate Harvester (Tomtec, Hamden, CT) or equivalent.
12. Printed Filter Mats, filter mat sample bags, heat sealer, and scintillation fluid: (Perkin Elmer) or equivalent.
13. Scintillation Counter capable of reading 96-well filtermats: (Wallac Microbeta) or similar.
14. Gamma-ray Irradiator: for irradiating PBMC to be used as stimulators: ^{137}Cs source GammaCell-1000 (or similar) (Best Theratronics, Ottawa, Canada) (*see* **Note 5**).
15. Tissue culture incubator set to 37 °C/5%CO_2/80% humidity.
16. Red Blood Cell Lysis Buffer (Lonza Corp.), or equivalent, commercially available, (Sigma #R7757)), or your lab's own recipe for ACK buffer.
17. Peripheral blood collected into heparinized vacutainers or plateletpheresis/leukopheresis-derived blood products: two separate donors are sufficient for an experiment consisting of two different donor:stimulator pairings, each pair consisting of one responder and one first party (FP) stimulator; a third donor blood would be required for testing alloresponses to a third party (TP) stimulator (*see* **Note 6**).
18. Freezing medium part 1: RPMI-30% heat inactivated fetal bovine serum, 1× pen/strep, 1× HEPES, 1× L-glutamine.
19. Freezing medium part 2: 80% heat inactivated fetal bovine serum plus 20% tissue culture grade dimethyl sulfoxide, or equivalent.
20. Passive Freezing container, e.g., Nalgene® Mr. Frosty, or equivalent: −1 °C/min cooling rate required for successful cryopreservation of viable PBMC. Alternately, a programmable, cooling rate-controlled freezer can be used (Planer PLC, Middlesex, UK) or equivalent.
21. (optional) CFSE, carboxyfluorescein diacetate succinimidyl ester from the CellTrace™ CFSE Cell Proliferation Kit, Cat # C34554 or Vybrant CFDA-SE Cell Tracer Kit Cat#V12883 (Molecular Probes/Life Technologies), as well as fluorescently conjugated monoclonal antibodies for costaining responder $CD4^+$ and $CD8^+$ T cells and (optional) anti-HLA antibodies for gating out residual stimulator cells in flow cytometric assays. See the specifications for your lab's particular flow cytometer for the fluorochromes that may be used for this type of assessment.

3 Methods

3.1 Isolation of Peripheral Blood Mononuclear Cells from Whole Blood or Blood Products

All procedures involving the use of human blood, blood products, and cells should be handled using Universal Precautions and all manipulations done within a laminar-flow biosafety cabinet using good aseptic technique.

3.1.1 Blood Collection and Processing

1. Blood should be collected directly into a container with preservative-free heparin (using Vacutainer®) or by pheresis or similar.
2. Platelet reduction spin: Dilute blood volume 1:2 with sterile DPBS in a 50 mL conical centrifuge tube. Use multiple tubes if necessary.
3. Centrifuge at at 240–300 × *g* for 10 min at room temperature (RT) with BRAKE OFF.
4. Carefully aspirate off top plasma layer (this contains a large majority of the platelets) leaving 5 mL or less of diluted plasma above the packed cells. Take care not to disturb or aspirate off any of the white layer of leukocytes on the top of the packed red cells.

3.1.2 Ficoll-Hypaque Density Gradient Centrifugation

1. Gently resuspend blood in 2–3 volumes of DPBS.
2. Fill 50 mL Falcon conical tubes with 15 mLs of lymphocyte separation medium, e.g., Ficoll-Hypaque (at RT; stored in dark, check expiry).
3. Gently and very slowly overlay a maximum of 30 mL of blood/DPBS onto the Ficoll-Hypaque using only gravity to drain a 10 mL pipette. The object is to layer blood on slowly in order to maintain a clean interface between the Ficoll and the blood/PBS mixture.
4. Centrifuge at 400 × *g* for 25 min at RT with the BRAKE OFF.
5. The PBMC should appear as a pale cloudy layer at the DPBS/Ficoll interface. Harvest this layer from the interface with a sterile serological pipette after first removing some of the liquid above the cell layer without disrupting the floating cells.
6. Transfer cells to a fresh 50 mL tube and dilute with DPBS to a volume of up to 40–45 mL.
7. Centrifuge at 400 × *g* for 10 min at RT with the BRAKE ON.
8. Aspirate DPBS from the cell pellet. Resuspend the cells in 40 mL DPBS and repeat step g for a total of 2 washes.

3.1.3 RBC Lysis

1. Discard DPBS supernatant from second wash (*see* **Note** 7). Gently, but thoroughly resuspend cell pellet in 5–6 mL of red blood cell lysis buffer, mixing by pipette for about 5 s.
2. Incubate at RT for 5 min while periodically swirling the tube contents. Immediately after the 5 min incubation has lapsed, add 40 mLs of DPBS. Overlysis can affect cell yield and viability. Do not lyse cells for more than 5 min.
3. Centrifuge at 400 × *g* for 10 min at RT with the BRAKE ON.

3.1.4 Cell Enumeration and Cryopreservation

1. Dispose of top liquid layer and dilute remaining cell pellet with additional Complete Medium or DPBS (for a total of 2 washes) to 40 mL while gently resuspending them.
2. Remove a small aliquot of cells and perform a cell count using a hemocytometer and trypan blue exclusion by microscopy (or other system) for determining the viable cell count.
3. Centrifuge samples at 400 × *g* for 10 min at RT with the BRAKE ON.
4. Discard top layer and resuspend cells at a 2× concentration: typically 20–100 × 1 × 10^6 cells per mL in freezing medium part 1 (RPMI-30% FBS) for a final concentration of 10–50 × 10^6 cells per vial. Keep the cells on ice until well chilled.
5. Remove Mr. Frosty container from 4 °C to RT just before use, making sure it has a sufficient amount of isopropyl alcohol in it (see side of Mr. Frosty container for fill line and instructions).
6. Prepare cryovials labeled with the donor designation, cell concentration, date.
7. Add an equivalent amount of chilled freezing medium part 2 (80% FBS-20% DMSO) to the tube containing cells already resuspended freezing medium part 1, add it *very slowly, drop by drop* while making sure to *gently agitate the solution* gently mix the two components, diluting cells to a final concentration of 10–50 × 1 × 10^6 cells/mL.
8. Then, working quickly (*see* **Note 8**), pipet 1 mL aliquots of cells using a 5 mL pipette into cryovial vials. Be sure to keep cells in the conical centrifuge tube well suspended during the aliquotting process in order to reduce cell settling that affects the accuracy of vial-to-vial cell numbers. Keep cells chilled on ice until they are ready for placement into the passive freezer, e.g., Nalgene Mr. Frosty.
9. Cap the vials tightly to avoid the cells becoming contaminated during the waterbath thawing process, and to avoid liquid nitrogen from seeping into the vials, causing them to explode upon warming.

10. Place ampules in a passive freezer, e.g., Nalgene® Mr. Frosty. Place at −80 °C overnight to 24 h. After this point, cells can either remain at −80 °C storage for use within 3 months or switched to liquid nitrogen vapor phase storage indefinitely.

3.1.5 Thawing PBMC

1. Vials of cells are thawed in a 37 °C waterbath with gentle agitation just until the last ice crystals thaw.
2. Vials should then be wiped down upon transfer from the water bath with 70% alcohol disinfection, and then immediately pipeted into conical centrifuge tubes containing at least 10 volumes of pre-warmed RPMI-10% HuAB serum Complete Medium. The goal of steps a and b above is to get the freshly thawed cells into warm medium as soon as possible to dilute out the DMSO cryoprotectant, which is toxic to cells over time.
3. Centrifuge at 400 × *g* for 10 min at RT with the BRAKE ON.
4. Decant supernatant, resuspend PBMC in fresh pre-warmed RPMI-10% HuAB serum Complete Medium, and use a hemocytometer and trypan blue exclusion for determining the viable cell count.

3.2 Alloanergization of PBMC

Setting up Bulk RS and RSB Culture Flasks: PBMCs from two separate donors are necessary to set up both the control culture that includes responder (R) PBMC + stimulator (S) PBMC as APC, termed the RS control culture, and the Anergy culture that contains responder PBMC + stimulator PBMC as APC + the CSB agent, belatacept, which is called the RSB flask culture. Cells from one donor will serve as the responder and cells from another donor will serve as the stimulator in each of the cultures. The RS and RSB cultures are set up identically except for the inclusion of belatacept in the RSB culture. The PBMC used can either be freshly ficoll-isolated or previously frozen and thawed, as in the two preceding sub-protocols.

3.2.1 RSB Culture Setup

1. Place a total of 10×10^6 PBMC, to serve as stimulator PBMC at a concentration of 1×10^6/mL in RPMI-10% HuAB serum Complete Medium into a 15 mL conical centrifuge tube and add 40 μL of the 10 mg/mL belatacept stock for costimulatory blockade; the final concentration is 40 μg/mL. In case of setting up multiple flasks, set up one 15 mL tube for flask, or scale up all volumes accordingly and use 50 mL tubes.
2. Gently invert the closed tube several times to mix, or mix by pipet, then incubate for 30 min in a 37 °C/5%CO_2/80% humidified tissue culture incubator.

3. While the RSB stimulators are incubating, aliquot 10 × 10^6 PBMC to serve as the RSB responders at a concentration of 1 × 10^6/mL in RPMI-10% HuAB serum Complete Medium into an upright T-25 cm^2 cell culture flask with a filtered gas-permeable cap. Add 40 μL of the 10 mg/mL belatacept stock for costimulatory blockade; the final concentration is 40 μg/mL. Incubate for 30 min in a 37 °C/5%CO_2/80% humidified tissue culture incubator.
4. Irradiate RSB stimulator PBMC to 35 Gy/3500 rads, and then add these irradiated cells to the RSB flask containing responder PBMC + belatacept. Mix gently.
5. Incubate flask in an upright position for 72–96 h (*see* **Note 9**).

3.2.2 RS Culture Setup

1. The RS culture flask is set up with the same responder and stimulator PBMC in exactly the same manner as the RSB, with the exception that *no belatacept is added to either the RS flask or the tube containing the stimulator PBMC.*
2. If there are any remaining responder cells left over after setting up the RS and RSB flasks, these can be kept at 0.5 × 10^6/mL in RPMI-10% HuAB serum Complete Medium in a 37 °C/5% CO_2/80% humidified tissue culture incubator for use as a control in the MLR assay. Similarly, if stimulator PBMC are limiting, any unirradiated cells left over can also be held in culture at the cell concentration above for use in the secondary MLR (*see* **Note 10**).

3.2.3 Primary MLR Setup

Costimulatory blockade efficacy is measured in the primary MLR which uses PBMC from both the RS and RSB flasks. It is an important distinction to note that the Primary MLR is a continuation of the conditions existing in the RS and RSB flasks, and the plate format permits the evaluation of alloproliferation by ^{3}H-thymidine incorporation. Washed PBMC from these flasks will also be plated in the presence of anti-CD3/CD28 antibodies as a test of the overall ability of the cells to respond to a strong mitotic stimulus.

1. Three 96-well round-bottom tissue culture plates are needed for the Primary MLR assay, one for each of the three time points to be measured (Days 4, 5, and 6 after the flask cultures were first initiated).
2. The following conditions will be plated in triplicate in each of the three 96-well round-bottom tissue culture MLR plates, per the plate map shown in Fig. 1:
   (a) RS PBMC alone, 200 μL.
   (b) RSB PBMC alone, 200 μL.

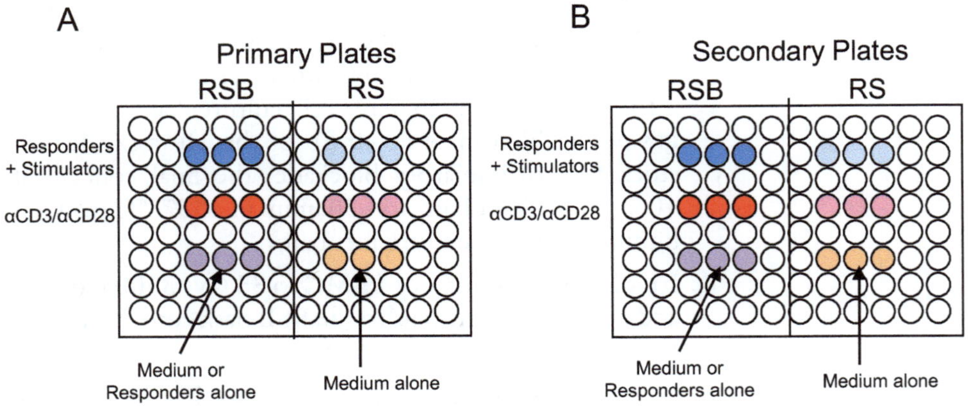

Fig. 1 Plate map

(c) Washed RS PBMC, 200 μL + αCD3 antibody (10 μL) + αCD28 antibody (10 μL).

(d) Washed RSB PBMC, 200 μL+ αCD3 antibody (10 μL) + αCD28 antibody (10 μL).

(e) (if available) Washed responder PBMC alone, 100 μL + 100 μL RPMI-10% HuAB serum Complete Medium

(f) RPMI-10% HuAB serum Complete Medium, 200 μL as negative control.

(g) Sterile DPBS is added to all remaining wells to prevent excessive evaporation.

3. Resuspend PBMC in the RS and RSB flasks well by pipetting and place 5 mL from each flask into separate 15 mL conical tubes.

   (a) From this tube, take out 1.8 mL of the cell suspensions and using a single or multichannel pipettor and reagent reservoir, if desired, aliquot 200 μL of RS PBMC and RSB PBMC, respectively, into triplicate wells on each of the three Primary Day 4, Day 5, Day 6 plates (9 wells altogether), as detailed in Subheading 3.3, **step 2** and as shown in Fig. 1a, taking care to keep cells well suspended in the process to maintain consistent well-to-well cell numbers.

   (b) Add 10 mL of RPMI-10% HuAB serum Complete Medium to the remaining ~3.6 mL of cells in the 15 mL conical tubes, spin at 400 × *g* for 5–10 min at RT with the centrifuge BRAKE ON.

   (c) Aspirate supernatant from the cell pellet, resuspend cell pellet and repeat above wash, for a total of 2 washes to remove residual belatacept.

(d) These washed RS and RSB cells are then resuspended. The cell concentration is adjusted to 1×10^6/mL in RPMI-10% HuAB serum Complete Medium and cells plated into the wells designated for washed RS and RSB cells.

(e) Add 10 μL each αCD3 antibody and αCD28 antibody to the appropriate wells.

(f) If available, responder cells can be washed, adjusted to 1.0×10^6/mL in RPMI-10% HuAB serum Complete Medium and plated as a further negative control.

(g) Medium and DPBS are added to remaining wells, where indicated.

(h) Plates are returned to the 37 °C/5%CO_2/80% humidified tissue culture incubator (*see* **Note 11**).

3.2.4 Secondary MLR Setup

Following the initial 72 h alloanergization process, the PBMC in the RS and RSB flasks are washed, and the alloproliferation in both cell populations is measured during a secondary MLR with the addition of another round of alloantigen exposure, but in the absence of costimulatory blockade by belatacept.

1. Three 96-well round-bottom tissue culture plates are needed for the Secondary MLR assay, one for each of the three time points to be measured (Days 6, 8, and 10 after the flask cultures were first initiated).
2. The following conditions will be plated in triplicate in each of the three 96-well round-bottom tissue culture MLR plates, per the plate map shown in Fig. 1b:

   (a) Washed RS PBMC, 100 μL + 100 μL 35 Gy-irradiated FP stimulators.

   (b) Washed RSB PBMC, 100 μL + 100 μL 35 Gy-irradiated FP stimulators.

   (c) (optional) Washed RS PBMC, 100 μL + 100 μL 35 Gy-irradiated TP stimulators

   (d) (optional) Washed RSB PBMC, 100 μL + 100 μL 35 Gy-irradiated TP stimulators

   (e) Washed RS PBMC, 100 μL + 100 μL RPMI-10% HuAB serum Complete Medium + αCD3 antibody (10 μL) + αCD28 antibody (10 μL).

   (f) Washed RS PBMC, 100 μL + 100 μL RPMI-10% HuAB serum Complete Medium + αCD3 antibody (10 μL) + αCD28 antibody (10 μL).

   (g) (if available) Washed responder PBMC alone, 100 μL + 100 μL RPMI-10% HuAB serum Complete Medium

(h) RPMI-10% HuAB serum Complete Medium, 200 μL as negative control.

(i) Sterile DPBS is added to all remaining wells to prevent excessive evaporation.

3. Resuspend PBMC in the RS and RSB flasks well by pipetting and then aliquot 8–10 mL into separate 50 mL conical tubes.
4. Spin at 400–450 × *g* for 5–10 min at RT with the BRAKE ON.
5. Aspirate the supernatant carefully, then disrupt the PBMC pellets and resuspend PBMC well by adding 20 mL RPMI-10% HuAB serum Complete Medium.
6. Spin at 400–450 × *g* for 5–10 min at RT with the BRAKE ON. Repeat this washing step for a total of two washes.
7. Aspirate pellet, resuspend each cell pellet in 1–2 mL of RPMI-10% HuAB serum Complete Medium.
8. Perform a cell count using a hemocytometer by trypan blue exclusion for determining the viable cell count. Adjust washed RS and RS PBMC to 1×10^6/mL in RPMI-10% HuAB serum Complete Medium.
9. Aliquot 100 μL of washed RS PBMC and washed RSB PBMC into triplicate wells on each of the three Secondary Day 6, Day 8, Day 10 plates (9 wells altogether), as detailed in Subheading 3.4, **step 2** and as shown in Fig. 2, taking care to keep cells well suspended in the process to maintain consistent well-to-well cell numbers.
10. Prepare irradiated FP (and TP *optional*, *see* **Note 12**), stimulator PBMC by isolating ficolled PBMC from fresh blood,

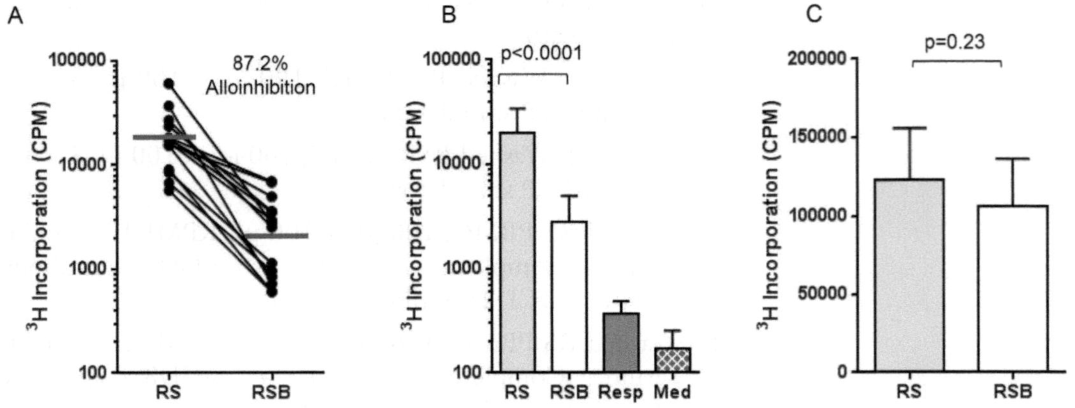

Fig. 2 Primary MLRs were established in the absence (RS) and presence (RSB) of belatacept (40 μg/mL) with cryopreserved PBMC (n = 14 HLA-mismatched unrelated donor pairs). (**a**) Alloproliferation measured by 3H-thymidine incorporation was reduced by a median of 87.2% at Day 6 (range 61–98%). (**b**) Composite mean and standard deviation for 3H-thymidine incorporation in the RS, RSB, responders alone (Resp) in complete medium, and medium alone (Med). (**c**) Global stimulation by αCD3/αCD28 activating antibodies was not significantly decreased in RSB PBMC cultures

thawing cryopreserved PBMC, both per the previous sub-protocols, or use remaining, unirradiated stimulator PBMC held in culture from the RS and RSB culture set-up procedure.

11. You will need approximately 2.5 mL of FP or TP stimulators adjusted to 1×10^6/mL in RPMI-10% HuAB serum Complete Medium to set up triplicate secondary MLR plates.
12. Irradiate FP and TP stimulator PBMC to 35 Gy and then add these irradiated cells to RS and RSB responder PBMC as detailed in Subheading 3.4, **step 2** and as shown in Fig. 2, taking care to keep cells well suspended in the process to maintain consistent well-to-well cell numbers.
    (a) Add 10 μL each αCD3 antibody and αCD28 antibody to the appropriate wells.
    (b) If available, responder cells can be washed, adjusted to 1.0×10^6/mL in RPMI-10% HuAB serum Complete Medium and plated as a further negative control.
    (c) Medium and DPBS are added to remaining wells, as indicated.
    (d) Incubate plates in a 37 °C/5%CO_2/80% humidified tissue culture incubator.

3.3 Measuring Alloproliferation in the Primary and Secondary MLR Plates by Tritiated Thymidine Incorporation

Responder cell alloproliferation in the RS and RSB cultures is measured by ^{3}H-thymidine uptake. Alloproliferation is measured at Days 4, 5, and 6 from the Primary MLR plates, and at Days 6, 8, and 10 in the Secondary MLR plates.

1. 16–20 h prior to desired harvest time point, the plate is pulsed by adding 1 μCi of ^{3}H-thymidine to each well of the appropriate MLR plate by adding 25 μL of the 1:25 diluted ^{3}H-thymidine stock (*see* **Note 13**).
2. Incubate pulsed plate(s) for 16–20 h.
3. Harvest plate(s) onto a filter mats using a Tomtec cell harvester.
4. Allow the filter mats to air dry for at least 1 h before packaging them into sample bags with enough scintillation fluid to fully saturate and cover the mat (generally 5–7 mL depending on the size of the filter mats).

3.4 Optional Protocol for Staining RS and RSB Responder PBMC to Enable Flow Cytometric Assessment of Suppression of Alloproliferation by Costimulatory Blockade

If facilities do not exist for performing alloproliferation assays by radionucleotide incorporation, CFSE labeling of cells is a useful alternate assay for assessing alloproliferation by flow cytometry [7] and also provides the opportunity to measure cell proliferation in specific PBMC cell subsets. If the CFSE method is used, responder cells should be CFSE labeled just prior to set up in 72 h alloanergization and control bulk cultures.

1. Thaw purified DMSO "Component B" for about 20 min before use. Keep sterile and return to storage at −20 °C immediately after use.
2. Take one vial of dye labeled "Component A" from the freezer just prior to use. It contains lyophilized dye and may look like a yellow film or a few yellowish grains inside the vial. Bring to RT only briefly and keep away from light.
3. Prepare a 10 mM stock by dissolving one vial (Component A) with 90 μL of DMSO (Component B). Recap and vortex for about 5 s after addition of DMSO.
4. Make Working Stock by diluting 10 mM stock with DPBS to obtain a final concentration of 10 μM (i.e., 1 in 1000); Ex: 10 μL Stock CFSE at 10 mM + 9990 μL DPBS.
5. Vortex well and keep CFSE and the working dilutions in the dark. Use only freshly prepared reagents, discard remainder.
6. Wash 10–50 million PBMC in DPBS and pellet the cells in a 50 mL conical centrifuge tube. It is important to remove serum proteins from the cells prior to labeling, as the presence of proteins inhibits dye uptake into cells. Gently resuspend the cell pellet with 500 μL DPBS by pipet tip such that there are no clumps. Gently vortex the cells.
7. Add 500 μL of Working Stock CFSE to PBMC to give a final volume of 1000 mL in the 50 mL tube.
8. Incubate cells in CFSE for 8 min at RT in the dark, *vortexing gently, but thorougly, for a few seconds every 90 s.*
9. Stop the staining by adding 5–10 mL *cold* FBS and mix gently. Place cells in 37 °C incubator for 20 min to allow further dye incorporation.
10. Centrifuge PBMC for 10 min at 400–300 × *g*.
11. Aspirate the supernatant carefully, then disrupt the PBMC pellets and resuspend PBMC well by adding 20 mL RPMI-10% HuAB serum Complete Medium.
12. Spin at 400–450 × *g* for 5–10 min at RT with the BRAKE ON. Repeat this washing step for a total of two washes.
13. Count cells; readjust to 1×10^6/mL in RPMI-10% HuAB serum Complete Medium, and proceed with using these cells as RS responder PBMC and RSB responder PBMC in 72 h alloanergization flask cultures (*see* **Notes 14** and **15**).

3.5 Calculating Allosuppression in the Primary and Secondary MLR

The percentage inhibition (PI) of alloresponses in the primary MLR can be calculated as below, where mean counts per min (cpm) from the RS and RSB triplicate wells are determined:

Primary MLR:

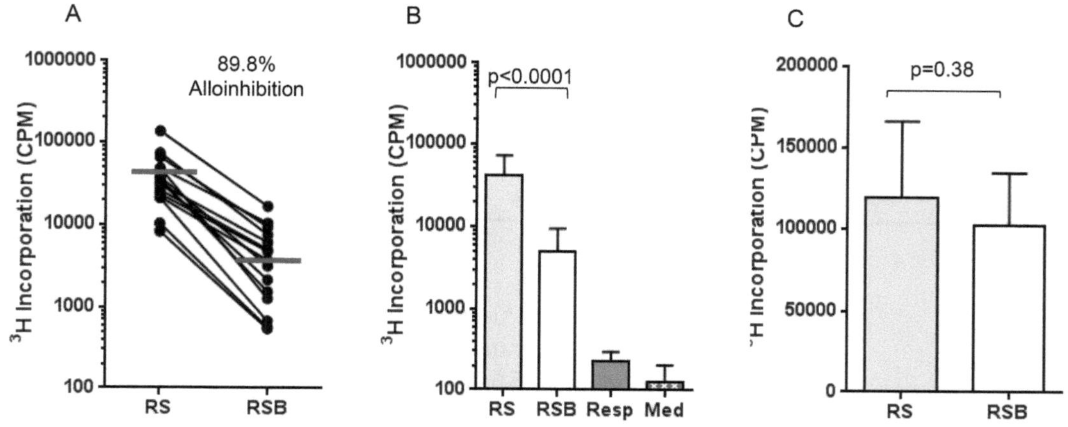

Fig. 3 Primary MLR cultures of RS and RSB PBMC were washed and restimulated with additional irradiated first party (FP) stimulators in a secondary MLR. (**a**) Alloproliferative responses were reduced by a median of 89.8% at Day 8 (range 79–97%). (**b**) Composite mean and standard deviation for 3H-thymidine incorporation in the RS, RSB, responders alone (Resp) in complete medium, and medium alone (Med). (**c**) Global stimulation by αCD3/αCD28 activating antibodies was not significantly decreased in RSB PBMC cultures

$$\mathrm{PI} = 100 - \left\{100 \times {}^{\text{cpm (primary MLR+CSB)}}\!/_{\text{cpm (primary MLR no CSB)}}\right\}$$

Secondary MLR:

$$\mathrm{PI} = 100 - \left\{100 \times {}^{\text{cpm (restimulated alloanergized PBMC)}}\!/_{\text{cpm (retimulated non-anergized PBMC)}}\right\}$$

3.6 Representative Results (See Note 16)

Anergization cultures established with a total of 14 different HLA-mismatched, unrelated donor pairs in the absence (RS) and presence (RSB) of belatacept at a dose of 40 μg/mL were set up using human cryopreserved PBMC, by 3 independent operators. Costimulatory molecule blockade with belatacept resulted in a median reduction of 87.2% at Day 6, range 61–98% (Fig. 2a) in proliferative alloresponses from primary MLRs. Data in Fig. 2b show the composite mean and standard deviation values measured in the RS and RSB cultures by ^{3}H-thymidine incorporation, as well as assay background levels measured in wells containing responders alone (Resp) in complete medium, and medium alone (Med). There was no significant decrease in the proliferation of RSB PBMC cultures responding to global stimulation by αCD3/α CD28 activating antibodies compared to the values measured in the RS cultures (Fig. 2c).

The RS and RSB PBMC were then washed and restimulated with a bolus of additional irradiated FP stimulators in a secondary MLR; alloproliferative responses were reduced by a median of 89.8% at Day 8, range 79–97% (Fig. 3a). Data in Fig. 2b show the aggregate mean and standard deviation values measured in the RS and RSB cultures by ^{3}H-thymidine incorporation, as well as assay background levels measured in wells containing responders alone (Resp) in complete medium, and medium alone (Med).

The anergization process resulted in marked allospecific tolerization without immunosuppression as response levels to mitotic stimulus by αCD3/αCD28 activating antibodies were not statistically different when RSB PBMC were compared to RS PBMC (Fig. 3c).

4 Notes

1. Human AB serum used in this medium should either be purchased heat inactivated from the vendor or inactivated by the user by heating to 56 °C for 1 h. If possible, screen multiple lots of pooled serum before proceeding with assays to ensure that the medium supports the culture of human PBMC without excessive background proliferation.
2. RPMI-10% HuAB serum Complete Medium older than 1 month should not be used for plating RS, RSB bulk cultures or MLR plates due to degradation of labile media supplements. Just expired medium can be used for wash steps provided that it remains sterile and pH stable.
3. Alternately other agents that block B7:CD28 binding/signaling may be used, such as individual monoclonal antibodies to human Anti-B7.1/B7.2, at concentrations of approximately 10 μg/mL each.
4. Alternately, the CFSE dye dilution method can be used, if desired. Other non-radioactive, non-flow cytometric assays such as Alamar Blue or MTT might be employed, but could result in a loss of sensitivity of detection.
5. If a γ-irradiation source is not available, x-ray irradiation, or mitomycin-C treatment of the APC population/stimulators could be alternatively used, although this would require additional testing and optimization of the procedure and/or dosimetry necessary to prepare the stimulator population. These have not been directly tested in our lab for these particular assays, but are commonly used for preventing the outgrowth of APC populations in similar assays that require APC antigen presentation to responding lymphocyte populations, without APC contributing significantly to background measurements, such as in ELISpot assays.
6. Depending on your particular institution's regulatory requirements, the collection of blood products may require an authorized protocol. Cells may also be obtained from commercial sources.
7. Prior to addition of RBC lysis buffer, all liquid must be well aspirated from the pellet completely with little to no residual

liquid remaining (which can affect the efficiency of the lysis step).

8. Cells should not be exposed to DMSO for more than 20–30 min prior to placing the freezing container into the freezer.
9. 72 h is the standard incubation time. Although incubating for up to 96 h tends to result in slightly better allosuppression, recovered cell yields are slightly reduced.
10. PBMC held in culture for 72–96 h can be used successfully as stimulators, however a proportion of the adherent APC population will be lost to binding.
11. It is essential to the success of the assay to minimize as much as possible the time that any of the PBMC preparations in tubes or plates are out of the incubator. During periods when the cells are not directly being manipulated, keep them in the incubator.
12. Using a third party stimulator (TP) control in the secondary MLR is optional, but useful for assessing the specificity of alloanergization. If specific alloanergization is induced, the alloresponse to TP stimulation should not be significantly different in RSB PBMC compared to RS PBMC. Using additional controls may require the use of additional 96-well tissue culture plates.
13. Since plates are pulsed for 16–20 h, it is usually convenient to add ^{3}H-thymidine to plates the night before the desired harvest time point. Thus, for harvesting a Day 4 MLR plate, add ^{3}H-thymidine at the end of the day on Day 3, for a Day 5 plate, add on Day 4, etc. Our lab uses ^{3}H-thymidine within 6 months of receipt to avoid potential decreases in signal associated with degradation during longer term storage.
14. When using CFSE labeled cells as RS and RSB responders, remember to hold some CFSE-labeled cells in culture for determining the basal control peak. Proliferation is observed as dye dilution by successive daughter cells and the basal peak represented by unstimulated responder cells is critical for gating the alloproliferative response.
15. When using the CFSE format, using multiple wells of 24 or 48-well plates or T-25 cm^{2} flasks may be used in lieu of 96-well plates for primary and secondary MLR assays, since cells will be removed for flow cytometry at intervals. In such cases, the suggested cell concentration and ratio of responders: stimulators should be adhered to in order to ensure proper allostimulation, which partly relies on adequate responder: stimulator ratio and close proximity.

16. Typical results in both primary and secondary MLRs should show increasing RS values and at least a 50% reduction in these values by RSB PBMC, commensurate with an increasing proliferative response to mitotic stimulus in both RS and RSB PBMC. Donor-specific factors, such as parity, blood transfusion occurrences, and other immune response and health factors, can cause variability in the rate of alloproliferation, especially as observed in RS PBMC. In general, it should be possible to observe increasing allo- and mitotic stimulus-mediated proliferation by RS cells on at least two of the three primary and secondary MLR time points. At times, most pronounced at later time points of the secondary (Day 8 or Day 10), culture wells show increased acidity (media no longer an orange-pink color, but instead yellow). This is often accompanied by markedly decreased cpms in affected wells, and is an indication of nutrient exhaustion of the medium due to cell proliferation over time. Should this occur, it may be necessary to read MLR plates on Days 6, 7, 8 instead. A lack of strong alloproliferation can occur if PBMC are in poor condition, were frozen incorrectly, are contaminated, are in the incorrect or expired media, or, very occasionally, there is a lack of sufficient HLA disparity to drive a proliferative alloresponse. In general, wells containing responders alone should have a mean value of ~800 cpm, or less, typically 400–600 cpm, or less.

References

1. Guinan EC, Boussiotis VA, Neuberg D et al (1999) Transplantation of anergic histoincompatible bone marrow allografts. N Engl J Med 340(22):1704–1714
2. Davies JK, Yuk D, Nadler LM et al (2008) Induction of alloanergy in human donor T cells without loss of pathogen or tumor immunity. Transplantation 86(6):854–864
3. Davies JK, Barbon CM, Voskertchian A et al (2012) In vitro allostimulation in the context of Co-stimulatory blockade with belatacept expands allospecific regulatory T cells with enhanced suppressive capacity. Cell Transplant 21(9):2047–2061 *ePub* PMID: 22507909
4. Bretscher PA (1970) A two-step, two-signal model for the primary activation of precursor helper T cells. Science 169:1042–1049
5. Bretscher P, Cohn M (1999) A theory of self-nonself discrimination. Proc Natl Acad Sci 96:185–190
6. Linsley PS, Brady W, Urnes M et al (1991) CTLA-4 is a second receptor for the B cell activation antigen B7. J ExpMed 174(3):561–569
7. Lyons AB, Parish CR (1994) Determination of lymphocyte division by flow cytometry. J Immunol Methods 171(1):131–137

Chapter 9

In Vitro Suppression of CD4$^+$ T-Cell Responses by Murine and Human Myeloid-Derived Suppressor Cells

Katerina Vlachou and Panayotis Verginis

Abstract

Myeloid-derived suppressor cells (MDSCs) are myeloid precursors of macrophages, dendritic cells, and neutrophils with a prominent role in the regulation of immune responses in cancer, infection, and autoimmunity. Herein, we describe a protocol for the isolation of murine and human MDSCs and the assessment of their ability to suppress CD4$^+$ T-cell responses in vitro.

Key words Myeloid-derived suppressor cells, Cell sorting, In vitro proliferation assay, CD4$^+$ T-cell isolation, Carboxyfluorescein succinimidyl ester (CFSE)

1 Introduction

Myeloid-derived suppressor cells (MDSCs) comprise a heterogeneous cell population of myeloid cells, with great plasticity and strong potential to regulate immune responses in cancer, infection, inflammation, and autoimmunity [1–3]. Murine MDSCs are characterized as CD11b$^+$Gr-1$^+$ and could be further divided into two distinct subsets according to the expression of two epitopes of Gr-1 as follows; the granulocytic-like (G-MDSCs) defined as CD11b$^+$Ly6G$^+$Ly6C^{low} and the monocytic-like (M-MDSCs) defined as CD11b$^+$Ly6G$^-$Ly6C^{high} [4]. MDSCs have been also studied in humans with M-MDSCs to be characterized as CD14$^+$CD11b$^+$HLA-DR$^{low/neg}$ [5] whereas G-MDSCs as HLA--DR$^{intermediate/low}$CD14$^-$CD15$^+$CD33$^+$ [6].

Despite heterogeneity, MDSCs share a common biological activity; they can potently suppress T-cell responses. Several mechanisms have been implicated to the MDSC-mediated suppression of the immune responses, including arginase, induced nitric oxide species (iNOS), reactive oxygen species (ROS) [7], and programmed cell death ligand 1 (PD-L1) [6]. However, the nature of the interaction between MDSCs and T cells is complex and depends

Ashleigh S. Boyd (ed.), *Immunological Tolerance: Methods and Protocols*, Methods in Molecular Biology, vol. 1899,
https://doi.org/10.1007/978-1-4939-8938-6_9, © Springer Science+Business Media, LLC, part of Springer Nature 2019

on the inflammatory microenvironment [8]. The design of in vitro suppression assays has provided a useful tool to investigate the mechanisms of MDSC-mediated suppression. MDSC suppressive activity on T-cell proliferation in vitro could be assessed either through [^{3}H]-thymidine uptake by proliferating T cells or by labeling cells with Carboxyfluorescein succinimidyl ester (CFSE) prior to coculture with MDSCs and measuring CFSE incorporation at the end of the culture [9].

Herein, we describe a protocol for the in vitro assessment of the MDSC-mediated suppression of CD4^{+} T-cell proliferation with the use of CFSE intracellular fluorescent dye. CFSE is highly membrane permeable and able to stain the cytoplasm of the cells. As cells divide, CFSE is progressively diluted within daughter cells and can be monitored with flow cytometry, correlated thus to T-cell proliferation.

2 Materials

2.1 Isolation of Murine MDSCs and T Cells

1. Spleen, bone marrow, and/or lymph nodes, from 6 to 12 weeks mice.
2. Forceps and small dissection scissors.
3. 60 × 15 mm sterile polystyrene petri dishes (PE-LD).
4. 10 ml Disposable Syringes and 25G$^{5/8}$ needles (NIPRO).
5. 40 μm cell strainers (BD FALCON).
6. 15 ml conical falcon tubes (Greiner).
7. Phosphate-buffered saline 1×, pH 7.4 without calcium chloride/magnesium chloride (PBS). You can use tablets and dilute according to manufacturer's protocol (Gibco). Store at 4 °C.
8. NH_4Cl_2 pH = 7.2–7.6 in order to perform erythrolysis. Store at 4 °C.
9. To isolate cells by flow cytometry sorting MDSCs were characterized according to the following markers and monoclonal antibodies; Fluorochrome-conjugated 7-Aminoactinomycin (7-AAD) from BD Biosciences. CD11c (clone N418); CD11b (clone M1/70); Ly6G/Ly6C (GR-1) (clone RB6-8C5); Ly6G (clone 1A8), Ly6C (cloneHK1.4); CD4 (clone RM4–5); CD25 (clone pc61) and CD44 (clone IM7), all from Biolegend.
10. 5 ml polystyrene round-bottom tubes with cell strainer cap (12 × 75 mm style), (BD Falcon).
11. Fetal Bovine Serum (FBS) (Gibco).
12. 5% PBS/FBS. Dilute FBS in PBS to a final concentration of 5% FBS. Use it as the diluent of the cell suspensions and as the

staining buffer for staining the cells with monoclonal antibodies. Keep on ice and do not store for long term use.

13. Flow Cytometer—Sorter.

2.2 Cell Culture

1. Sterile 96-well round bottom microplates (Costar).
2. Purified hamster anti-mouse CD3e (clone 145-2C11) (eBioscience).
3. Purified hamster anti-mouse CD28 (clone 37.51) (eBioscience).
4. Carboxyfluorescein diacetate succinimidyl ester (CFSE) (Invitrogen).
5. Bovine Albumin Fraction V Solution (BSA Fraction V) 7.5% (Gibco).
6. Humidified CO_2 incubator.
7. Complete DMEM culture medium (Gibco) containing 10% FBS, Penicilin (100 U/ml), Streptomycin (100 μg/ml), 2-mercaptoethanol (5×10^{-5} M) (Gibco).

2.3 Analysis of MDSCs Suppressive Activity

1. Fluorochrome-conjugated 7AAD (BD Biosciences) and CD4 (clone RM4-5), CD44 (clone IM7) antibodies from Biolegend.
2. 1.5 ml microcentrifuge tubes (Costar).
3. Flow Cytometer.
4. FlowJo software (Tree Star Inc.) version 8.7.

2.4 Human Subjects

1. Heparinized syringe.
2. Histopaque-1077 Ficoll density gradient (Sigma).
3. 5 ml polystyrene round-bottom tubes with cell strainer cap (12 × 75 mm style) (SarstedT).
4. For the characterization of human MDSCs the following were used; Fluorochrome-conjugated antibodies CD15 (clone 8OH5), CD33 (clone D3HL60.251), CD14 (clone RM052), CD25 (clone B1.49.9) from Beckman Coulter. HLA-DR (clone L243, G46-6) and CD4 (clone RPA-T4), (BD Pharmingen).
5. Sterile disposable transfer pipettes (SarstedT).
6. 15 ml conical falcon tubes (Greiner).
7. Fluorescence-Activated Cell Sorter.
8. Purified mouse anti-human anti-CD3 (clone OKT3) (BioLegend).
9. Purified mouse anti-human anti-CD28 (clone CD28.2) (BioLegend).

10. RPMI culture (Gibco) containing 10% FBS, Penicilin (100 U/ml), Streptomycin (100 μg/ml), 2-mercaptoethanol (5×10^{-5} M).
11. 5% PBS/FBS. Dilute FBS in PBS to a final concentration of 5% FBS. Use it as the diluent of the cell suspensions and as the staining buffer for staining the cells with monoclonal antibodies. Keep on ice and do not store for long term use.

2.5 Human T-Cell Proliferation and Activation

1. Fluorochrome-conjugated CD4 (RPA-T4) antibody (BD Pharminfen).
2. 1.5 ml microcentrifuge tubes (Costar).
3. Flow Cytometer.
4. FlowJob software version 8.7.

3 Methods

3.1 Isolation of Murine MDSCs

1. Sacrifice the animal by cervical dislocation to isolate the spleen and the bone marrow as follows;

   Spleen

   (a) Place the tissue in a 40 μm cell strainer, inside a petri dish containing 5 ml of 5% PBS/FBS medium. Homogenize the tissue with a syringe plunger to obtain single cell suspension. Collect the cells in a 15 ml falcon. Fill up to 15 ml with 5% PBS/FBS. Keep on ice.

   Bone Marrow

   (a) Use 70% ethanol to spray the animal at the ventral side. Make a lateral incision with the help of the scissors. Carefully remove the skin from the hind limbs and then dissect them away from body by cutting above the femur. Remove tissue from limbs with the help of the scissors. Detach the femur from the shinbone.

   (b) Keep the bones in PBS 1x until you flush the bone marrow.

   (c) Cut the proximal and distal ends of the bones. Fill the 10 ml syringe with 5% PBS/FBS. Place the syringe at one of the cut ends to flush the bone marrow in a sterile petri dish. Repeat procedure for both bone ends (*see* **Note 1**).

   (d) After flushing all bones in the petri dish, homogenize the tissue suspension by passing it through a $25G^{5/8}$ needle 10–12 times. Transfer the cell suspension in a 15 ml falcon tube. Fill up to 15 ml with 5% PBS/FBS. Keep samples on ice.

   (e) Centrifuge for 10 min, at $400 \times g$, RT and discard the supernatant.

Continue now processing the spleen- and bone-marrow-derived cells the same way.

2. Resuspend the pellet in 2 ml NH_4Cl_2 pH = 7.2–7.6 to lyse the erythrocytes. Leave the cells in NH_4Cl_2 for 2 min (*see* **Note 2**). Stop the erythrolysis by adding 8 ml cold PBS 1×.
3. Centrifuge for 10 min, at 400 × *g*, at room temperature (RT) and resuspend the pellet in 1 ml of 5% PBS/FBS. Keep at 4 °C until next step.
4. Label the cells with the proper antibodies to sort total MDSCs, G-MDSCs or M-MDSCs. For total MDSCs; 7-AAD, CD11c, CD11b, Gr-1 at an optimal concentration. For the two subsets; 7-AAD, CD11c, CD11b, Ly6G, Ly6C at an optimal concentration (*see* **Note 3**).
5. Leave at 4 °C for 20 min in the darkness for the cells to be labeled.
6. Stop the reaction by adding cold PBS 1× up to 10 ml.
7. Centrifuge for 10 min, at 400 × *g*, at 4 °C.
8. Resuspend the cells in 500 μl of 5% PBS/FBS.
9. Transfer the cells in a 5 ml polystyrene round-bottom tube by filtering the suspension through a cell-strainer cap.
10. Use FACS sorting to isolate MDSCs as follows. For isolation of total MDSCs, first gate on 7-AAD and CD11c. Exclude dead cells (7-AAD^{+}) and dendritic cells (CD11c^{+}). Then gate for Gr-1 and CD11b expression. The 7-AAD^{-}CD11c^{-}Gr-1^{+}CD11b^{+} cell population constitutes the total MDSCs compartment. For G-MDSC and M-MDSC cell sorting do the following; gate on 7-AAD and CD11c to exclude again dead and dendritic cells (7-AAD^{+}CD11c^{+}). Then gate on CD11b^{high} and distinguish G-MDSCs and M-MDSCs according to expression of Ly6G and Ly6C respectively (*see* Fig. 1).
11. Collect sorted cells in a 1.5 ml polystyrene round-bottom tube containing 5% PBS/FBS.
12. Centrifuge for 10 min, at 400 × *g*, RT and resuspend the pellet in 1 ml complete DMEM medium in order to use them for the suppression assay.

3.2 Isolation and Preparation of Murine T Cells from Lymph Nodes

1. Collect the inguinal, branchial, or axillary lymph nodes. Detach them from the body with the help of a pair of forceps. Carefully clean away any fat remainants that could increase cell death.
2. Place the lymph nodes in a 40 μm cell strainer in a petri dish, containing 5 ml of 5% PBS/FBS medium. Prepare single cell suspension with the help of a syringe plunger and collect in a 15 ml falcon tube. Fill up to 15 ml with 5% PBS/FBS.

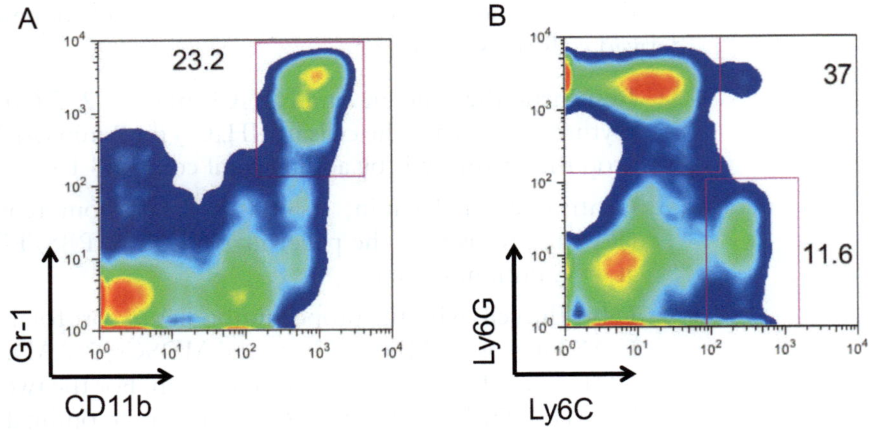

Fig. 1 Phenotypic characterization of total and granulocytic/monocytic MDSCs. Flow cytometric analysis of MDSCs in the spleen of Myelin Oligodendrocyte Glycoprotein (MOG 35-55) emulsified in Complete Freund's Adjuvant (CFA) injected mice. (**a**) Total Gr1^{+}CD11b^{+} MDSCs (gated on 7-AAD^{-}CD11c^{-} CD3^{-}CD19^{-} cells). (**b**) CD11b^{high}Ly6G^{+}Ly6C^{-} G-MDSCs (top left gate) and CD11b^{high}Ly6G^{-}Ly6C^{+} M-MDSCs (bottom right gate) both gated on 7AAD^{-}CD3^{-}CD19^{-}CD11c^{-}. Numbers indicate the frequency of MDSCs in the respective gates

3. Centrifuge for 10 min, at 400 × *g*, RT and resuspend the pellet in 1 ml of 5% PBS/FBS in order to label the cells with fluorescent labeled monoclonal antibodies.
4. Label the cells using 7-AAD and CD4, CD25 monoclonal antibodies for 20 min at 4 °C, in the darkness.
5. Wash the cells by adding 1 ml cold PBS 1× and centrifuge for 10 min, at 400 × *g*, 4 °C.
6. Resuspend the cell pellet in 500 μl of 5% PBS/FBS and transfer the cells in a 5 ml polystyrene round-bottom tube by passing the suspension through a cell-strainer cap.
7. Use FACS sorting to isolate T cells. Set up the gates as described below:
8. Exclude 7-AAD^{+} cells (dead cells) and plot the 7-AAD^{-} gated cells for CD4 and CD25 expression. Select the CD4^{+} cells that are negative for CD25 expression (*see* **Note 4**).
9. Collect cells in a sterile, 5% PBS/FBS coated polystyrene round-bottom and centrifuge for 10 min, at 400 × *g*, RT.
10. Count the sorted cells and adjust to 10^6 cells/1 ml. Label CD4^{+}CD25^{-} T cells with 1 μM CFSE/10^6 cells/1 ml. Resuspend the cells in pre-warmed (RT) 0.1% PBS/BSA and transfer maximum 5 × 10^6 T cells in a 15 ml falcon tube. Mix and vortex.
11. Place the tube at 37 °C for 20 min, in the darkness.
12. Wash the cells 5 ml of cold 5% PBS/FBS and centrifuge at 400 × *g*, 10 min, RT.
13. Resuspend the pellet in complete DMEM medium to set the culture.

3.3 Cell Culture

1. Use U-bottom 96-well culture plates to coculture T cells with MDSCs, in 200 μl final culture volume.
2. Coat the plate with 10 μg/ml anti-CD3 diluted in 50 μl PBS 1× per well. Leave anti-CD3 coating overnight at 4 °C or for 4 h at 37 °C.
3. Wash twice the plate with 200 μl PBS 1× per well to remove the unbound anti-CD3 molecules.
4. Set the culture. Plate 4×10^4–10×10^4 sorted T cells per well and add titrated number of sorted MDSCs (*see* **Notes 5** and **6**).
5. Add soluble anti-CD28 to a final concentration of 1 μg/ml in a final culture volume of 25 μl (*see* **Note** 7).
6. Culture the cells in the incubator, at 37 °C, 5% CO_2. The day when setting the culture is defined as day 0.
7. Monitor the proliferation of T cells starting from day 3 of culture until day 7. Follow the protocol described right after.

3.4 Analysis

1. Collect the cells in a 1.5 ml eppendorf and centrifuge for 10 min, at 400 × *g*, RT. Resuspend the pellet in 200 μl of 5% PBS/FBS to label T cells with the CD44 activation marker. Collect culture supernatants and store at −20 °C (*see* **Note 8**).
2. Label the cells with the following antibodies; 7AAD, CD4, CD44 using the aforementioned method used to label the cells prior to sorting.
3. To assess T-cell activation, analyze the $7AAD^-CD4^+$ T cells for CD44 expression. Activated T cells upregulate the expression of CD44.
4. To assess T-cell proliferation monitor the CFSE dilution in $7AAD^-CD4^+$ T cells. Cell proliferation can be measured, as each cell division results in halving of the fluorescence intensity of CFSE (*see* Fig. 2).

3.5 Human Assay

In this section we highlight modifications of the murine protocol for the assessment of human MDSCs-mediated suppression of $CD4^+$ T cells.

3.5.1 Isolation of Human PBMCs

1. Collect 5 ml peripheral blood in a heparinized syringe.
2. Mix the blood with 5 ml PBS 1× layer and overlay the mix on top of 5 ml ficoll gradient in a 15 ml falcon tube (*see* **Note 9**).
3. Centrifuge at 600 × *g*, for 30 min, RT, without break.
4. Collect the peripheral blood mononuclear cells (PBMCs) with the help of a plastic poir and transfer into a 15 ml falcon tube.
5. Wash the cells twice by adding PBS 1× up to 15 ml each time.

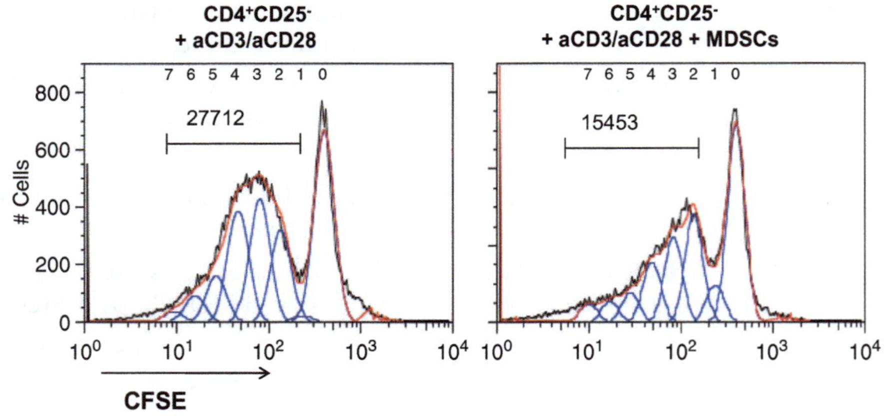

Fig. 2 In vitro MDSC-mediated suppression of CFSE-labeled $CD4^+$ T-cell proliferation. Gr-1^+CD11b^+ cells (gated on 7-AAD^-CD11c^-) were cocultured with polyclonally stimulated CFSE-labeled $CD4^+CD25^-$ T cells. MDSCs were isolated from spleen of MOG/CFA-injected C57BL/6 mice. CFSE dilution was assessed by flow cytometry after 5 days of coculture. Representative histograms of CFSE dilution of anti-CD3, anti-CD28 stimulated T cells cultured in the absence (left panel) or presence (right panel) of MDSCs. The numbers indicate the cell divisions

6. Centrifuge at 400 × *g*, for 10 min. Discard the supernatant and resuspend the pellet in 1 ml of 5% PBS/FBS to label the cells with the respective antibodies.
7. Split the cell suspension into two parts to label for MDSCs and T cells separately. Use the same staining protocol as described for murine cells, to label with HLA-DR, CD14, CD15, CD33 antibodies for MDSCs and CD4, CD25 antibodies for T cells. Afterwards, use FACS sorting to isolate the following subsets; HLA-$DR^{intermediate/low}CD14^-CD15^+CD33^+$ (G-MDSCs), $CD14^+CD11b^+$HLA-$DR^{low/neg}$ (M-MDSCs) and $CD4^+CD25^-$ (T cells).

3.5.2 In Vitro Suppression Assay

1. Coat the culture plate with 2 μg/ml anti-CD3 (OKT3).
2. Label T cells using the same protocol as with murine cells, despite leaving the cells to be labeled with CFSE for 10 min.
3. Set up the coculture as in murine cells by adding 1 μg/ml anti-CD28 (CD28.2).

4 Notes

1. The use of PBS/FBS to flush the bone marrow will form some foam bubbles. To avoid this inconvenience use plain PBS and add FBS afterward to a final solution of 5%. PBS/FBS. Additionally, to avoid breaking the bones while flushing, use a $25G^{5/8}$ needle.

2. To eliminate cell death during erythrolysis, do not exceed 2 min of NH_4Cl_2 treatment.
3. A titration assay of the fluorochrome-conjugated antibodies is suggested prior to cell labeling in order to determine the antibody concentration needed for optimal detection.
4. Gating out the $CD4^+CD25^+$ cell subset is necessary in order to minimize the presence of T regulatory cells (CD25 is mostly expressed on T regulatory cells) that could also exert a suppressive function and interfere with the results.
5. Several MDSCs: T-cell ratios should be performed (i.e., 1:0, 1:1, 1:4, 1:16) so as to demonstrate the specificity of MDSCs-mediated suppression of T-cell proliferation. This way, titrating out the MDSCs should result in restoration of T-cell proliferation.
6. Always include positive and negative controls for the proper interpretation of the results. Thus, culture of T cells alone or only in the presence of anti-CD3 could serve as negative control. On the other hand, addition of another regulatory cell subset (i.e., T regulatory cells) could be used as a positive control.
7. Alternatively, MDSC-mediated suppressive ability could be monitored in an antigen-specific T-cell proliferation system. To this end, draining lymph nodes from antigen-challenged mice could be CFSE labeled and then cultured in vitro in the presence of the respective antigen. This allows only antigen-specific $CD4^+$ T cells to proliferate.
8. An additional evidence of the MDSC suppressive capacity could be obtained by performing cytokine ELISA in culture supernatants. For this reason, IL-2 and IFNγ cytokines could be monitored.
9. Add the blood solution over the ficoll gradient slowly and carefully, to prevent mixing with the ficoll gradient layer.

Acknowledgment

This work was supported by grant from the Greek General Secretariat of Research and Technology (Synergasia 09SYN-12-1074 to P.V.).

References

1. Gabrilovich DI, Nagaraj S (2009) Myeloid-derived suppressor cells as regulators of the immune system. Nat Rev Immunol 9 (3):162–174
2. Cripps JG, Gorham JD (2011) MDSC in autoimmunity. Int Immunopharmacol 11 (7):789–793

3. Nagaraj S, Collazo M, Corzo CA et al (2009) Regulatory myeloid suppressor cells in health and disease. Cancer Res 69(19):7503–7506
4. Youn JI, Nagaraj S, Collazo M et al (2008) Subsets of myeloid-derived suppressor cells in tumor-bearing mice. J Immunol 181 (8):5791–5802
5. Poschke I, Mougiakakos D, Hansson J et al (2010) Immature immunosuppressive CD14 +HLA-DR−/low cells in melanoma patients are Stat3hi and overexpress CD80, CD83, and DC-sign. Cancer Res 70(11):4335–4345
6. Ioannou M, Alissafi T, Lazaridis I et al (2012) Crucial role of granulocytic myeloid-derived suppressor cells in the regulation of central nervous system autoimmune disease. J Immunol 188(3):1136–1146
7. Kusmartsev S, Nefedova Y, Yoder D et al (2004) Antigen-specific inhibition of CD8+ T cell response by immature myeloid cells in cancer is mediated by reactive oxygen species. J Immunol 172(2):989–999
8. Nagaraj S, Youn JI, Gabrilovich DI (2013) Reciprocal relationship between myeloid-derived suppressor cells and T cells. J Immunol 191(1):17–23
9. Ioannou M, Alissafi T, Boon L et al (2013) In vivo ablation of plasmacytoid dendritic cells inhibits autoimmunity through expansion of myeloid-derived suppressor cells. J Immunol 190(6):2631–2640

Chapter 10

Disassembling and Reaggregating the Thymus: The Pros and Cons of Current Assays

Elia Piccinini and Paola Bonfanti

Abstract

This review briefly describes the last decades of experimental work on the thymus. Given the histological complexity of this organ, the multiple embryological origins of its cellular components and its role in carefully regulating T lymphocyte maturation and function, methods to dissect and understand this complexity have been developed through the years. The possibility to study ex vivo the thymus organ function has been achieved by developing Fetal Thymus Organ Cultures (FTOC). Subsequently, the combination of organ disaggregation and reaggregation in vitro represented by Reaggregate Thymus Organ cultures (RTOC) allowed mixing cellular components from different genetic backgrounds. Moreover, RTOC allowed dissecting the different stromal and hematological components to study the interactions between Major Histocompatibility Complex (MHC) molecules and the T-cell receptors during thymocytes selection. In more recent years, prospective isolation of stromal cells and thymocytes at different stages of development made it possible to explore and elucidate the molecular and cellular players in both the developing and adult thymus. Finally, the appearance of novel cell sources such as embryonic stem (ES) cells and more recently induced pluripotent stem (iPS) cells has opened new scenarios in modelling thymus development and regeneration strategies. Most of the work described was carried out in rodents and the current challenge is to develop equivalent or even more informative assays and tools in entirely human model systems.

Key words Fetal thymus organ culture, Progenitor/stem cells, Pluripotent stem cells, Thymus bioengineering

1 Introduction

The thymus was the last organ whose function was elucidated by the pioneering work of Jacques Miller approximately 50 years ago [1]. Because of its anatomical and histological complexity, the thymus remains a difficult organ to study and the difficulty is increased by the developmental changes it undergoes during fetal and perinatal life, followed by involution during adulthood.

Several in vitro models and organotypic cultures were developed through the years and helped to study some aspects of T-cell development and selection in partially simplified systems; however

Ashleigh S. Boyd (ed.), *Immunological Tolerance: Methods and Protocols*, Methods in Molecular Biology, vol. 1899, https://doi.org/10.1007/978-1-4939-8938-6_10, © Springer Science+Business Media, LLC, part of Springer Nature 2019 the thymic microenvironment is organized in a 3D meshwork [2] where different stromal components such as thymic epithelial cells (TECs) and dendritic cells (DCs) organize a unique instructing environment that allows T-cell precursor migration and maturation [3]. In addition to the stromal components and maturing thymocytes, many different cell types contribute to the cellular and extracellular matrix (ECM) complexity of the thymus: nerve and myoid cells; macrophages, natural killer (NK), and B cells; mesenchymal cells and reticular fibroblasts which organize trabeculae, specific reticulin fibers, blood vessels and perivascular space. The specific role of each component, and the complex network of interactions within this cellular diversity remain largely unknown.

Throughout a diversity of approaches to recapitulate in vitro the functionality of the thymus, the relevance of certain aspects of this complexity became more apparent, e.g., the arrangement of TEC in three-dimensional (3D) structures to preserve TEC phenotype and functionality, and the need of engrafting thymic grafts in vivo to maintain long term lymphopoiesis.

This review focuses on the protocols and methods for thymic organ models and summarizes the different in vitro and in vivo approaches developed in the last three decades underlying their advantages and limitations, and showing the possibility of expanding, to a different extent, TECs ex vivo.

2 T-Cell Development In Vitro in Fetal Thymus Organ Cultures (FTOC)

Following the seminal report of Miller, a conspicuous amount of work addressed the role of thymus on T-cell development [4, 5]. In the 1970s, Doherty and Zinkernagel clarified the biological role of major histocompatibility (MHC) antigens [6]. Although this was a major breakthrough in the field, recognized by the Nobel Prize award, the cellular basis of this process remained elusive for much longer and the central role of thymus in T-cell ontogeny controversial [7, 8].

An approach to understanding the function of any organ and tissue is represented by the possibility to dissect the various components (e.g., different cell types, extra cellular matrix—ECM, released cytokines, and circulating factors) and trying to reconstruct them, ideally, in vitro. The group of John Owen in Birmingham carried out a first attempt in this direction. They realized that organ cultures of embryonic thymic lobes preserve better the 3D structure of the stroma and therefore support T-cell development in vitro [5, 9] while other attempts of growing thymic stromal components in 2D able of maintaining thymopoiesis were not successful [10]. Accordingly, thymic lobes were isolated from mice at embryonic day 13 (E13) to E14 and placed on gelatin foam sponge resting on Nuclepore membrane filters (pore size

0.8 μm) that were cultured in RPMI-1640 containing 10% FCS [11]. This technique, known as Foetal Thymus Organ Culture (FTOC), allows cultivating thymic lobes up to 1 week at the air/-liquid interface. In 1982, Owen's group cultured embryonic thymic lobes in the presence of 2′-deoxyguanosine (dGuo) that kills virtually all the thymocytes while allowing survival of the stroma [12]. dGuo treatment had been previously shown to inhibit proliferation and has a cytotoxic effect on intra-thymic thymocytes [13]. Importantly, the surviving structures could be recolonized by lymphoid precursors of a different mouse strain, thus creating chimeric thymuses that offered the possibility to study in vitro T-cell development and MHC restriction mechanisms. Repopulation of these "empty" structures was possible by optimizing the trans-filter culture technique developed by the group of Nicole Le Douarin in Paris and published in 1981 [14]. Briefly, the dGuo-treated AKR thymic rudiments (recipient thymuses expressing Thyl.1 antigen) were placed over a 3 μm filter that separated them from the donor thymic lobes isolated from C57 or CBA mouse embryos, which express Thyl.2 antigen. This sandwich structure was cultivated for 5 days over a Nuclepore membrane (0.8 μm) before transferring the recipient thymuses to normal FTOC for additional 7 days [10]. The thymocytes analysis at this time point proved that AKR thymic rudiments, cultivated in association with C57 or CBA donor ones, were repopulated and supported the development of thymocytes carrying the Thyl.2 antigen. The absence of Thyl.1 antigen confirmed also the specificity of the toxic effect of dGuo on immature T cells [10].

This method allowed obtaining a-lymphoid thymic lobes that could be repopulated in vitro with defined progenitor populations through trans-filter cultures; the experiment in vitro could be carried out for an additional week to study T-cell development as stromal cells could not survive for much longer time in FTOC conditions. However, the dGuo-treated lobes could also be transplanted under the kidney capsule and repopulated in vivo demonstrating they could be then functional for longer periods [15]. The characterization of a-lymphoid thymic rudiments in the mouse revealed that also dendritic cells (DCs) had been eliminated, with survival of mainly the epithelial populations that allowed investigating their specific role in detail. However, the same approach using rat thymic rudiments yielded a different result since DCs were not eliminated by this treatment, thus uncovering a possible difference between the two species [16].

Cultures of intact murine thymus lobes require low amounts of media and reagents and are also quite easy to manipulate; therefore, they have been largely used to address the role of secreted factors on T-cell development. An example is represented by the studies of exogenous Interleukin (IL)-7 on T-cell precursors and their development [17]. In addition to cytokines, FTOC with intact lobes also provided a useful strategy to explore the molecular mechanisms mediating the interactions between stromal cells and lymphoid precursors: in fact, the availability of specific knock-out (KO) and transgenic mice with mutations in molecules involved in cell-cell interactions and of antibodies blocking or mimicking ligand-specific binding offered additional applications for the FTOC technique [18–22].

As an example, mice deficient for a transporter associated with antigen processing (TAP-1) were used to investigate the specific role of peptide/MHC interaction in supporting T-cell differentiation and restriction for MHC class I (Positive Selection) as well as central tolerance by deletion (Negative Selection) in the FTOC setup [23–25]. Similarly, reconstituting dGuo-treated FTOC with single hematopoietic progenitors at different stages of differentiation allowed defining the lineage relationship of hematopoietic progenitors. These "multi-lineage progenitor assays" have already been reviewed [26].

Notably, the use of retroviral vector transduction of mouse thymocytes in FTOC has allowed elucidating the role of intracellular signaling molecules (e.g., ZAP-70) in T-cell development and function [27]. This combined methodology has been facilitated also by the possibility of introducing fluorescent reporter proteins to follow the fate of specific thymocyte subtypes [27–31]. A novel, serum-free system, denominated ATO (Artificial Thymic Organoid) able to generate mature T cells with TCR diversity has been developed [30].

Nowadays FTOC represents a still widespread used technique, which offers the possibility of studying T-cell development as well as stroma-thymocytes interactions using novel available transgenic mice, cytokines, and gene targeting methods. Nevertheless, FTOC allow only limited dissection/reconstitution of the various thymic components.

3 Thymus Bioengineering: Multidisciplinary Approaches to Reconstruct a Lymphopoietic Organ

A further development of thymic in vitro models derived from the capacity to disaggregate enzymatically the stromal component of the thymus to single cell level, and applying different techniques to isolate TEC or other accessory cells. As a result, epithelial, stromal, and lymphoid components could be assembled in form of reaggregated thymic organ cultures, commonly referred to as RTOC, in defined proportions. For example, RTOC were originally exploited to explore the role of non-epithelial mesenchyme in ex vivo thymic organoids by G. Anderson [32–33]. Magnetic bead depletion and enrichment allowed the separation of CD45+ cells for the lymphoid compartment and MHC II+/A2B5-/CD45- cells for the epithelial compartments, which were then reaggregated by centrifugation with or without mesenchymal cells to demonstrate a supporting role of the stromal cells in T-cell development. The concept of this seminal experiment, coupled with an increased capacity to isolate specific cell types by fluorescence-activated flow cytometry (FACS), set the path for increasingly refined models aimed at understanding the biological role of specific cell subsets and recapitulating the organotypic complexity of the thymus. As of today, many protocols and techniques are available to isolate TEC and relative subpopulations [34–37]. However, it was observed that TEC in monolayer culture lose expression of functional molecules as Notch ligands, Foxn1 and AIRE, during in vitro expansion [2, 38]. Thus, it was proposed that modulating a 3D culture environment could support the development of novel thymic models able to sustain T-cell maturation in vitro. In an early attempt, TEC were seeded on a biocompatible scaffold constituted of tantalum-coated carbon matrix, and were able to support limited lymphopoiesis [39]. More recently, hydrogels able to form 3D TEC aggregates and suitable for injection in vivo demonstrated to maintain the molecular and functional properties of TEC in a bioengineered thymic graft. Although these approaches provide, to a certain extent, the necessary 3D architecture to TEC, they neglect the important role provided by the complex chemo-physical composition of the surrounding ECM. Histological analysis of thymic ECM shows an intricated thread of collagen type IV, fibronectin, and laminin [40]. Experimental conditions confirmed the crucial role of ECM components, like CYR61 and laminin-211, in determining TEC morphology, functionality, and the interactions with the developing T cells [41, 42]. Although the constitutive components of thymic ECM and their respective roles in supporting TEC identity have not been systematically dissected, tissue engineering has devised an approach based on organ decellularization that has shown various practical, and even clinical, applications [43, 44]. A recent report has explored the use of decellularized mouse thymic tissue in combination with TEC to generate a thymic organoid, suggesting the opportunity to exploit the naturally occurring ECM composition and architecture of the native thymus to improve our current limited ability to maintain functional TEC in culture [45].

Improvement of technologies to isolate and sort single cells allows the fabrication of thymic organoids with defined cellular composition, and approaches aimed at integrating 3D cell cultures with relevant ECM components. However, models aimed at maintaining functional TEC in vitro for prolonged periods need to take into account the maintenance of a more primitive pool of TEC able, to a certain extent, to self-renew and generate a differentiated progeny. These features are normally associated with stem and progenitor cells.

4 Stemness of TECs: In Vitro Expansion and 3D Reassembling

TECs represent the major component of the thymus stroma that supports differentiation of hematopoietic precursors into mature functional T cells. TECs are endodermal in origin and derive from the third pharyngeal pouch [46]. They are organized in different compartments classified as medullary, cortical, and subcapsular region respectively. The existence of TEC progenitors and/or stem cells is the topic of a long lasting debate in the field. However, more and more evidence accumulates supporting that multipotent epithelial progenitors arise during development and are maintained also in post-natal life. A 2006 report demonstrated that single E12 TECs from eYFP reporter mice—sorted on the basis of the expression of EpCAM1 and YFP—were able to give rise to both medullary and cortical differentiated TECs [47]. Interestingly, the authors used embryonic intact wild-type thymic recipient explants that were microinjected each with a single YFP^+ TEC. The microscope visualization allowed monitoring the microinjections and assured that only one single cell was injected into a single lobe. In order to allow better and longer development of the explants, they were grafted under the kidney capsule of adult mice and analyzed by immunohistochemistry after 4 weeks in vivo [47].

More recently, clonal cultures of TECs with long term expansion potential were derived from thymus of embryonic, postnatal, and adult rats that constitutively express eGFP reporter protein. Clonogenic TECs were of both cortical and medullary origin, expressed keratin 5/14 (K5/14) and K8/18 in culture and could expand for more than 50 doublings while maintaining a normal rat karyotype [38]. These TECs expressed stably marker genes that demonstrated their thymic identity but downregulated functional markers such as MHC-class II and AIRE1 while expanding in culture. In order to demonstrate the capacity to re-express these markers after clonal long term expansion, a whole organ thymic reaggregation assay was used to assess the differentiation potential of cultivated clonal rat TECs: embryonic E13 mouse or E14 rat thymic lobes were dissected, dissociated, and mixed in vitro with the progeny of clonal TECs from eGFP rats at defined ratios. They were then transplanted in vivo for 4 or 5 weeks before analysis [38]. The $eGFP^+$ rat TECs consistently integrated in the developing thymus under the kidney capsule and differentiated as demonstrated by upregulation at protein level of both MHC-class II and AIRE1, thus proving their capacity to maintain thymic potential after extensive clonal expansion. Importantly, extra-thymic potency was shown by the ability of clonal TECs to generate all the cell types of the skin (i.e., epidermis, hair follicle, and sebaceous gland) when transplanted on the back skin of *nude* athymic mice. Clones recovered from this in vivo assay were shown to be able to contribute to both thymus and epidermis. Possible fusion between eGFP$^+$ rat cells and mouse tissue was excluded by fluorescent in situ hybridization (FISH), thus proving unequivocally stemness and multipotency of rat TECs that were maintained after serial transplantation [38, 48].

More recently, thymic epithelial cells with progenitor phenotype (TECPs) were isolated from the adult mouse thymus on the basis of surface marker characterization [37]. The authors used a multi-parameter flow cytometry approach to define several epithelial subpopulations that were then purified, characterized, and classified mainly on the basis of the level of MHC-class II (MHCII), the known medullary marker *Ulex Europaeus* agglutinin-1 (UEA-1) and the cortical Ly51 marker expression: TEC^{lo} (MHCII^{lo}UEA-1$^-$Ly51^{lo}), cTEC^{hi} (MHCII^{hi}UEA-1$^-$Ly51^{hi}), mTEC^{lo} (MHCII^{lo}UEA-1$^+$Ly51$^-$), and mTEC^{hi} (MHCII^{hi}UEA-1$^+$Ly51$^-$). These four populations were further characterized for the expression of other known fetal TECP cells such as CD205, beta-5t, alpha-6, and Sca-1 epithelial surface markers which were differentially distributed among them. Importantly, the expression of Foxn1 transcription factor essential for further TEC differentiation was detected in all four subpopulations. When the proliferation capacity was evaluated in vivo in young mice that were exposed to 5-bromo-20-deoxyuridine (BrdU) for 12 days pulse period and 6 months chasing, a quiescent label-retaining (LRC) cell subset (~1%) was observed mainly (~70%) within the TEC^{lo} population. These data suggest the possibility of LRC cells representing putative TECP, however the low numbers isolated did not allow direct functional analysis of these progenitors and therefore a functional demonstration of stemness could not be reached [37]. In a next step, the authors reaggregated the four subpopulations derived from eGFP$^+$ mice with fetal wild-type thymic lobes and engrafted them under the kidney capsule of nude recipient mice in a similar assay used for rat eGFP$^+$ cultivated clonal TECs [38] and this assay further supported that the TEC^{lo} population harbor the cells with the highest integration capacity (~1.7%) within the thymus microenvironment after 6 weeks in vivo while a eGFP$^+$TEC^{lo} population was still detectable after 12 weeks indicating long term survival under these conditions. Finally, the in vitro growth potential of the different epithelial subsets was tested in 3D cultures that had the advantage of maintaining the expression of transcription factor Foxn1 up to 1 week in vitro. Again, the TEC^{lo} subpopulation demonstrated the highest colony-forming efficiency (CFE, ~0.3%) and the capacity of giving rise to secondary cultures while the other three epithelial subsets did not [37]. Despite the short-term capacity of TEC^{lo} to expand in vitro, this report further supports the existence of a progenitor subpopulation among the epithelial cells of the adult rodent thymus.

5 Novel Sources of TECs and Stromal Cells: ESC- or iPS-derived TECs

Exploiting the differentiation potential and self-renewal properties of adult stem cells represents a currently available approach for certain clinical applications, e.g., hematopoietic, skin, cornea, and other stem cell-based transplants [49–52]. However, limited availability of biological material, immunological barriers, and a restricted range of attainable therapeutic indications has fostered research toward the use of pluripotent stem cells (PSC). Pluripotency is defined as the capacity of a cell to differentiate into virtually any cell type of the body, including germ cells. As a result, PSC supposedly possess the potential to regenerate any damaged tissue and thus trigger novel approaches for the treatment of a wide range of medical conditions. Current sources of PSC include somatic nuclei transfer, derivation of human embryonic stem cells (hESC), and induced pluripotent stem cells (iPSC) [53–55], although most of the current scientific efforts of relevance in this article are focused on the use ESC and iPSC. While ESC, obtained from the inner cell mass of human blastocysts, remain the golden standard for studies involving developmental aspects, iPSC pose far less ethical issues, and possibly solve immunological compatibility when derived from the perspective recipient.

The use of PSC for regenerating tissues and organs with limited endogenous regenerative potential is extremely enticing, and the thymus is no exception. With the thymus functionality being affected by a number of factors like aging, malnutrition, infection, ablative treatments in cancer therapy, and congenital diseases, current remedies aimed at restoring lymphopoiesis—intended as the thymus principal role in developing adaptive immunity—are still suboptimal or limited to specific applications [56–60]. Moreover the existence, and the persistence throughout life, of human thymic epithelial stem/progenitor (hTEPC) cells that could sustain tissue regeneration, has still to be demonstrated and their potential harnessed. Thus, scientists recently started to explore the avenue of PSC differentiation, aiming at overcoming the limitations of current therapies.

Initially, mouse ESC were differentiated into TEC-like progenitors that could generate thymic structures and supported limited lymphopoiesis when transplanted in vivo [61, 62]. More recently, a handful of reports described similar results with the use of hESC [63, 64]. Following the principle of developmental engineering, PSC differentiation was guided by the temporal recapitulation of tissue-specific morphogenetic cues in vitro. The first phase of differentiation required obtaining definitive endoderm, defined by the expression of the transcription factors FOXA2 and SOX17, by administering Activin A and activating WNT3a signaling. Subsequently, the protocols diverge, but overall both rely on the same exogenous signals including retinoic acid (RA), bone morphogenetic protein 4 (BMP4), WNT3A, and TGF-ß inhibitors. After 12 days, cells had further differentiated into "anterior foregut endoderm-like tissue," then third pharyngeal pouch, and finally human thymic epithelial cell progenitors (hTEPC). These hTEPC show upregulation of early TEC transcription factors like FOXN1, HOXA3, EYA1, but do not display typical mature TEC markers like MHC II, DLL4, or AIRE. Indeed, functional validation of the graft required transplantation in vivo, with the purpose of tracking de novo lymphopoiesis derived by TEPC constructs. Newly generated mouse T cells [63] and human T cells [64] were observed, although with limited efficiency, confirming that at least some cells in the hTEPC graft possessed the ability to mature into functional TEC. Following these seminal differentiation protocols, Soh and collaborators proposed a different approach where hESC are aggregated in embryoid bodies before undergoing differentiation [65]. Interestingly, after an initial priming with Activin A, culture conditions did not require the manipulation of specific pathway through exogenous factors until day 14 when KGF was provided, possibly implying the capacity of differentiating embryoid bodies to secrete chemokines and cytokines in a para/autocrine fashion. In combination with a GFP-FOXN1 reporter system, this work allowed the identification of a EpCAM^{+}/HLA-DR^{+}/ Integrin-ß4^{+} subpopulation that is highly enriched in FOXN1 expressing cells. However, in vitro tests failed to confirm the functionality of hESC-derived TEC-like cells.

Finally, another recent report exploited the exogenous delivery of recombinant FOXN1 and HOXA3 to increase the efficiency of the in vitro differentiation into K5^{+}/K8^{+} TEPC, a more mature phenotype. These cells displayed then in vivo competence to recapitulate a certain degree of architectural organization in the mTEC and cTEC compartments, and sustained lymphopoiesis from both human and mouse hematopoietic progenitors.

So far, differentiation protocols for hESC have generated immature cells that require in vivo transplantation to acquire competent functionality. These partial results might be due to a differential need for lymphostromal or mesenchymal interactions when compared to rodent models [26, 66–68], and more in general with the current limited knowledge of molecular events occurring throughout human thymic development. Moreover, no attempts were made to recapitulate the morphogenetic events determining cortical or medullary identity and architecture of the thymus, advocating for deeper investigations and possibly the introduction of scaffolding devices that could support proper cell dissemination in a 3D environment.

Overall, the development of strategies aimed at creating in vitro hTEC from PSC may represent a pivotal complement to the currently limited regenerative strategies and possibly an alternative, but many aspects need to be strengthened beforehand. These aspects include a better understanding of developmental dynamics, an efficient generation of sufficiently committed hTEPC able to generate the necessary epithelial/stromal components, the capacity of TEC to sustain competent T-cell formation with a wide affinity repertoire, and finally safety related to the risk of creating teratomas due to contaminating, undifferentiated PSC.

6 Conclusions

Since Miller's seminal discovery of its immunological function less than 6 decades ago, enormous strides have been achieved in understanding the complex mechanisms regulating the thymus. The dynamic cross-talk between lymphoid precursors, TEC, mesenchymal-stromal cells, and other tissue-resident cells described so far, portrays an intricate network of interactions. However, crucial mechanisms related to thymus physiology like its age-related involution have not been elucidated yet; similarly, the development of effective treatments to restore its impaired functionality has only partially tackled current clinical needs. In this regard, the contribution of the in vitro models described so far has been invaluable, but further advancements are required.

FTOC was the first model able to provide ex vivo thymic lymphopoiesis, but its use is restricted by ineffective mass transport of oxygen, nutrients, and waste, that limits the size of FTOC that remain viable. Moreover, with the notable exception of the use of dGuo, manipulation of the relative cellular fractions of FTOC to assess their contribution has not been described yet. This drawback was overcome with the use of RTOC, which support a higher degree of manipulation and arrays of different cellular compositions. As a consequence of disaggregating the thymus at the single cell level, the complex 3D architecture of the thymus, i.e., the topological information of the single cell, is disrupted and substituted with a random, but still 3D, arrangement. For these reasons, some approaches were recently described which aimed at better capturing the native structure of the thymus. Recapitulating the main aspects of architectural and molecular complexity of native tissues requires a multidisciplinary approach that encompasses, among others, material sciences and bioprocess engineering [69]. Biomaterials properties like composition, architecture, elasticity, porosity, and biodegradability can be tuned to match the desired experimental parameters, uncovering a tremendous array of possible conditions to be examined [70]. Decellularized tissues provide an interesting paradigm for the development of scaffold-based approaches: depending on the decellularization protocol, key architectural, chemical, or physical parameters could be directly related to the native tissue representing a close match of its physiological properties.

Additionally, adopting advanced platforms that can precisely control the chemo-physical conditions of culture environment and upscale the size of cultured thymic organoids, namely bioreactors, could support the development of multicellular niches and thus constitute a valuable model for in vitro investigations. Moreover, bioreactors could also represent a necessary resource for the translation of research into viable clinical products for the long term restoration of thymus function [71, 72].

Due to the invasive harvesting procedure, most of the scientific work carried over has heavily relied on the use of animal models. Similarly, our knowledge related to the existence of TEC stem/progenitor cells is restricted to rodents. Similarities between rats and mice might suggest a conserved inter-species mechanism encompassing the presence of stem/progenitor cells in the adult thymus; however, further investigation is required to assess whether human TEC contain a population with self-renewal and multilineage differentiation properties. The need of a better understanding of the human thymus, in fact, advocates an increased attention to developing hTEC-based models that can recapitulate important aspects of the thymus structure and function.

In this regard, the recent introduction of hPSC-derived TEC offers a powerful resource that will likely move the field forward once current limitations of PSC differentiation, e.g., efficiency and safety, will have been addressed.

Acknowledgments

We thank Giulio Cossu, Peter W. Zandstra, Anna Cariboni and Sara Campinoti for critical reading.

P.B. is supported by the European Research Council (ERC-2014-Stg), the Rosetrees Trust Foundation, the UCL Excellence Fellowship Program and the NIHR Biomedical Research Centre at Great Ormond Street Hospital for Children NHS Foundation Trust; E.P. was supported by the New Ideas Grant provided by the Ontario Institute for Regenerative Medicine (OIRM). S.C. is supported by a GOSH Charity studentship (V6116).

References

1. Miller J (1961) Immunological function of the thymus. Lancet 278:748–749
2. Mohtashami M, Zúñiga-Pflücker JC (2006) Three-dimensional architecture of the thymus is required to maintain delta-like expression necessary for inducing T cell development. J Immunol 176:730–734
3. Takahama Y et al. (2017) Generation of diversity in thymic epithelial cells. Nature Reviews Immunology 17:295–305
4. Robinson JH, Owen JJT (1978) Transplantation tolerance induced in foetal mouse thymus in vitro. Nature 271:758–760

5. Robinson JH, Owen JJ (1977) Generation of T-cell function in organ culture of foetal mouse thymus. II. Mixed lymphocyte culture reactivity. Clin Exp Immunol 27:322–327
6. Doherty PC, Zinkernagel RM (1975) Enhanced immunological surveillance in mice heterozygous at the H-2 gene complex. Nature 256:50–52
7. Zinkernagel RM (1982) Selection of restriction specificities of virus-specific cytotoxic T cells in the thymus: no evidence for a crucial role of antigen-presenting cells. J Exp Med 156:1842–1847
8. Owen JJ, Jordan RK, Robinson JH et al (1976) In vitro studies on the ontogeny of lymphocyte populations. Ann Immunol 127:951–956
9. Robinson JH, Owen JJT (1976) Generation of T-cell function in organ culture of foetal mouse thymus. I. Mitogen responsiveness. Clin Exp Immunol 23:347
10. Röpke C (1997) Thymic epithelial cell culture. Microsc Res Tech 38:276–286
11. Jenkinson EJ, Van Ewijk W, Owen JJ (1981) Major histocompatibility complex antigen expression on the epithelium of the developing thymus in normal and nude mice. J Exp Med 153:280–292
12. Jenkinson EJ, Franchi LL, Kingston R et al (1982) Effect of deoxyguanosine on lymphopoiesis in the developing thymus rudiment in vitro: application in the production of chimeric thymus rudiments. Eur J Immunol 12:583–587
13. Cohen A, Lee JW, Dosch HM et al (1980) The expression of deoxyguanosine toxicity in T lymphocytes at different stages of maturation. J Immunol 125:1578–1582
14. Fontaine-Perus JC, Calman FM, Kaplan C et al (1981) Seeding of the 10-day mouse embryo thymic rudiment by lymphocyte precursors in vitro. J Immunol 126:2310–2316
15. Plum J, De Smedt M, Verhasselt B et al (2000) Human T lymphopoiesis. In vitro and in vivo study models. Ann N Y Acad Sci 917:724–731
16. Martín-Fontecha A, Schuurman HJ, Zapata A (1994) Role of thymic stromal cells in thymocyte education: a comparitive analysis of different models. Thymus 22:201–213
17. Plum J, De Smedt M, Leclercq G (1993) Exogenous IL-7 promotes the growth of CD3-CD4-CD8-CD44+CD25+/− precursor cells and blocks the differentiation pathway of TCR-alpha beta cells in fetal thymus organ culture. J Immunol 150:2706–2716
18. Levelt CN, Carsetti R, Eichmann K (1993) Regulation of thymocyte development through CD3. II. Expression of T cell receptor beta CD3 epsilon and maturation to the CD4 +8+ stage are highly correlated in individual thymocytes. J Exp Med 178:1867–1875
19. Müller KP, Kyewski BA (1993) T cell receptor targeting to thymic cortical epithelial cells in vivo induces survival, activation and differentiation of immature thymocytes. Eur J Immunol 23:1661–1670
20. Jones LA, Izon DJ, Nieland JD et al (1993) CD28-B7 interactions are not required for intrathymic clonal deletion. Int Immunol 5:503–512
21. Jenkinson EJ, Anderson G, Moore NC et al (1994) Positive selection by purified MHC class II+ thymic epithelial cells in vitro: costimulatory signals mediated by B7 are not involved. Dev Immunol 3:265–271
22. Jenkinson EJ, Anderson G (1994) Fetal thymic organ cultures. Curr Opin Immunol 6:293–297
23. Hogquist KA, Gavin MA, Bevan MJ (1993) Positive selection of CD8+ T cells induced by major histocompatibility complex binding peptides in fetal thymic organ culture. J Exp Med 177:1469–1473
24. Ashton-Rickardt PG, Van Kaer L, Schumacher TN et al (1993) Peptide contributes to the specificity of positive selection of CD8+ T cells in the thymus. Cell 73:1041–1049
25. Ashton-Rickardt PG (2007) Studying T-cell repertoire selection using fetal thymus organ culture. Methods Mol Biol 380:171–184
26. Anderson G, Jenkinson EJ (2001) Lymphostromal interactions in thymic development and function. Nat Rev Immunol 1:31–40
27. Sugawara T, Di Bartolo V, Miyazaki T et al (1998) An improved retroviral gene transfer technique demonstrates inhibition of CD4-CD8- thymocyte development by kinase-inactive ZAP-70. J Immunol 161:2888–2894
28. Owens BM, Hawley RG, Spain LM (2005) Retroviral transduction in fetal thymic organ culture. Methods Mol Med 105:311–322
29. Travers H, Anderson G, Gentle D et al (2001) Protocols for high efficiency, stage-specific retroviral transduction of murine fetal thymocytes and thymic epithelial cells. J Immunol Methods 253:209–222
30. Takahama Y (2001) Genetic modulation of immature T lymphocytes and its application. J Med Investig 48:25–30
31. Seet CS et al. (2017) Generation of mature T cells from human hematopoietic stem/progenitor cells in artificial thymic organoids. Nature Methods 14:521–530

32. Anderson G, Jenkinson EJ, Moore NC et al (1993) MHC class II-positive epithelium and mesenchyme cells are both required for T-cell development in the thymus. Nature 362:70–73
33. Deng Z, Liu H, Rui J, Liu X (2016) Reconstituted Thymus Organ Culture. Methods in Molecular Biology 1323:151–8
34. Xing Y, Hogquist KA (2014) Isolation, identification, and purification of murine thymic epithelial cells. J. Vis. Exp. (Issue 90), e51780
35. Stoeckle C, Rota IA, Tolosa E et al (2013) Isolation of myeloid dendritic cells and epithelial cells from human thymus. J. Vis. Exp. (Issue 79), e50951
36. Seach N, Hammett M, Chidgey A (2013) Epithelial cell culture protocols, vol 945. Humana Press, Totowa, NJ, pp 251–272
37. Wong K, Lister NL, Barsanti M et al (2014) Multilineage potential and self-renewal define an epithelial progenitor cell population in the adult thymus. Cell Rep 8(4):1198–1209
38. Bonfanti P, Claudinot S, Amici AW et al (2010) Microenvironmental reprogramming of thymic epithelial cells to skin multipotent stem cells. Nature 466:978–982
39. Poznansky MC, Evans RH, Foxall RB et al (2000) Efficient generation of human T cells from a tissue-engineered thymic organoid. Nat Biotechnol 18:729–734
40. Lannes-Vieira J, Dardenne M, Savino W (1991) Extracellular matrix components of the mouse thymus microenvironment: ontogenetic studies and modulation by glucocorticoid hormones. J Histochem Cytochem 39:1539–1546
41. Emre Y, Irla M, Dunand-Sauthier I et al (2013) Thymic epithelial cell expansion through matricellular protein CYR61 boosts progenitor homing and T-cell output. Nat Commun 4:2842
42. Ocampo JSP, de Brito JM, Corrêa-de-Santana E et al (2008) Laminin-211 controls thymocyte--thymic epithelial cell interactions. Cell Immunol 254:1–9
43. Macchiarini P, Jungebluth P, Go T et al (2008) Clinical transplantation of a tissue-engineered airway. Lancet 372:2023–2030
44. Benders KEM, van Weeren PR, Badylak SF et al (2013) Extracellular matrix scaffolds for cartilage and bone regeneration. Trends Biotechnol 31:169–176
45. Fan Y, Tajima A, Goh SK et al (2015) Bioengineering thymus organoids to restore thymic function and induce donor-specific immune tolerance to allografts. Mol Ther 23 (7):1262–1277
46. Gordon J, Wilson VA, Blair NF et al (2004) Functional evidence for a single endodermal origin for the thymic epithelium. Nat Immunol 5:546–553
47. Rossi SW, Jenkinson WE, Anderson G et al (2006) Clonal analysis reveals a common progenitor for thymic cortical and medullary epithelium. Nature 441:988–991
48. Amici AW, Onikoyi FO, Bonfanti P (2014) Lineage potential, plasticity and environmental reprogramming of epithelial stem/progenitor cells. Biochem Soc Trans 42:637–644
49. Copelan EA (2006) Hematopoietic stem-cell transplantation. N Engl J Med 354:1813–1826
50. Ronfard V, Rives JM, Neveux Y et al (2000) Long-term regeneration of human epidermis on third degree burns transplanted with autologous cultured epithelium grown on a fibrin matrix. Transplantation 70:1588–1598
51. Rama P, Matuska S, Paganoni G et al (2010) Limbal stem-cell therapy and long-term corneal regeneration. N Engl J Med 363:147–155
52. Daley GQ (2012) The promise and perils of stem cell therapeutics. Cell Stem Cell 10:740–749
53. Gurdon JB, Elsdale TR, Fischberg M (1958) Sexually mature individuals of Xenopus laevis from the transplantation of single somatic nuclei. Nature 182:64–65
54. Thomson JA (1998) Embryonic stem cell lines derived from human blastocysts. Science 282:1145–1147
55. Takahashi K, Tanabe K, Ohnuki M et al (2007) Induction of pluripotent stem cells from adult human fibroblasts by defined factors. Cell 131:861–872
56. Savino W, Dardenne M, Velloso LA et al (2007) The thymus is a common target in malnutrition and infection. Br J Nutr 98 (Suppl 1):S11–S16
57. Holländer G a, Krenger W, Blazar BR (2010) Emerging strategies to boost thymic function. Curr Opin Pharmacol 10:443–453
58. Baksh D, Davies JE, Zandstra PW (2003) Adult human bone marrow-derived mesenchymal progenitor cells are capable of adhesion-independent survival and expansion. Exp Hematol 31:723–732
59. Markert ML, Devlin BH, McCarthy EA (2010) Thymus transplantation. Clin Immunol 135:236–246
60. Davies EG (2013) Immunodeficiency in Digeorge syndrome and options for treating cases with complete athymia. Front Immunol 4:322

61. Lai L, Jin J (2009) Generation of thymic epithelial cell progenitors by mouse embryonic stem cells. Stem Cells 27:3012–3020
62. Lai L, Cui C, Jin J et al (2011) Mouse embryonic stem cell-derived thymic epithelial cell progenitors enhance T-cell reconstitution after allogeneic bone marrow transplantation. Blood 118:3410–3418
63. Parent AV, a Russ H, Khan IS et al (2013) Generation of functional thymic epithelium from human embryonic stem cells that supports host T cell development. Cell Stem Cell 13:219–229
64. Sun X, Xu J, Lu H et al (2013) Directed differentiation of human embryonic stem cells into thymic epithelial progenitor-like cells reconstitutes the thymic microenvironment in vivo. Cell Stem Cell 13:230–236
65. Soh C-L, Giudice A, Jenny RA et al (2014) FOXN1GFP/w reporter hESCs enable identification of integrin-β4, HLA-DR, and EpCAM as markers of human PSC-derived FOXN1+ thymic epithelial progenitors. Stem Cell Rep 2:1–13
66. Jenkinson WE, Rossi SW, Jenkinson EJ et al (2005) Development of functional thymic epithelial cells occurs independently of lymphostromal interactions. Mech Dev 122:1294–1299
67. Zuklys S, Balciunaite G, Agarwal A et al (2000) Normal thymic architecture and negative selection are associated with Aire expression, the gene defective in the autoimmune-polyendocrinopathy-candidiasis-ectodermal dystrophy (APECED). J Immunol 165:1976–1983
68. Holländer G, Gill J, Zuklys S et al (2006) Cellular and molecular events during early thymus development. Immunol Rev 209:28–46
69. Tajima A, Pradhan I, Trucco M, Fan Y (2016) Restoration of Thymus Function with Bioengineered Thymus Organoids. Current stem cell reports 2(2):128–139
70. Discher DE, Mooney DJ, Zandstra PW (2009) Growth factors, matrices, and forces combine and control stem cells. Science 324:1673–1677
71. Di Maggio N, Piccinini E, Jaworski M et al (2011) Toward modeling the bone marrow niche using scaffold-based 3D culture systems. Biomaterials 32:321–329
72. Gosselin EA, Haleigh EB, Jonathan BS, Christopher JM (2018) Designing natural and synthetic immune tissues. Nature Materials 17(6): 484–498

Chapter 11

Isolation of Highly Viable Thymic Epithelial Cells for Use in In Vitro and In Vivo Experiments

Mi-Jeong Kim and Thomas Serwold

Abstract

Thymic epithelial cells (TECs) play multiple essential roles in T-cell development and the establishment of immune tolerance, but their isolation can be challenging, and their low viability upon isolation complicates downstream experiments. A method that allows TECs to be isolated easily and to survive afterward will be useful for elucidating key questions in TEC biology. Here, we demonstrate a simple method to isolate highly viable TECs. Primary TECs isolated using papain together with collagenase IV and DNase I survive and proliferate in vitro. Moreover, these primary TECs functionally engraft after intrathymic transplantation into recipient mice. Thus, the methods described herein will be useful for elucidating the roles of TECs and TEC subsets in T-cell development and immune tolerance.

Key words Thymic epithelial cells, Intrathymic transplantation, Papain, Thymus

1 Introduction

TECs, the major stromal component of thymus, are essential mediators of T-cell development [1]. The interaction between TECs and developing T-cells ensures the development of self-tolerant, functional T cells [2]. The thymus reaches its maximal size early in life, and then begins a poorly understood process of involution [3, 4]. Thymic involution is accompanied by decreased T-cell production, which contributes to immune dysfunction in aged individuals [5]. Loss of TECs likely contributes to age-associated thymic involution, though the mechanisms underlying TEC loss are not well understood [6]. Furthermore, there are multiple subsets of TECs, both in the cortex and in the medulla of the thymus. The functions of some of the TEC subsets have been characterized using genetic methods, but functional characterization of isolated subsets of TECs has been difficult to achieve, partly because of challenges associated with isolation of highly viable TEC subsets. Improvements in the isolation and manipulation of TEC subsets

Ashleigh S. Boyd (ed.), *Immunological Tolerance: Methods and Protocols*, Methods in Molecular Biology, vol. 1899, https://doi.org/10.1007/978-1-4939-8938-6_11,

have the potential to prospectively identify TEC subsets that play specific roles in T-cell development and immune tolerance.

TECs, unlike epithelial cells from other tissues such as the skin and intestine, form a three-dimensional mesh-like network which provides freedom of movement for highly migratory developing thymocytes, while still enabling extensive thymocyte-TEC contact [7]. This complex 3-D network of TECs occupies the entire thymus; however, TECs still comprise less than 1% of total thymic cells. The predominant cells within the thymus are developing T cells, but the thymus also contains multiple other hematopoietic lineages, most notably dendritic cells and B cells. The thymus also contains rare endothelial cells and mesenchymal cells. TECs form junctions with other TECs and are also supported by extracellular matrix (ECM) components, collagen type I, collagen type IV, fibronectin, and laminin [8, 9]. Thus, in contrast to developing T cells, which can be isolated from the thymus by simply dispersing the thymus (for example, by grinding between frosted slides), isolation of TECs requires an enzymatic digestion to break down TEC-TEC and TEC-ECM adhesions.

Many methods for TEC isolation have been described in the literature, however improved methods are needed for isolating highly viable TECs so that their functions can be assessed in vitro and in vivo. In this chapter, we demonstrate a simple, rapid TEC isolation method, which includes papain (a cysteine proteinase of the peptidase C1 family), collagenase IV and DNase I. Papain has been used to isolate various cell types including neurons, vascular smooth muscle cells, and ruminal epithelial cells [10–13], and we find papain facilitates the isolation of mouse TECs as well. This papain-based method is not only simple and fast, but also generates highly viable TECs; in vitro culture and intrathymic transplantation are shown here as examples of downstream applications.

2 Materials

2.1 Thymus Dissection

1. Mice of any age; in this chapter, green fluorescent protein (GFP) mice are used to visualize and track isolated TECs in vitro and in vivo.
2. Dissection board.
3. Dissection scissors.
4. Dissection forceps.
5. 70% ethanol.
6. 35 mm diameter petri dishes.
7. DMEM-F12 (Sigma), supplemented with sodium bicarbonate.

2.2 Enzymatic Dissociation of Thymic Epithelial Cells

1. DMEM-F12 (Sigma), supplemented with sodium bicarbonate.
2. 0.25–0.5 mg/ml Papain (Worthington Biochemicals); aliquots stored at −80 °C, do not repeat freezing and thawing.
3. 0.25 mg/ml Collagenase IV (Roche Life Science).
4. 0.1 mg/ml DNase I (Roche Life Science).
5. 35 mm diameter petri dishes.
6. 37 °C CO_2 incubator.
7. 5 ml round-bottom tubes.
8. 15 ml tubes.
9. 2% bovine calf serum/PBS (2% Buffer).
10. Scalpel.
11. Forceps.
12. 70 μm nylon mesh.
13. 1000 μl pipette tips with wide-bore ends (commercially available, and also can be prepared by simply cutting the end with scissors and autoclaving) and regular ends.

2.3 Fluorescence-Activated Cell Sorting of Thymic Epithelial Cells

1. 2% Buffer.
2. Ice.
3. 5 ml round-bottom tubes.
4. Anti-Cy7 MicroBeads (Miltenyi Biotec; catalogue number 130-091-652), MACS Separation MS or LS Columns (Miltenyi Biotech; catalogue number 130-042-201 (MS), 130-042-401 (LS)), MiniMACS or MidiMACS Separator (Miltenyi Biotec; catalogue number 130-042-102 (Mini), 130-042-302 (Midi)), and MACS MultiStand (Miltenyi Biotec; catalogue number 130-042-303) are used for the positive selection of $EpCAM^+$ TECs.
5. Antibodies against mouse antigens and lectin are as follows: CD16/32 (clone 93, Biolegend), CD45 (clone 30-F11, Biolegend), EpCAM (clone G8.8, Biolegend), Ly-51 (clone 6C3, BD Biosciences), *Ulex Europaeus* Agglutinin 1 (UEA1, Vector laboratories), MHCII I-A/I-E (clone M5/114.15.2, Biolegend), and CD80 (clone 16-10A1, Biolegend). Propidium iodide (PI, 1 μg/ml, Sigma) is used to distinguish live and dead cells.
6. FACSAria (BD Biosciences) or a similar cell sorter.
7. FlowJo software (Tree Star) or a similar software to analyze flow cytometry data.
8. 1.5 ml tubes for cell collection.
9. 10% bovine calf serum/PBS (10% Buffer) to collect sorted cells for in vivo experiments.

10. MCDB153 medium containing 10% fetal calf serum (Hyclone), 50 units/ml penicillin (Life Technologies), 50 μg/ml streptavidin (Life Technologies), 2 mM L-glutamine (Life Technologies), 1 mM sodium pyruvate (Life Technologies), and 10 μM p160ROCK inhibitor Y-27632 (TOCRIS Bioscience) is used to collect sorted cells for in vitro culture pH adjusted to 7.2.

2.4 In Vitro Culture of Sorted Thymic Epithelial Cells

1. Tissue culture (TC) treated plates.
2. Mouse embryonic fibroblasts (MEFs): prepared from fetuses of embryonic stage ~13.5 (E13.5), and aliquots of propagated MEFs (passage 1 or 2) are stored at ≤−80 °C. Irradiated MEFs are prepared by exposing MEFs to 60 Gray of irradiation, before freezing or after thawing MEFs.
3. The same medium described in Subheading 2.3, **step 10** is used to culture TECs in vitro.
4. Inverted fluorescence microscope (Olympus) is used to observe GFP-positive TECs growing in plates.
5. 4% paraformaldehyde (PFA) in PBS, freshly prepared.
6. 1% Rhodamine B (Sigma) in PBS is used to stain fixed TECs in plates.
7. Heating plate or a similar device, which can incubate PFA-fixed and Rhodamine B-stained TECs in plates.
8. PBS.
9. A camera to capture Rhodamine B-stained TECs in plates.

2.5 Intrathymic Transplantation of Sorted Thymic Epithelial Cells

1. Sterile Saline (0.9% sodium chloride in water, autoclaved).
2. A centrifuge with swinging buckets to spin down sorted cells in 1.5 ml microcentrifuge tubes.
3. Hamilton syringe (Hamilton Company; catalogue number 7654-01, model 1702RN).
4. Hamilton 30 gauge needle (Hamilton Company; catalogue number 7803-07, Small Hub RN; needle length of 1 in.).
5. 1.5 ml tubes that can fit a Hamilton syringe (the outer barrel diameter of Hamilton syringe 1702RN is 7.75 mm (0.305 in.)).
6. 10% Buffer to resuspend spun down cells in microcentrifuge tubes for intrathymic transplantation. AUTOCLIP 9 mm Wound Clips (Becton Dickson; catalogue number 427631).
7. AUTOCLIP 9 mm Wound Clip Applier (Becton Dickson; catalogue number 427630).
8. 2,2,2,-Tribromoethanol (Avertin, Sigma).
9. Ice.
10. 27-gauge needle for intraperitoneal injection.
11. 1 ml syringe.

12. Surgical board (styrofoam or any appropriate board).
13. Rubber bands and needles to fix anesthetized animals on the surgical board.
14. Blunt-end dissection scissors (Fisher; catalogue number 08-950).
15. Forceps.
16. Buprenorphine hydrochloride (Sigma).
17. Headlight to aid the surgery.
18. Heating pad.
19. Sterile alcohol prep pads (Fisher; catalogue number 06-669-62).
20. Inverted fluorescence microscope (Olympus) is used to track down intrathymically transplanted GFP donor cells ex vivo.

3 Methods

3.1 Isolation of Mouse Thymus

1. Euthanize a mouse according to institutional guidelines.
2. Place the animal's dorsal side onto the dissection board, and fix four limbs using needles or appropriate pins.
3. Spray the ventral surface with 70% ethanol.
4. Using forceps, lift up the midline skin right under the rib cage, and cut through the skin longitudinally, starting from the center of the midline all the way up to the neck. Make two more cuts from the center of the midline to left and right, and peel the skin over. This exposes the peritoneum and rib cage.
5. While holding the bottom tip of sternum with forceps, use scissors to cut through the peritoneum and thoracic diaphragm. Cut the far left and right sides of the rib cage longitudinally, and lift up the loosened rib cage all the way to expose thoracic viscera. The two-lobed thymus is located just above heart.
6. Use forceps to carefully remove any surrounding connective tissue (especially adipose tissue) around thymus.
7. Hold the middle part of thymus using a dissection blunt-end forceps, and then place another forceps with strong tips at the top end of thymus and gently pull out thymus towards you. Place the organ in a 35 mm petri dish containing DMEM/F12 medium (*see* **Note 1**).

3.2 Dissociation of Thymic Epithelial Cells

1. Using a scalpel, dice thymus into small pieces (0.1–0.2 cm in length and width) in 3 ml of DMEM/F12 medium (from Subheading 2.1, **step** 7, room temperature) in a 35 mm petri dish.

2. Transfer tissue fragments and medium into a 15 ml tube, and add DMEM/F12 medium up to 15 ml.
3. Rock the tube at room temperature for 3 min.
4. Stand the tube for 3 min, until tissue fragments settle down to the bottom.
5. Discard released thymocytes.
6. Add fresh DMEM/F12 medium up to 15 ml.
7. Rock the tube at room temperature for another 3 min.
8. Stand the tube for 3 min, until tissue fragments settle down to the bottom.
9. Discard the supernatant (*see* **Note 2**).
10. Transfer the remaining tissue fragments into a new 35 mm petri dish.
11. Add 500 μl of fresh DMEM/F12 medium (*see* **Note 3**).
12. Add enzymes to the dish: final concentrations at papain 0.25–0.5 mg/ml, collagenase IV 0.25 mg/ml, and DNase I 0.1 mg/ml.
13. Incubate tissue fragments with enzymes at 37 °C CO_2 incubator, for 30 min (Fig. 1; *see* **Note 4**).
14. Add 1 ml of 2% Buffer to stop the enzymatic reaction.
15. Pipet up and down using first a wide-bore end 1 ml tip and then a regular end 1 ml tip.
16. Filter the dissociated cells in medium through 70 μm nylon mesh and transfer to a 5 ml round-bottom tube (*see* **Note 5**).
17. Add 2% Buffer up to 5 ml.

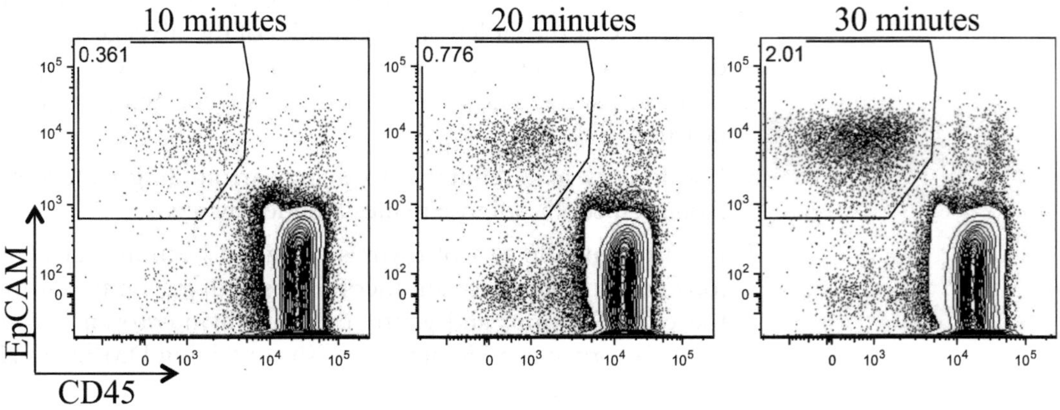

Fig. 1 The time course of papain digestion on thymic epithelial cells. Three of half thymuses (~35 mg net mass/a half thymus) from 3-week old male C57BL/6 mice were digested in 250 μl of DMEM/F12 medium with 0.25 mg/ml papain/0.25 mg/ml collagenase IV/0.1 mg/ml DNase I, for 10, 20, and 30 min. Cells were pre-gated on live, PI− cells, and further gated on EpCAM vs. CD45 (hematopoietic cells). The percentage of EpCAM+ TECs increases as the digestion time increases

18. Centrifuge at 300 × *g* for 5 min.
19. Discard the supernatant.
20. Resuspend cells in ~200 μl of 2% Buffer and keep cells on ice.

3.3 Fluorescence-Activated Cell Sorting of Thymic Epithelial Cells (See Note 6)

1. Add EpCAM-APC/Cy7 antibody (1 μl per 10^8 cells) and Fc blocking antibody (CD16/CD32) to cells in 2% Buffer (prepared in Subheading 3.2, **step 14**) and vortex the tube briefly (*see* **Note 7**).
2. Incubate cells on ice for 15 min, and protect cells from light.
3. Add 2% Buffer up to 5 ml.
4. Centrifuge at 300 × *g* for 5 min.
5. Resuspend cells in ~200 μl of 2% Buffer.
6. Add anti-Cy7 microbeads (5 μl per 10^8 cells) to cells and vortex the tube briefly (*see* **Note 7**).
7. Incubate cells on ice for 15 min, and protect cells from light.
8. Add 2% Buffer up to 5 ml.
9. Centrifuge at 300 × *g* for 5 min.
10. Resuspend cells in 1 ml of 2% Buffer.
11. Set up MACS Separation Columns following the manufacturer's (Miltenyi Biotech) instructions.
12. Apply cells in solution from Subheading 3.3, **step 10** onto a MACS column.
13. Collect $EpCAM^+$ cells into a new 5 ml tube.
14. Add 2% Buffer up to 5 ml.
15. Centrifuge at 300 × *g* for 5 min.
16. Resuspend cells in ~200 μl of 2% Buffer.
17. Make a master mixture of antibodies in 20 μl of 2% Buffer (listed in Subheading 2.3, **step 5**) (*see* **Note 7**).
18. Add the antibody mixture to cells in solution (from Subheading 3.2, **step 16**) and vortex the tube briefly.
19. Incubate cells on ice for 15 min, and protect cells from light.
20. Add 2% Buffer up to 5 ml.
21. Centrifuge at 300 × *g* for 5 min.
22. Resuspend cells in ~200 μl of 2% Buffer.
23. Add secondary antibody to cells and vortex the tube briefly (*see* **Note 7**).
24. Incubate cells on ice for 15 min, and protect cells from light.
25. Add 2% Buffer up to 5 ml.
26. Resuspend cells in 2% Buffer containing 1 μg/ml PI (the concentration of cells is up to 10^7/ml).
27. Filter cells in solution through 70 μm nylon mesh.

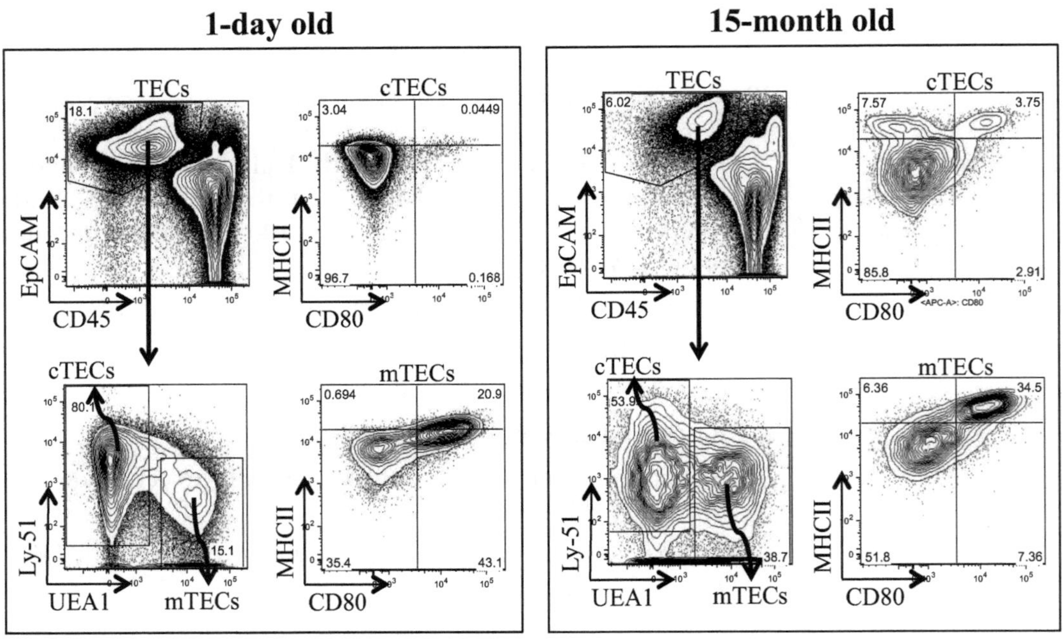

Fig. 2 Flow Cytometry and cell sorting of thymic epithelial cells. Thymuses from 1-day old ($n = 6$) and 15-month old ($n = 1$) GFP mice were digested by 0.25 mg/ml papain/0.25 mg/ml collagenase IV/0.1 mg/ml DNase I, followed by EpCAM-positive selection through MACS columns. Positively selected cells were further stained with TEC markers and subjected to analysis and sorting. Live cells were divided into cTECs and mTECs based on Ly-51 and UEA1 expressions, respectively. cTECs and mTECs show different expression levels for functional markers such as CD80 and MHCII. This analysis also shows differences in cTECs and mTECs between 1-day old and 15-month old mice

28. Run and sort cells on a FACSAria, using a 70 μm nozzle, at speed of ~3000 cells per second. Gate PI^- live cells and then select $CD45^-$ $EpCAM^+$ cells. TECs are divided using UEA1 anti-Ly-51, which stain medullary TECs (mTECs) and cortical TECs (cTECs), respectively. mTECs and cTECs are further gated based on MHCII and CD80 expression (Fig. 2). The yield of sorted TECs varies depending on the age of the mouse: from one 3-day old mouse, 80,000 cTECs and 20,000 mTECs can be sorted; from one 3-month old mouse, 60,000 cTECs and 170,000 mTECs can be sorted.
29. Sort cTECs and mTECs into collection tubes containing 1 ml of 10% Buffer for in vivo or MCDB153 medium (from Subheading 2.3, **step 10**) for in vitro culture.

3.4 In Vitro Culture of Sorted Thymic Epithelial Cells

1. Prior to cell sorting, prepare irradiated MEFs in MCDB153 medium (from Subheading 2.3, **step 10**, without Y-27632) onto a tissue-treated 96 flat-bottom plate, at a density around 3×10^4–4×10^4 per well (*see* **Note 8**).

2. Plate sorted TECs (from Subheading 3.3, **step 29**) onto the MEFs layer, and add 200 μl of MCDB153 medium (from Subheading 2.3, **step 10**) per well (*see* **Note 9**).
3. Change medium every 2–3 days (*see* **Note 10**).
4. Stop the culture when TECs are confluent or at a desired time point (*see* **Note 11**) (Fig. 3).
5. Remove medium and fix TECs in 4% PFA for 10 min.
6. Wash fixed TECs with PBS.
7. Stain fixed TECs with 1% Rhodamine B, at 60 °C for 15 min.
8. Remove Rhodamine B solution.
9. Capture the image of the entire plate (Fig. 3).

3.5 Intrathymic Transplantation of Sorted Thymic Epithelial Cells

1. Prepare all the tools described in Subheading 2.5 and sterilize by autoclaving or soaking in 70% ethanol.
2. One hour before the intrathymic transplantation, inject a mouse intraperitoneally with preoperative analgesic, buprenorphine (0.075 mg/kg body), prepared in Saline.
3. Centrifuge sorted cells in a 1.5 ml tube (from Subheading 3.3, **step 29**) at 300 × *g* for 5 min (*see* **Note 12**).
4. Resuspend cells in 10% Buffer (concentration up to 400,000 cells/10 μl) and keep on ice until injection. Use ~10 μl of cells per intrathymic injection (*see* **Note 13**).
5. Inject the mouse intraperitoneally with Avertin (250 mg/kg body weight), prepared in Saline.
6. When the mouse is unconscious, place it in the supine position onto the surgical board and fix it with rubber bands and pins. Place the mouse head toward you (Fig. 4a).
7. Wipe the chest area with a sterile alcohol prep pad.
8. Lifting up the skin around the neck with forceps, make a small perpendicular cut in the neck using a blunt-end scissors (Fig. 4b). Be careful not to puncture blood vessels. Using forceps, flip over salivary glands toward you (Fig. 4c).
9. Using one tip of forceps, make a small incision through the serous membrane, right above the top of sternum (Fig. 4d).
10. Using the same blunt-end scissors (Fig. 4e), cut ~0.5 cm of the manubrium and sternum perpendicularly (Fig. 4f).
11. Draw out ~10 μl of cells in suspension into Hamilton syringe attached with 30-gauge needle. To prevent the needle going through the entire thymus, epoxy can be applied to the bottom tip of the needle, based on the thymus thickness (Fig. 4g).

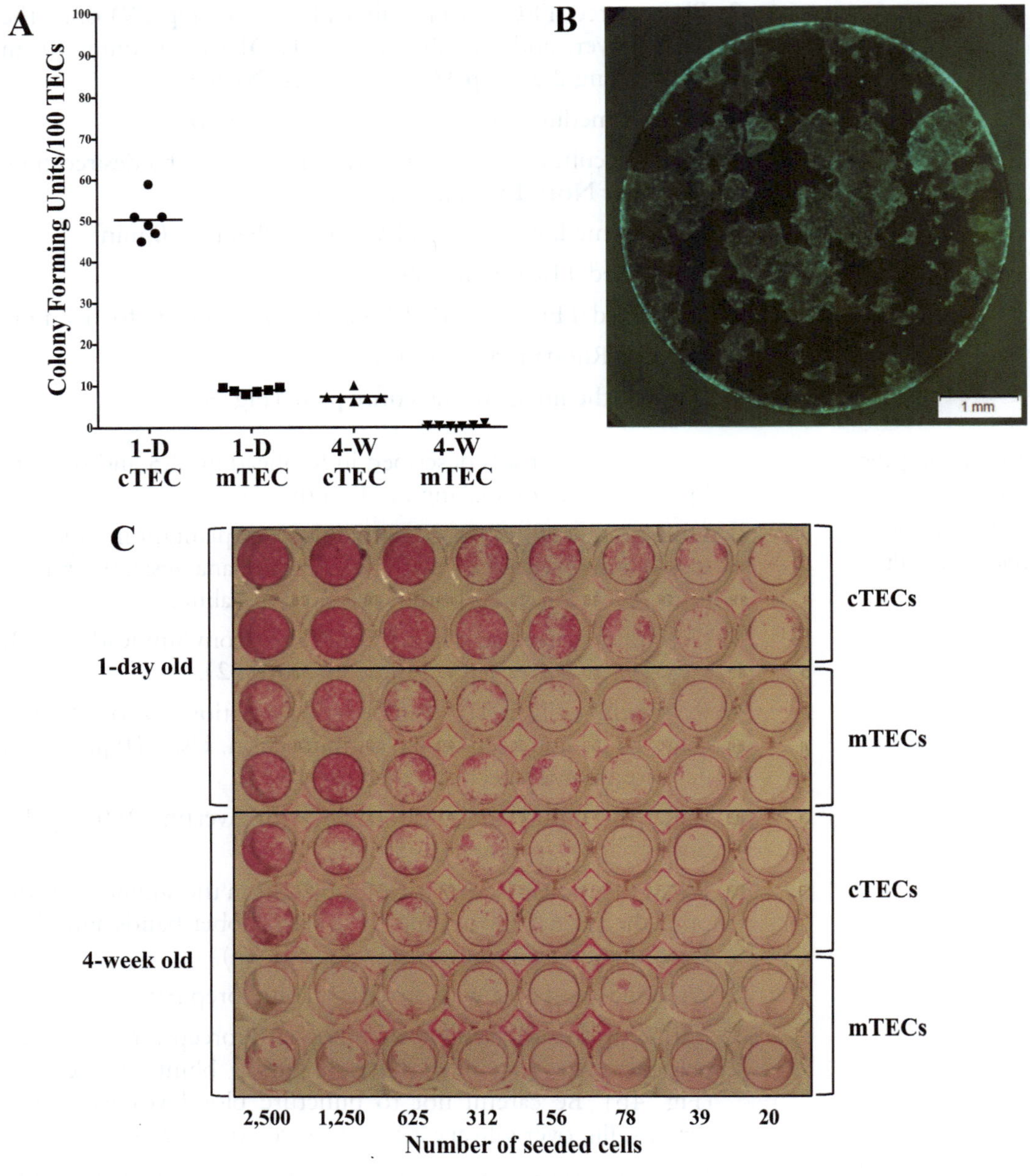

Fig. 3 Proliferation of thymic epithelial cells in vitro. cTECs and mTECs were sorted from 1-day old and 4-week old GFP mice and the indicated numbers of cells were plated onto a TC-treated 96-well plate. (**a**) At day 3 post-seeding, GFP+ TEC colonies were manually counted under a fluorescence microscope and plotted (1-D: 1-day old; 4-W: 4-week old). (**b**) At day 7 post-seeding, proliferating GFP cTECs (from 1-day old mice; 1000 cTECs were seeded) are seen under an inverted fluorescence microscope. (**c**) At day 10 post-seeding, TECs were fixed in 4% PFA and stained with Rhodamine B solution. This shows the difference in colony forming units between 1-day old and 4-week old, and also between cTECs and mTECs. This assay is useful to assess the differentiation and function of TECs in vitro

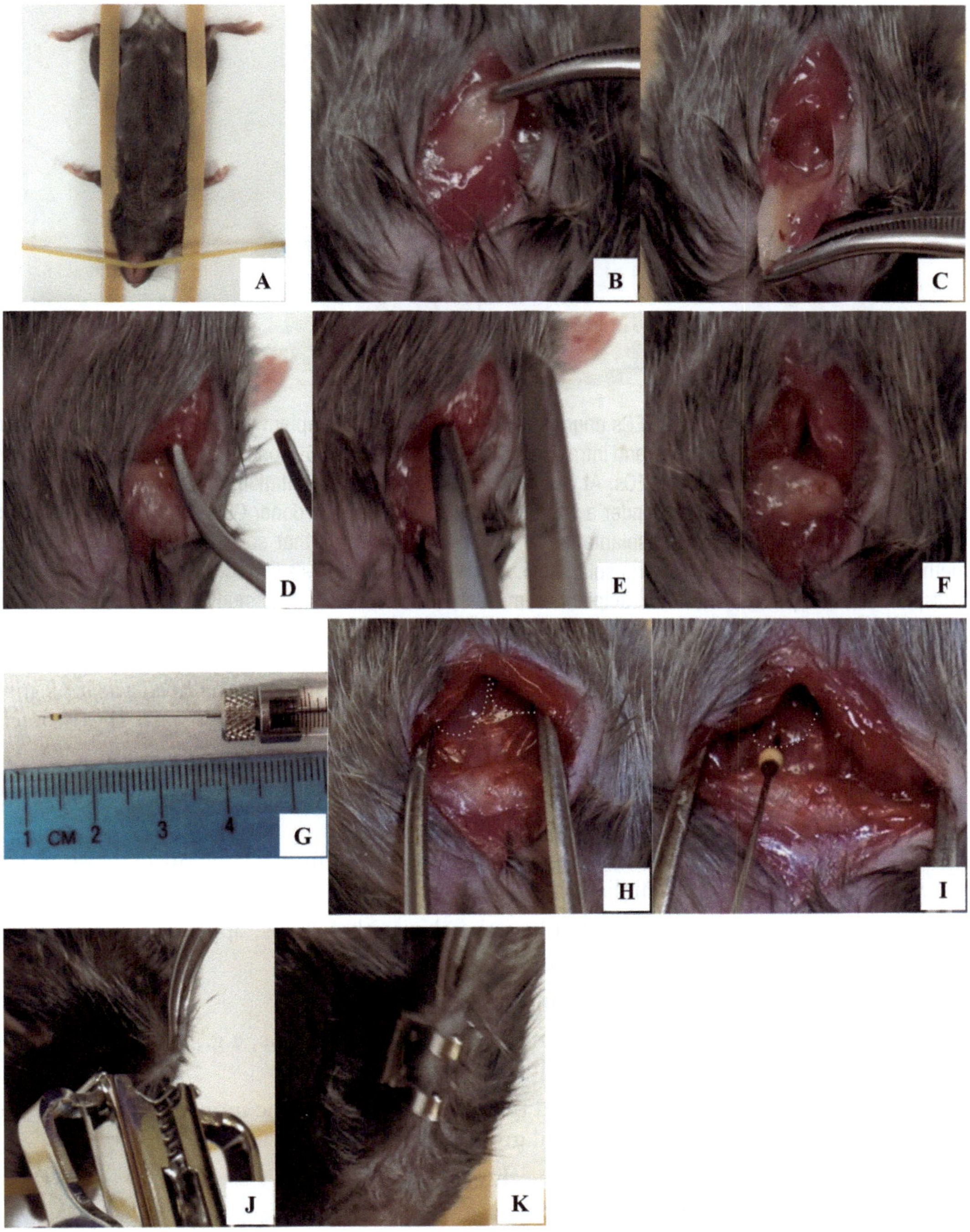

Fig. 4 Intrathymic injection of donor cells into a recipient thymus. As described in Subheading 3.5, an anesthetized mouse is placed on the surgical board (**a**), and a small incision is made in the thoracic area (**b–f**). TECs drawn into a Hamilton syringe and needle (**g**) are injected into a thymic lobe (**h** and **i** dotted lines indicate thymic lobes). After intrathymic injection, the wound is closed with wound clips

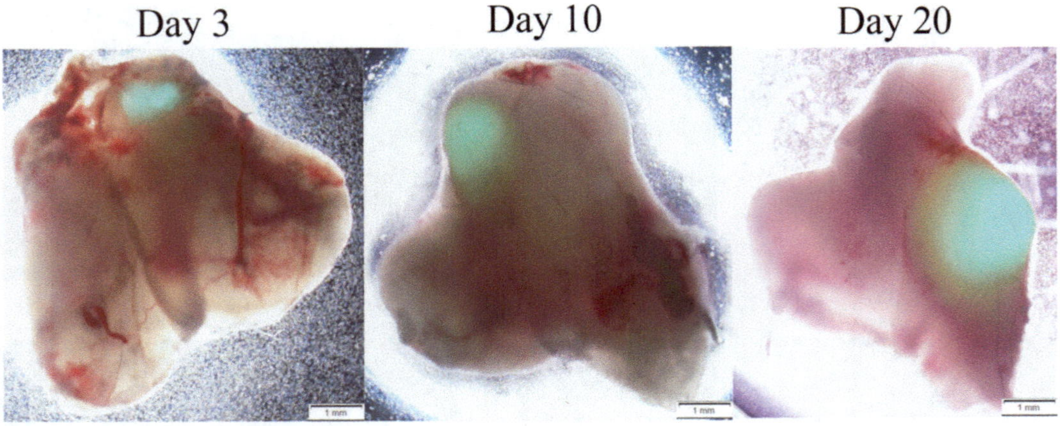

Fig. 5 Intrathymically transplanted TECs engraft and proliferate within recipient thymuses. cTECs were sorted from 3-day old GFP transgenic mice and intrathymically transplanted into 5-month old male mice. Each mouse thymic lobe received 110,000 of cTECs. At day 3, 10, and 20 posttransplantation, thymuses were recovered from recipient mice and examined under a fluorescence microscope. The donor GFP TECs are seen as green fluorescence. This intrathymic transplantation technique demonstrates that sorted TECs using the papain method are not only viable but also transplantable. According to our analysis by flow cytometry and histology, transplanted TECs proliferate within recipient thymuses. This will be useful to study TEC differentiation and function in vivo

12. Turn on the headlight (worn around your head) to look into the thoracic cavity better. Use forceps to keep the thoracic cavity area open (Fig. 4h).
13. While holding the tip of the rib cage, inject cells into a thymic lobe (Fig. 4i).
14. Put back salivary glands and bring back the divided skin to the midline.
15. While holding the skin with forceps, apply 1–2 wound clips perpendicularly (Fig. 4j k and k).
16. Place the mouse on the heating pad.
17. When the mouse becomes conscious, e.g., reflexes in eyes or limbs, put it back to its original cage.
18. At a desired time point, euthanize the mouse according to the institutional guideline.
19. Open up the thoracic cavity.
20. Remove thymus as described in Subheading 3.1 and place it in a 35 mm petri dish with PBS.
21. Using a fluorescence microscope, check for donor fluorescent cells within the recipient thymus (Fig. 5).
22. Process the organ for further analysis, e.g., flow cytometry and histology.

4 Notes

1. If thymus mass needs to be measured, weigh thymus before putting it into medium.
2. Repeat the thymocyte releasing step if the supernatant is still turbid.
3. For one adult thymus of ~50 mg mass (measured upon tissue harvest from a mouse), use 500 μl of medium. The medium volume is adjusted depending on the tissue mass.
4. For fetal thymuses, incubate tissue fragments in enzyme solution for 10 min. Do not exceed the enzymatic digestion time over an hour; it will lead to cell death.
5. Thymus from mice of age older than 2–3 weeks old leaves undigested tissue remnants. Make sure to filter out them before adding antibodies.
6. Keep all the reagents, cells, and centrifuge at 4 °C for Subheading 3.3.
7. Antibodies need to be titrated in each laboratory. If EpCAM-positive selection is not necessary, skip **steps 1–14** and proceed to the cell staining at **step 15** and include EpCAM antibody to the antibody mixture at **step 17**.
8. The cell seeding density can be adjusted based on the surface area of the culture plate. TECs can be plated onto a TC-treated plate without MEFs layer, although the survival and growth decrease without MEFs.
9. Instead of dividing 1 ml of sorted cells into a 96-well plate (10 μl per well), it is more accurate to divide a larger volume of cells in solution; e.g., MCDB153 medium is added to 1 ml of sorted TECs up to 20 ml, and then 200 μl of medium that contains sorted cells can be plated into each well. Prepare at least two wells of each TEC type (e.g., cTEC and mTEC) as a technical replicate. In this system, TEC proliferation and function can be measured.
10. A p160ROCK inhibitor, Y-27632, is only necessary for the first 2–3 days of TEC culture after sorting and plating.
11. During the culture, observe the growth of TECs in plates under a fluorescence microscope, if TECs are of GFP or other fluorescence.
12. It is better to spin down cells using a centrifuge with swing buckets so that cells form a nice pellet at the bottom tip of the tube.
13. All the steps from enzymatic digestion to cell sorting reduce the number of viable TECs; therefore for the successful readout after intrathymic injection, sorted TECs of at least 50,000 need to be injected into each thymic lobe. The younger the

donor mice are, the better the transplantation works. Authors found that sorted TECs of mice aged from E13 (embryonic stage 13) up to P14 (post-natal 14) transplant well and they are also recoverable.

Acknowledgments

MJK was funded by a Mary K. Iacocca Foundation Research Fellowship. TS received funding from a seed grant from the Harvard Stem Cell Institute. The authors gratefully acknowledge the Joslin Diabetes Center Flow Cytometry Core supported by an NIH Diabetes Research Center grant (NIH award P30DK036836) and the Harvard Stem Cell Institute. The authors acknowledge the excellent support of the Joslin Animal Facility.

References

1. Anderson G, Jenkinson EJ (2001) Lymphostromal interactions in thymic development and function. Nat Rev Immunol 1:31–40
2. Palmer E (2003) Negative selection–clearing out the bad apples from the T-cell repertoire. Nat Rev Immunol 5:383–391
3. Steinmann GG, Klaus B, Müller-Hermelink HK (1985) The involution of the ageing human thymic epithelium is independent of puberty. A morphometric study. Scand J Immunol 22:563–575
4. Hale JS, Boursalian TE, Turk GL, Fink PJ (2006) Thymic output in aged mice. Proc Natl Acad Sci U S A 103:8447–8452
5. Sempowski GD, Gooding ME, Liao HX, Le PT, Haynes BF (2002) T cell receptor excision circle assessment of thymopoiesis in aging mice. Mol Immunol 38:841–848
6. Chinn IK, Blackburn CC, Manley NR, Sempowski GD (2012) Changes in primary lymphoid organs with againg. Semin Immunol 24:309–320
7. van Ewijk W, Wang B, Holländer G, Kawamoto H, Spanopoulou E, Ito M, Amagai T, Jian YF, Germeraad WTV, Chen WF, Katsura Y (1999) Thymic microenvironments, 3-D versus 2-D? Semin Immunol 11:57–64
8. Berrih S, Savino W, Cohen S (1985) Extracellular matrix of the human thymus: immunofluorescence studies on frozen sections and cultured epithelila cells. J Histochem Cytochem 33:655–664
9. Lannes-Vieira J, Dardenne M, Savino W (1991) Extracellular matrix components of the mouse thymus microenvironment: ontogenetic studies and modulation by glucocorticoid hormones. J Histochem Cytochem 39:1539–1546
10. Huettner JE, Baughman RW (1986) Primary culture of identified neurons from the visual cortex of postnatal rats. J Neurosci 6:3044–3060
11. Sarthy PV, Balkema GW (1981) Retrograde labeling and dissociation of mouse retinal ganglion cells. Neurosci Lett 25:205–208
12. Bolzon BJ, Cheung DW (1989) Isolation and characterization of single vascular smooth muscle cells from spontaneously hypertensive rats. Hypertension 14:137–144
13. Weekes TE (1974) The preparation of a viable suspension of epithelial cells from the rumen mucosa of cattle. Comp Biochem Physiol 49:407–413

Part IV

Transplantation Tolerance

Chapter 12

Immune Tolerance and Rejection in Organ Transplantation

Jessica Stolp, Masaaki Zaitsu, and Kathryn J. Wood

Abstract

In this chapter, we describe the history of transplantation, the multiple cell types, and mechanisms that are involved in rejection and tolerance of a transplanted organ, as well as summarize the common and promising new therapeutics used in transplant patients.

Key words Organ transplant, Transplant tolerance, Immune mechanisms of rejection, T cells, B cells, Regulatory cells, Clinical symptoms of rejection, Immunosuppression, Cell therapy

1 Introduction

The importance of a well-balanced and functioning immune system is crucial for the eradication of pathogens as well as the protection of self-tissues. While organ transplantation is one of the greatest achievements in modern medicine, the challenge of balancing immunity to foreign pathogens and protection of transplanted organs from a genetically dissimilar individual (allogeneic) remains elusive. Current therapeutics administered to protect the transplanted organ from rejection, initiate general immunosuppression in patients, which leads to serious complications such as chronic infections, malignancies, and organ failure. As a consequence, thorough understanding of the immune mechanisms involved in tolerance and rejection of transplanted organs are crucial for the development of better therapeutics and improved patient outcomes. In this chapter, we describe the history of transplantation, the multiple cell types, and mechanisms that are involved in rejection and tolerance of a transplanted organ, as well as summarize the common and promising new therapeutics used in transplant patients.

Ashleigh S. Boyd (ed.), *Immunological Tolerance: Methods and Protocols*, Methods in Molecular Biology, vol. 1899, https://doi.org/10.1007/978-1-4939-8938-6_12,

2 History of Transplantation

Transplantation attempts date back as far as 600 BC. However, skin transplants performed by Medawar on burn victims during World War II gave the first scientific explanation of transplant tolerance and/or rejection [1]. They observed that when a patient received skin from himself or herself (autograft, now commonly also known in experimental settings as a syngeneic graft), the skin was tolerated with no complications. However, if the skin came from another individual (allogeneic graft), it was rejected. In addition, these integral experiments confirmed the involvement of an "actively acquired immune reaction" in rejection. They observed that recipients of a second skin allograft from the same donor rejected this graft more rapidly than the initial one [2, 3]. Further experiments by Medawar and colleagues confirmed that rejection could be caused by cellular components of the immune system. Mice that received a skin graft closely followed by cells from the allograft-draining lymph node of a transplanted mouse, rejected the allograft with accelerated kinetics, similar to mice transplanted for a second time [4].

These and other integral experimental results [5–7] in addition to advances in surgical techniques [8] lead to Joseph E. Murray performing the first successful kidney transplant from one identical twin to another [9, 10]. While this was a great moment for medicine, the immense challenge of controlling immune rejection in transplants between nonidentical individuals still remained.

Many different therapeutics have been developed that force the immune system into an immunosuppressed state, allowing for the continued function of an allogeneic transplanted organ. Azathioprine was the immunosuppressant used on the first patient to survive after receiving a cadaveric allograft in 1962 [11, 12]. This recipient survived for one year after the procedure. Cyclosporine A (CsA) was approved for use in transplantation in the 1980s [13]. This therapeutic revolutionized transplantation and substantially improved the survival of allogeneic transplanted organs and patients. Even today, lifelong immunosuppression is essential to prevent rejection for the vast majority of transplant recipients.

3 Tolerance

3.1 Overview of Mechanisms of Immune Tolerance (Central and Peripheral)

The immune system has evolved many efficient mechanisms through which to achieve immunity against foreign pathogens without mounting unwanted responses to self-antigens. The challenge in transplantation is to induce these or similar mechanisms to allo-antigens, resulting in allo-specific T cells being deleted or deemed nonresponsive to the transplanted organ. The first of these mechanisms a developing T cell will encounter is central tolerance.

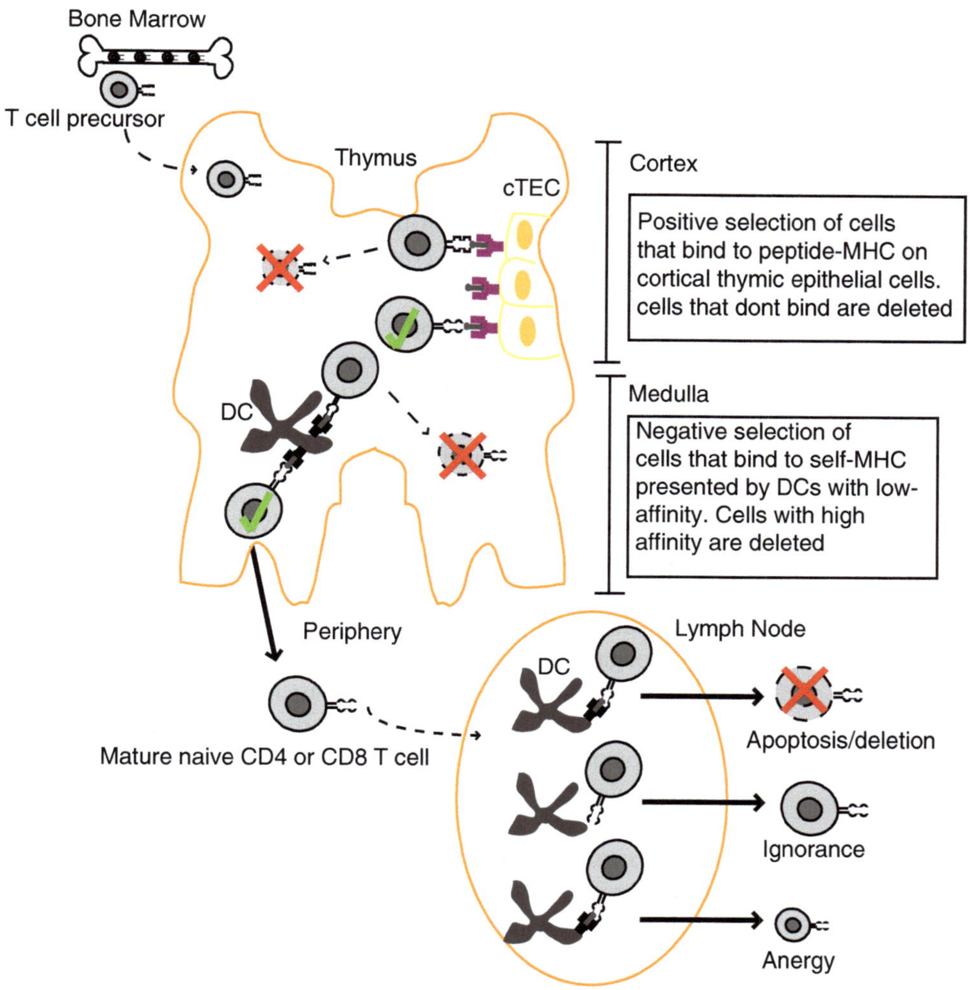

Fig. 1 Central and peripheral T-cell tolerance. (**a**) T-cell precursors travel from the bone marrow to the thymus. In the thymic cortex, T-cell precursors that bind to peptide-MHC on cortical thymic epithelial cells are positively selected, while those that do not bind are deleted. Negative selection occurs in the medulla of the thymus, where cells that bind to self-MHC presented by DCs with low-affinity are selected for maturation and occupation of the peripheral tissues. T cells that bind to self-MHC with a high affinity are deleted. (**b**) Some T cells with specificities for self-antigen will be allowed to mature and enter peripheral tissues. Peripheral tolerance mechanisms such as apoptosis/deletion, Ignorance, and anergy ensure that unwanted immune responses do not occur

The generation of T-cell receptors (TCR) with different specificities is a random process. Consequently, the proportion of T cells that can recognize self-antigen is quite substantial. Central tolerance occurs in the thymus and ensures the deletion of autoreactive thymocytes prior to antigen exposure in the periphery (Fig. 1a). Positive selection occurs in the cortex and thymocytes that possess a low or intermediate affinity for self-antigen are selected. Negative selection in the medulla then ensures the clonal deletion of high-affinity TCR. Negative selection is mediated by the expression of tissue-specific antigens (TSA) on medullary thymic epithelial cells (mTEC) [14, 15]. Recent advances in the understanding of central tolerance have been attributed to the role played by the transcription factor Aire (autoimmune regulator). Anderson and colleagues were the first to propose that Aire controlled self-tolerance by enabling ectopic expression of TSAs on the mTECs [16]. The ability of Aire to control thymic tolerance by regulating expression of TSAs was formally demonstrated when hen egg lysozyme (HEL) was expressed under the control of the rat insulin promoter (RIP) [17]. Aire regulated expression of HEL within the thymus was vital for the deletion of HEL-specific thymocytes and prevention autoimmunity. Using another transgenic model, Aschenbrenner et al. [18] have more recently provided evidence that Aire-expressing mTECs may also participate in the thymic selection of regulatory T cells (Treg), although this effect has been disputed by others [19]. People and mice deficient in Aire develop an autoimmune disease referred to as autoimmune polyglandular syndrome type I or autoimmune polyendocrinopathy-candidiasis-ectodermal dystrophy [20, 21]. This disease is associated with circulating tissue-specific autoantibodies that contribute to the destruction of many target organs, mainly endocrine glands [22].

T cells that are successful at passing the positive and negative selection central tolerance checkpoints in the thymus are permitted to occupy peripheral lymphoid tissues. Despite the stringency of the central tolerance mechanisms, some T cells with specificities for self-antigens are still able to exit the thymus and have the potential to initiate autoimmunity [23–26] (Fig. 1b). As a result of the presence of self-reactive T cells in the periphery, peripheral tolerance mechanisms are another checkpoint imposed to control unwanted immune responses. These involve T-cell anergy, ignorance, and deletion. T-cell anergy is the functional inactivation of a T cell, usually through reduced TCR signaling and/or suboptimal co-stimulation. Some forms of anergy also result in regulatory cell activity [27]. Ignorance involves the ability of a T cell with affinity for a peripheral self-antigen to ignore tissues with the cognate antigen due to their anatomical separation and low avidity for the antigen, which allowed the T cell to evade thymic negative selection. Deletion of autoreactive T cells is very important in peripheral tolerance and has been shown to prevent autoimmunity [28, 29]. Deficiency of co-stimulation is one method which triggers deletion of peripheral T cells, T cells recognizing allo-antigen can be deleted using co-stimulation blockade [30].

3.2 Cell Subsets Involved in Peripheral Tolerance

Characterization of the immune system in transplant patients who have discontinued with their immunosuppressive medication has identified various cell subsets that are involved in operational tolerance. These originate from both the innate and adaptive arms of the immune system.

3.2.1 Regulatory Macrophages

Macrophages can have both regulatory and immunogenic properties. In transplantation they are often associated with early graft damage, with activation occurring as a result of tissue injury or ischemia [31]. Regulatory macrophages have been identified in human peripheral blood with a surface marker phenotype of $CD14^{-/low}CD16^{-/low}CD64^{+}CD80^{-/low}CD86^{+}CD163^{-/low}HLA\text{-}DR^{+}TLR2^{-}$. These regulatory macrophages have the ability to suppress T-cell proliferation in vitro [32]. A pilot clinical trial in kidney transplant recipients showed that adoptively transferred regulatory macrophages reduced the need for immunosuppressive drugs [32]. Other studies have linked the induction of regulatory macrophages with interactions with Tregs [33].

3.2.2 Dendritic Cells

While dendritic cells (DC) are more known for their ability to prime the immune system, some studies have shown they can also promote tolerance to alloantigen. Both myeloid and plasmacytoid DCs (pDC) can participate in tolerance to alloantigens. Immature myeloid DCs have been identified as the subtype of DC that can promote tolerance to solid-organ allografts, as they express low levels of major histocompatibility complex (MHC) class II and co-stimulatory molecules on their surface [34]. Experiments in mice have shown that a single injection of immature donor-derived DCs 7 days before an allo-heart transplant can prolong the survival of the graft [35, 36]. In addition, the injection of donor-derived DCs prevents the rejection of allo-skin grafts [37] as well as graft versus host disease (GVHD) [38]. More recently, pDCs have also been shown to promote tolerance in transplantation [39]. In a mouse model, alloantigen experienced pDCs have been shown to migrate to the draining lymph nodes where they induced Tregs [40]. It has been observed that human liver transplant patients receiving little or no immunosuppression had higher ratios of pDCs to myeloid DCs [41]. A similar trend was observed between patients receiving low-dose immunosuppressive therapy during prospective weaning and patients on maintenance immunosuppression [41]. Interestingly, higher levels of programmed death (PD) ligand 1 (PDL1) and CD86 on pDCs correlated with increased numbers of CD4 + CD25+FOXP3+ Tregs in immunosuppressive drug-free liver transplant recipients [42].

3.2.3 Myeloid-Derived Suppressor Cells

Myeloid-derived suppressor cells (MDSC) are a heterogeneous population of cells that have been associated with regulatory function in both humans and mice. In humans most MDSCs express CD11b, CD33, CD34 and low levels of MHC class II [43], while in mice GR1 and CD11b are expressed [44]. The first description of these cells in transplantation was in a renal allograft tolerance model in rats [45]. An accumulation of CD3-ClassII-CD11b +CD80/86+ cells was observed in the blood and graft of tolerant recipients. These MDSCs inhibited proliferation of effector T cells and caused inducible nitric oxide synthase (iNOS)-dependent apoptosis. Numerous other mechanisms of tolerance by MDSCs have been identified in mouse transplant models of islet [46] and cardiac grafts [47]. Hock and colleagues [48] have observed increased numbers of MDSCs in renal kidney recipients, especially in those that have squarmous cell carcinoma. While some evidence suggests that MDSC act through the expression of haem oxygenase1, which prevents DC maturation, promotes IL-10 production, and has cytoprotective properties [49]. The exact tolerance mechanism(s) elucidated by MDSCs in transplantation need further investigation.

3.2.4 Mesenchymal Stromal Cells

Mesenchymal stromal cells (MSC) are a population of multipotent cells that reside in the bone marrow supporting haematopoiesis; they also possess immunomodulatory and reparative properties. MSC can migrate to sites of inflammation, where they are capable of regulating many immune effector functions. MSC have been shown to promote the generation of Tregs both in vitro and in vivo through E2, transforming growth factor (TGF) β and cell-cell contact [50, 51]. In transplant recipients, the retrieval and transplant surgery of the allograft initiates ischemia-reperfusion injury resulting in an inflammatory site, thus recruiting MSC. This recruitment could potentially induce the generation of Tregs at the allograft site [52]. MSC may also promote allograft tolerance through the secretion of matrix metalloproteinases [53] and the prevention of allo-antibody production [54].

3.2.5 Regulatory B Cells

B cells have numerous functions within the immune system, mainly as stimulators of immune responses, predominantly in their ability to produce antibodies. However, B cells can also present antigen, produce multiple cytokines, and suppress immune responses through the production of IL-10 [55, 56]. Regulatory B cells have been identified in humans and mice, both of which possess an immature phenotype and secrete IL-10 (Fig. 2a). Regulatory B cells in mice express high levels of CD1d, CD5, CD21, CD24, and IgM, although some heterogeneity exists in this population [57]. Human regulatory B cells are identified by their expression of CD19, CD24, and CD38. These B cells can suppress inflammatory responses in experimental autoimmune encephalomyelitis (EAE), collagen-induced arthritis (CIA), and colitis [58–60]. Recently, the role that B cells play in controlling various immune responses has been increased, with studies showing the importance of IL-10 in combination with different co-stimulatory molecules for the differentiation and maintenance of Treg and for the inhibition of T helper (Th) 17 and Th1 responses [61, 62] (Fig. 2a). Furthermore, a strong B-cell signature has been observed in tolerant kidney transplant recipients receiving no immunosuppression.

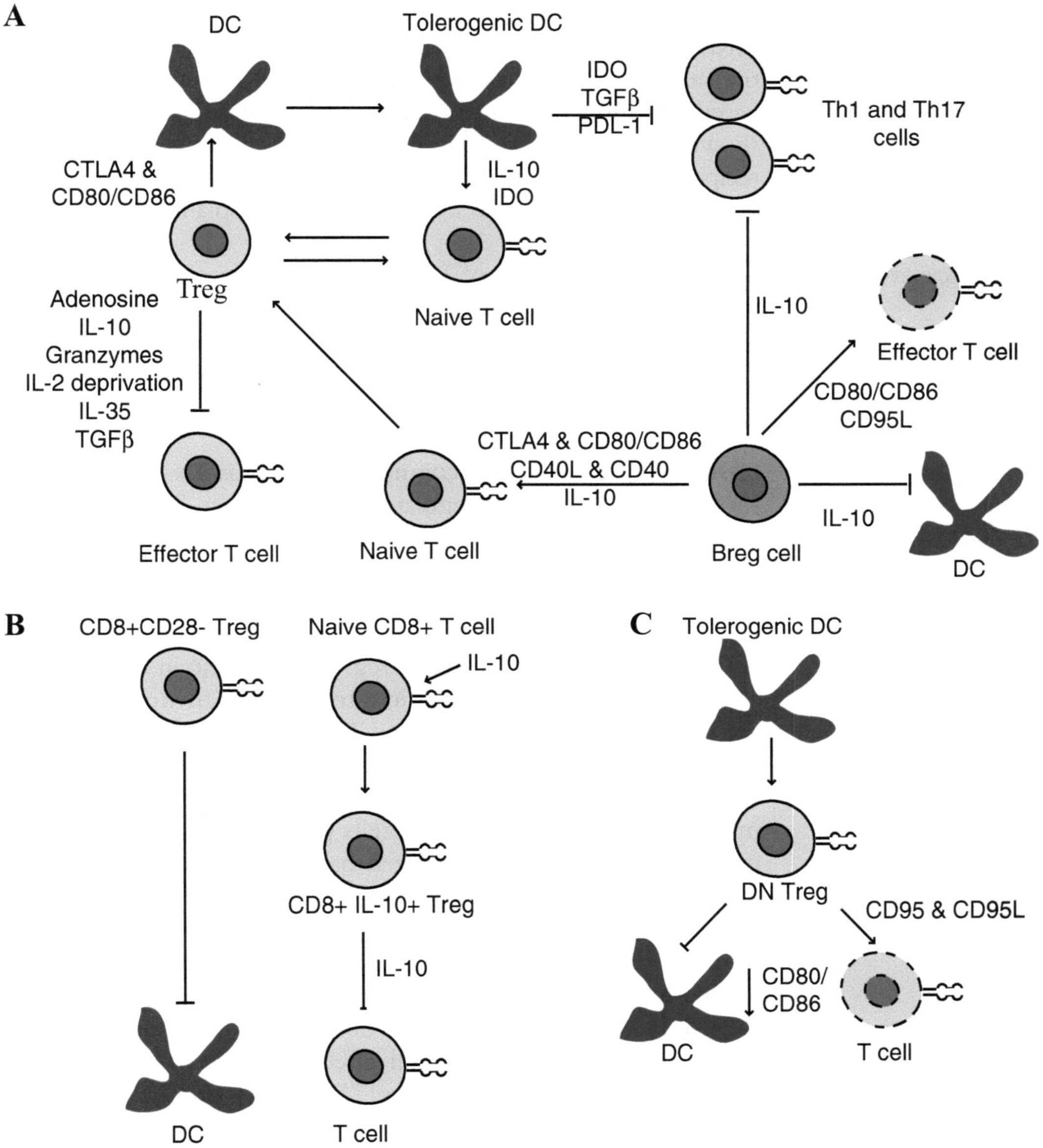

Fig. 2 Regulatory immune cell mechanisms in transplantation. (**a**) In the draining lymphoid tissue, Treg cells inhibit T-cell proliferation. Regulatory B cells and tolerogenic dendritic cells can promote the development of Treg cells from naive T cells. These Treg cells promote tolerance to the allograft through various mechanisms, including the production of IL-10 and TGFβ, the inhibition of antigen-presenting cell (APC) function, and effects on amino acid availability and energy metabolism. (**b**) $CD8^{+}CD28^{-}$ cells can inhibit APC function to promote immune regulation. In the presence of IL-10, naive $CD8^{+}$ T cells can be converted into $CD8^{+}$ Treg cells that function in a similar manner to IL-10 producing CD4+Treg cells. (**c**) Double-negative ($CD4^{-}CD8^{-}$) T cells function by downregulating the expression of co-stimulatory molecules by DCs, thus inhibit the pro-inflammatory DC responses. Double-negative T cells can acquire alloantigens through trogocytosis. This enables them to present antigens to effector T cells in a manner that promotes T-cell apoptosis

This B-cell signature was associated with the upregulation of *CD20* mRNA in urine sediment cells and increased numbers of naive and transitional B cells in the peripheral blood of tolerant patients compared with those receiving immunosuppression [63]. Other work has shown a transient increase in regulatory B cells in kidney transplant recipients treated with alemtuzumab [64]. These data highlight the possibility that B cells play a crucial role in transplant tolerance.

3.2.6 Regulatory T Cells

Numerous populations of T cells have been identified to play a role in transplant tolerance. These include CD4+ T cells [65–67] (Fig. 2a), CD8+ T cells [68, 69] (Fig. 2b), CD4−CD8− T cells [70] (Fig. 2c), natural killer (NK) T cells [71, 72], and γδ T cells [73].

CD4+ Regulatory T Cells

CD4+ regulatory T cells (commonly known as Treg) are the most thoroughly investigated regulatory T-cell subset. Treg can control both allograft rejection and GVHD in vivo [52]. Thymus derived or naturally occurring Treg are selected in the thymus and function in the periphery to suppress responses to self-antigens [67]. These cells express high levels of transcription factor forkhead box P3 (FOXP3). FOXP3 expressing Treg can also arise in the periphery after encounter with antigens in a tolerogenic environment, these are known as adaptive or induced Treg [74]. Both thymic-derived and induced Treg can contribute to the overall pool of Treg cells that can recognize and respond to alloantigen [75]. However, it is more likely that induced Treg cells generated in response to the persistent presence of alloantigen have a more important role in transplant tolerance [76].

The precise balance between graft destruction by the high numbers of alloantigen reactive T cells and regulation through the much smaller numbers of Tregs is critical. This balance can be shifted in several ways, either before or after transplantation, using strategies that either alter effector T cells or the frequency and/or functional ability of Tregs [75, 77, 78]. Immunosuppressive therapies that promote Treg cell generation and function are one effective approach [79]. Thymus-derived and induced Treg use numerous mechanisms to inhibit the activity of immune cells. Treg expression of cytotoxic T lymphocyte antigen 4 (CTLA4) can inhibit antigen presenting cell function, and prohibit T-cell proliferation through binding to CD80 and CD86 [80] (Fig. 2a). Treg can also produce immunosuppressive cytokine IL-10, which can inhibit antigen presenting cell function and induce conversion of T cells into Treg, aiding the regulatory activity in the draining lymphoid tissue and the allograft (Fig. 2a). Blocking the activity of CTLA4 or IL-10 in animal models of transplantation prevents Treg-mediated regulation [81, 82]. The location of these Treg is also very important; they initially function in the draining lymph node to inhibit the activation of naïve T cells and an allo-targeted response [83]. They also have the capacity to travel into the allograft where they can prevent ischemia-reperfusion injury [84] as well as establish a tolerant allograft environment [85, 86]. In animal models adoptive transfer of Treg is able to control acute [87–90] and chronic [90, 91] allograft rejection. However, the challenge of defining the human Treg populations and optimizing the expansion strategy remains. One of the concerns surrounding the use of Treg in the clinical arena is whether general immunosuppression will occur, thus offering no advantage to current immunosuppressive regimens.

CD8+ Regulatory T Cells

CD8+CD28− regulatory T cells inhibit antigen presenting cell (APC)-mediated T-cell activation by direct cell contact-dependent mechanisms [92] (Fig. 2b). These cells have been identified in renal transplant recipients who received alemtuzumab as an induction therapy, suggesting these cells may have a role in suppressing the immune response to donor alloantigens [93]. Another CD8+ regulatory T-cell population has been identified that can be generated from naïve CD8+ T cells and can inhibit T-cell responses through an IL-10 dependent mechanism [94] (Fig. 2b). IL-10 producing CD8+ regulatory T cells have been identified in a patient with long term acceptance of an allogeneic kidney transplant [95]. These studies suggest that there may be at least two different subsets of CD8+ regulatory T cells which utilize distinct mechanisms of action.

CD4−CD8− Regulatory T Cells

CD4−CD8− regulatory T cells express CD3 and the αβ TCR, however do not express CD4, CD8, or NK1.1. These cells have been shown to prevent immune responses mediated by CD4+ and CD8+ T cells and the rejection of allografts in animal models [96–98]. These CD4−CD8− regulatory T cells can induce suppression in numerous ways. Utilizing the CD95−CD95L pathway they can kill T cells, also can cause the DCs to downregulate the co-stimulatory molecules CD80 and CD86, induce DC apoptosis and sequester alloantigen from DCs by trogocytosis (Fig. 2c). In human recipients of hematopoietic stem cell transplantation, a deficiency of double negative T cells with regulatory activity can aid in the development of peripheral tolerance [99]. Thus there is some evidence that these cells may play a role in the development of peripheral tolerance, although the role they play in solid-organ transplantation remains to be observed.

γδ T Cells

γδ T cells are a subset of nonconventional T cells that have established roles in anti-tumour and anti-viral immunity. Interestingly, altered proportions of Vγ1- and Vγ2-expressing γδ T cells have been observed in tolerant liver transplant recipients compared with age-matched healthy controls [100, 101]. However, the role they have in protecting allograft destruction or mediating transplant tolerance has not been described.

Natural Killer T Cells

Due to the varied cytokine production by NK T cells, they have been associated with both transplant tolerance and rejection [102]. In a mouse model of hematopoietic stem cell transplantation, the adoptive transfer of highly purified NK T cells suppressed GVHD and decreased the production of interferon (IFN)-γ and tumor necrosis factor (TNF) by donor-derived T cells [103].

3.3 Co-stimulation in Peripheral Tolerance

Co-stimulation pathways play a central role in immune tolerance, with the major players being CD28, inducible T-cell co-stimulator (ICOS), CTLA4, and programmed cell death-1 (PD-1). CD28 is crucial for the development and survival of thymic-derived Treg [104, 105], as well as T-cell activation, proliferation, and survival upon T-cell interaction with APCs presenting their cognate antigen [106, 107]. Blockade of CD28 with its B7-ligands (CD80 and CD86) inhibits an effective T-cell response as well as promotes transplantation tolerance that initially depends on massive T-cell deletion [30, 108].

ICOS is a member of the CD28/B7 family and is expressed on activated T cells, while its ligand B7H/B7RP-1 is expressed on B cells and other non-immune tissues.

The effects of recipient ICOS deficiency or ICOS blockade have been tested in many transplant models. Prohibition of ICOS with B7RP-1 prolonged survival of heart, liver, and islet allografts in full MHC-mismatched rodent models [109–114]. This prolonged survival was associated with the decreased expansion of donor-reactive T cells and with lower serum titers of allo-antibody [115]. Interestingly, ICOS blockade also assists in long term allograft survival when used in combination with other graft-prolonging treatments, such as anti-CD154 mAb, CTLA4-Imunoglobulin (Ig), CsA, and rapamycin, making it an attractive therapeutic candidate [109, 111, 113, 114].

CTLA4 can affect tolerance by directing the immune system toward immunoregulation. Mice deficient in CTLA4 develop a chronic lymphoproliferative disease, illustrating the central role of CTLA4 in the controlling of T-cell immune responses. CTLA4 has been shown to enforce tolerance by enforcing the suppressive function of Treg and altering the function of DC through decreasing the expression of B7 molecules and increasing the production of immunosuppressive enzyme Indoleamine 2,3-dioxygenase (IDO) [82, 116]. The mechanism(s) behind the inhibitory effects on CTLA4 involve the competition with CD28 for the CD80 and CD86 ligands and blockade of TCR proximal and distal signaling. However, this is further complicated by the many splice variant isoforms, including a secreted soluble and a ligand independent form.

PD-1 is another member of the CD28 family that is expressed on activated B and T cells. While its functions in the thymus are important for both positive and negative selection, it also has a crucial role as a negative regulator for the maintenance of peripheral tolerance [117]. Mouse models of autoimmunity have highlighted the crucial role of PD-1 in autoimmune diseases such as Type-1 Diabetes and EAE [118]. While targeting of PD-1 signaling using a ligand-Ig (PD-L1.Ig) in a mouse cardiac allograft model could block allograft rejection and modulate T and B-cell dependent immune responses in vivo [119].

4 Rejection

4.1 Clinical Rejection

While many advances have been accomplished in transplant tolerance, the mechanisms behind allograft rejection have not been completely elucidated. Clinical rejection of an allograft can occur any time after transplantation and therefore these events are classified according to when after transplant they occur.

Hyperacute rejections occur within the first minutes to hours after transplantation, as a result of preformed allo-antibodies within the transplant recipient. These antibodies are against MHC antigens, or ABO blood group antigens which migrate into the allograft causing recruitment of inflammatory cells that trigger platelet aggregation and tissue necrosis. Modern crossmatch techniques have made hyperacute rejection through human leukocyte antigen reactive antibodies extremely rare.

Acute rejection occurs in the days to months after the transplant. This form of rejection is conducted by both allo-antibodies and allo-reactive T cells. Allo-reactive CD8+ T cells directly attack and destroy the transplanted organ through cytotoxic mechanisms (Fig. 4a). Allo-antibodies also have a role in this form of rejection (Fig. 4c). These alloantigen specific antibodies induce complement activation and neutrophil recruitment, which results in thrombotic ischemia of the transplanted organ. Therapies that deplete peripheral leukocytes, including T cells, are effective in preventing and reversing acute rejection, as well as improving the long-term outcomes for both patient and allograft [120].

Chronic rejection occurs in the months to years following transplantation. The secretion of cytokines by activated T cells and the production of allo-antibodies that activate the classical complement pathway, lead to chronic damage and failure of the transplanted organ [121] (Fig. 4b, c). This form of rejection still remains a challenge, and new strategies and therapeutics need to be developed.

4.2 Immune Mechanisms of Rejection

4.2.1 Ischemic-Reperfusion Injury

The physical process of removing, transplanting, and reperfusing organs initiates injury and stress responses. This results in alteration of gene and protein expression within the organ [122–124], which has a significant effect on the immune response of the recipient [125].

Cells of the immune system express pathogen-associated pattern recognition receptors (PRR) that allow them to detect structural units on pathogens as well as markers of tissue injury (damage-associated molecular patterns (DAMPS)). Ischemic-reperfusion injury generates many DAMPS such as reactive oxygen species, heat shock proteins, and heparin sulphate, which can all bind to PRRs. The detection of DAMPS by PRRs results in an inflammatory response including the production of IL-1, IL-6, TNF, type-1 interferon's, and chemokines [126]. These factors highlight the transplanted organ as a site of injury and inflammation, as well as initiate the alteration of the endothelial cells lining the vessels, triggering the release of antigens and antigen presenting cells [127] from the graft, culminating in the recruitment of inflammatory leukocytes into the graft.

Activation of the innate immune system through these mechanisms in the early stages after transplantation is predominantly a nonspecific response, occurring regardless of whether there is a genetic difference between the donor and the recipient [126]. While recent advances in organ preservation and perfusion have ameliorated some of these events [128, 129], it is currently impossible to prevent all tissue damage.

4.2.2 Allo-Recognition by T Cells

The priming of recipient T cells with antigen can occur by three different pathways (Fig. 3). Direct presentation is the interaction of the TCR on recipient T cells with donor-derived MHC complexes presented by donor APCs (Fig. 3a). This method of presentation is responsible for acute rejection; when donor APCs migrate to the draining lymph nodes and prime recipient T cells. Natural death of cells results in a limited time frame for this allo-recognition pathway to occur. Indirect presentation is the presentation of donor-derived MHC peptides by recipient APCs to recipient T cells (Fig. 3b). This form of antigen presentation is the dominant model of allo-recognition long term, as it persists for the life of the graft. The third mechanism of allo-recognition is called semi-direct presentation, where donor membrane fragments of MHC molecules are transferred to recipient APCs [130] (Fig. 3c). The significance of the semi-direct pathway of allo-recognition in the context of rejection remains to be elucidated [131].

Cytotoxic T-Cell Responses

After activation by an APC and a CD4+ Helper cell, CD8+ cytotoxic T cells migrate to the graft where they are able to identify their target cells through expression of MHC class I molecules (Fig. 4a). They kill their target cells by apoptosis through the release of

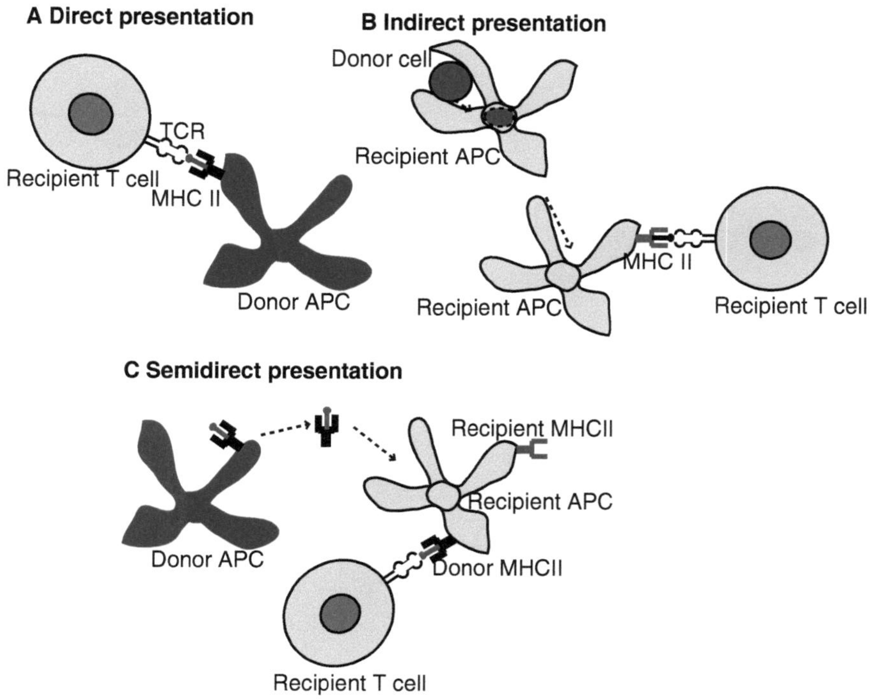

Fig. 3 Allorecognition pathways by T cells. (**a**) Direct allorecognition is the interaction of recipient T cells through the T cell receptor (TCR) with intact allogeneic major histocompatibility complex (MHC)-peptide complexes presented by donor-derived APCs, including DCs. (**b**) Indirect allorecognition occurs when peptides derived from donor MHC are degraded by antigen processing pathways and presented by recipient APCs. (**c**) Semi-direct allorecognition is the capture of donor MHC-peptide complexes by recipient APCs

granules containing cytotoxic molecules such as perforin and granzyme B, upregulating Fas ligand, and secreting soluble factors such as TNF-α. Increased levels of perforin and granzyme B mRNA can be detected in the urine of kidney transplant recipients experiencing rejection [132].

Helper T-Cell Responses

Alloantigen-specific CD4+ T-cell responses contribute to the effector phase of allograft rejection by a nonspecific effector mechanism referred to as the delayed-type hypersensitivity (DTH) response (Fig. 4b). This response consists of the release of multiple soluble mediators including IL-1, IFN-γ, and TNF-α. These soluble mediators attract infiltrating monocytes, macrophages, and eosinophils and the production of nitric oxide, reactive oxygen species, and arachidonic acid derivatives which cause damage to the graft. Activated CD4+ T cells also provide help to alloantigen-specific B cells assisting in proliferation and differentiation, as well as antibody class switching and affinity maturation (Fig. 4c).

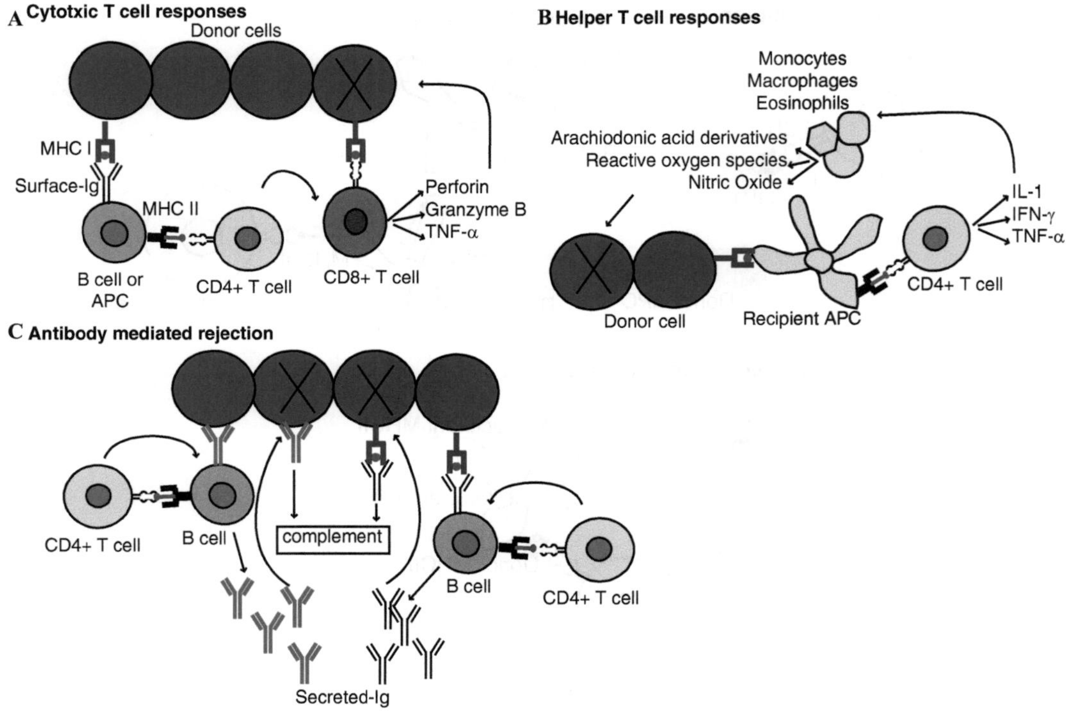

Fig. 4 Immune mechanisms of rejection. (**a**) APC and CD4+ helper cells activate CD8+ cytotoxic T cells. They then migrate to the graft where they are able to identify their target cells through expression of MHC class I molecules. Target cells are killed by apoptosis through the release of perforin and granzyme B, and secretion of soluble factors such as TNF-α. (**b**) After activation of allo-specific CD4+ T cells by APC, they secrete pro-inflammatory factors such as IL-1, IFN-γ, and TNF-α. These attract infiltrating monocytes, macrophages, and eosinophils which produce nitric oxide, reactive oxygen species, and arachidonic acid derivatives which cause damage to the graft. (**c**) B cells are responsible for antibody-mediated rejection. B cells can specifically recognize allo-antigens presented on MHC class I molecules of donor cells or other cellular components. With CD4+ T cell help, these B cells then produce antibodies that are specific to these proteins. The binding of these allo-antibodies to the graft induces complement fixation leading to graft damage

B Cells and Antibody-Mediated Rejection

B cells are responsible for antibody-mediated rejection that can begin within days after transplantation, but can also contribute to late graft loss [133] (Fig. 4c). The specificity of these allo-antibodies can range from MHC molecules and endothelial cells to blood group antigens [134], with the occurrence of antibody-mediated rejection being most dramatic in patients with pre-formed allo-antibodies. Complement fixation is most likely the predominant cause of antibody-mediated damage. Histologic staining of renal allograft biopsies with complement 4d is used for the identification of antibody-mediated rejection [135]. Antibodies can also utilize the Fc receptors present on NK cells and macrophages to elicit antibody-dependent cellular cytotoxicity inducing donor cell death. The humoral immune response is increasingly being implicated in the pathogenesis of both acute and chronic allograft responses [135].

5 Therapeutics and Clinical Strategies to Induce Long Term Graft Tolerance

The advances in immunosuppression regimens utilized in the clinic have significantly reduced the occurrence of acute rejection. However, there has been little change in the incidence of late graft loss, often referred to as chronic rejection. Moreover, current therapeutics cause general immunosuppression that can affect the ability of patients to fight malignancies and infections. Research is focused on promoting allograft specific immune tolerance as a means to reduce or replace current immunosuppressive therapeutics. This will allow the patient to react to potential pathogens and malignancies without injuring their allograft.

Most transplant recipients are currently treated with a combination of immunosuppressive drugs and biological agents to control the rejection of the transplanted organ. The exact immunosuppressants used vary depending on the type of transplant, as well as on the protocols used by individual transplant centers. Some centers employ induction therapy using a monoclonal antibody such as alemtuzumab or anti-thymocyte globulin. These treatments deplete most of the leukocytes in the peripheral blood and lymphoid organs. In the peripheral blood of alemtuzumab-treated transplant patients, Treg and regulatory B cells are present among the earliest re-populating leukocytes, which has the potential to tip the balance in favor of regulation, preventing the rejection of the allograft [64, 136]. Transplant patients are also treated with other immunosuppressive drugs, usually a calcineurin inhibitor such as a tacrolimus or CsA, in addition to an anti-proliferative agent such as mycophenolate mofetil. These drugs prevent the action of T cells, both activation of effector T cells as well as the generation and function of Treg. Rapamycin is another immunosuppressive drug used in transplant patients. This drug targets the mammalian target of rapamycin pathway and has been shown to support the generation of Treg ex vivo [137] and their function in vivo [79].

A more recent therapeutic approach to promote allograft tolerance is cell therapy, through the infusion of regulatory immune cells into transplant recipients. The transfer of regulatory immune cells shortly before or at the time of transplantation has the potential to inhibit the activity of effector cells and promote graft acceptance [76, 138]. Treg therapy has been shown to be very effective in controlling acute [87–90] and chronic [90, 91] rejection in numerous animal models of transplantation. These studies have provided strong evidence that such a therapy may work in the clinical setting. A multi-center Phase I/II study investigating the safety of infusing ex vivo expanded Treg cells into kidney transplant recipients is currently underway. Regulatory macrophages isolated from the organ donor have been administered to kidney recipients. In one of these studies, these patients had comparable graft function and the dose of tacrolimus was successfully reduced within the first 24 weeks after transplantation [32]. Strikingly, one year after transplantation the patterns of gene expression in the peripheral blood of these patients were similar to those described in the immunosuppression-free kidney transplant patients [139]. MSCs are another cell type to have been utilized in kidney transplant recipients. The infusion of autologous MSCs resulted in a lower incidence of acute rejection and opportunistic infection as well as better than estimated renal function at one year after transplant [140]. While all these therapeutics have shown promise, the route of administration, timing, dosing, and combination with other therapeutics still remain to be completely elucidated.

6 Conclusion

Mechanisms of graft tolerance and rejection consist of complex processes that entail many different functions of the immune system. Many effector and regulatory cell types play important roles in the survival of allografts. Current transplant recipients are usually treated with immunosuppressive therapeutics that ablate all of the actions of the immune system, leaving the patient with general immunosuppression. These therapeutics may also inadvertently alter the regulatory action of cells, thus further compromising the viability of the graft. More investigation is required to fully unravel all aspects behind immune tolerance and rejection in transplant recipients; however, current studies are showing lots of promise for the future of this field.

Acknowledgments

The work from the authors' own laboratory described in this review was supported by grants from The Wellcome Trust, Medical Research council, BBSRC, British Heart Foundation, and European Union through the ONE Study, Bio-DrIM and TRIAD projects. The authors would like to thank all members of TRIG past and present for their valuable contributions to the data reviewed herein. The authors have no conflict of interest.

References

1. Gibson T, Medawar PB (1943) The fate of skin homografts in man. J Anat 77 (299–310):294
2. Medawar PB (1944) The behaviour and fate of skin autografts and skin homografts in rabbits: a report to the War Wounds Committee of the Medical Research Council. J Anat 78:176–199
3. Medawar PB (1945) A second study of the behaviour and fate of skin homografts in

rabbits: a report to the War Wounds Committee of the Medical Research Council. J Anat 79(157–176):154
4. Billingham RE, Brent L, Medawar PB (1954) Quantitative studies on tissue transplantation immunity. II. The origin, strength and duration of actively and adoptively acquired immunity. Proc R Soc Lond B Biol Sci 143:58–80
5. Owen RD (1945) Immunogenetic consequences of vascular anastomoses between bovine twins. Science 102:400–401
6. Billingham RE, Brent L, Medawar PB (1953) Actively acquired tolerance of foreign cells. Nature 172:603–606
7. Mitchison NA (1953) Passive transfer of transplantation immunity. Nature 171:267–268
8. Hume DM, Merrill JP, Miller BF et al (1955) Experiences with renal homotransplantation in the human: report of nine cases. J Clin Invest 34:327–382
9. Guild WR, Harrison JH, Merrill JP et al (1955) Successful homotransplantation of the kidney in an identical twin. Trans Am Clin Climatol Assoc 67:167–173
10. Merrill JP, Murray JE, Harrison JH et al (1956) Successful homotransplantation of the human kidney between identical twins. J Am Med Assoc 160:277–282
11. Merrill JP, Murray JE, Takacs FJ et al (1963) Successful transplantation of kidney from a human cadaver. JAMA 185:347–353
12. Murray JE, Merrill JP, Harrison JH et al (1963) Prolonged survival of human-kidney homografts by immunosuppressive drug therapy. N Engl J Med 268:1315–1323
13. Thiel G, Harder F, Lortscher R et al (1983) Cyclosporin A used alone or in combination with low-dose steroids in cadaveric renal transplantation. Klin Wochenschr 61:991–1000
14. Egerton M, Scollay R, Shortman K (1990) Kinetics of mature T-cell development in the thymus. Proc Natl Acad Sci U S A 87:2579–2582
15. Surh CD, Sprent J (1994) T-cell apoptosis detected in situ during positive and negative selection in the thymus. Nature 372:100–103
16. Anderson MS, Venanzi ES, Klein L et al (2002) Projection of an immunological self shadow within the thymus by the aire protein. Science 298:1395–1401
17. Liston A, Lesage S, Wilson J et al (2003) Aire regulates negative selection of organ-specific T cells. Nat Immunol 4:350–354
18. Aschenbrenner K, D'Cruz LM, Vollmann EH et al (2007) Selection of Foxp3+ regulatory T cells specific for self antigen expressed and presented by Aire+ medullary thymic epithelial cells. Nat Immunol 8:351–358
19. Mathis D, Benoist C (2009) Aire. Annu Rev Immunol 27:287–312
20. Consortium F.-G (1997) An autoimmune disease, APECED, caused by mutations in a novel gene featuring two PHD-type zinc-finger domains. Nat Genet 17:399–403
21. Nagamine K, Peterson P, Scott HS et al (1997) Positional cloning of the APECED gene. Nat Genet 17:393–398
22. Ahonen P, Myllarniemi S, Sipila I et al (1990) Clinical variation of autoimmune polyendocrinopathy-candidiasis-ectodermal dystrophy (APECED) in a series of 68 patients. N Engl J Med 322:1829–1836
23. Goverman J, Woods A, Larson L et al (1993) Transgenic mice that express a myelin basic protein-specific T cell receptor develop spontaneous autoimmunity. Cell 72:551–560
24. Liu GY, Fairchild PJ, Smith RM et al (1995) Low avidity recognition of self-antigen by T cells permits escape from central tolerance. Immunity 3:407–415
25. Bouneaud C, Kourilsky P, Bousso P (2000) Impact of negative selection on the T cell repertoire reactive to a self-peptide: a large fraction of T cell clones escapes clonal deletion. Immunity 13:829–840
26. Bianchi T, Pincus LB, Wurbel MA et al (2009) Maintenance of peripheral tolerance through controlled tissue homing of antigen-specific T cells in K14-mOVA mice. J Immunol 182:4665–4674
27. Lombardi G, Sidhu S, Batchelor R et al (1994) Anergic T cells as suppressor cells in vitro. Science 264:1587–1589
28. Hao Z, Hampel B, Yagita H et al (2004) T cell-specific ablation of Fas leads to Fas ligand-mediated lymphocyte depletion and inflammatory pulmonary fibrosis. J Exp Med 199:1355–1365
29. Hildeman D, Jorgensen T, Kappler J et al (2007) Apoptosis and the homeostatic control of immune responses. Curr Opin Immunol 19:516–521
30. Wells AD, Li XC, Li Y et al (1999) Requirement for T-cell apoptosis in the induction of peripheral transplantation tolerance. Nat Med 5:1303–1307
31. Li XC (2010) The significance of non-T-cell pathways in graft rejection: implications for transplant tolerance. Transplantation 90:1043–1047

32. Hutchinson JA, Riquelme P, Sawitzki B et al (2011) Cutting edge: immunological consequences and trafficking of human regulatory macrophages administered to renal transplant recipients. J Immunol 187:2072–2078
33. Tiemessen MM, Jagger AL, Evans HG et al (2007) CD4+CD25+Foxp3+ regulatory T cells induce alternative activation of human monocytes/macrophages. Proc Natl Acad Sci U S A 104:19446–19451
34. Lu L, McCaslin D, Starzl TE et al (1995) Bone marrow-derived dendritic cell progenitors (NLDC 145+, MHC class II+, B7-1dim, B7-2−) induce alloantigen-specific hyporesponsiveness in murine T lymphocytes. Transplantation 60:1539–1545
35. Fu F, Li Y, Qian S et al (1996) Costimulatory molecule-deficient dendritic cell progenitors (MHC class II+, CD80dim, CD86−) prolong cardiac allograft survival in nonimmunosuppressed recipients. Transplantation 62:659–665
36. Lutz MB, Suri RM, Niimi M et al (2000) Immature dendritic cells generated with low doses of GM-CSF in the absence of IL-4 are maturation resistant and prolong allograft survival in vivo. Eur J Immunol 30:1813–1822
37. Roelen DL, Schuurhuis DH, van den Boogaardt DE et al (2003) Prolongation of skin graft survival by modulation of the alloimmune response with alternatively activated dendritic cells. Transplantation 76:1608–1615
38. Sato K, Yamashita N, Yamashita N et al (2003) Regulatory dendritic cells protect mice from murine acute graft-versus-host disease and leukemia relapse. Immunity 18:367–379
39. Swiecki M, Colonna M (2010) Unraveling the functions of plasmacytoid dendritic cells during viral infections, autoimmunity, and tolerance. Immunol Rev 234:142–162
40. Ochando JC, Homma C, Yang Y et al (2006) Alloantigen-presenting plasmacytoid dendritic cells mediate tolerance to vascularized grafts. Nat Immunol 7:652–662
41. Mazariegos GV, Zahorchak AF, Reyes J et al (2005) Dendritic cell subset ratio in tolerant, weaning and non-tolerant liver recipients is not affected by extent of immunosuppression. Am J Transplant 5:314–322
42. Tokita D, Mazariegos GV, Zahorchak AF et al (2008) High PD-L1/CD86 ratio on plasmacytoid dendritic cells correlates with elevated T-regulatory cells in liver transplant tolerance. Transplantation 85:369–377
43. Pak AS, Wright MA, Matthews JP et al (1995) Mechanisms of immune suppression in patients with head and neck cancer: presence of CD34(+) cells which suppress immune functions within cancers that secrete granulocyte-macrophage colony-stimulating factor. Clin Cancer Res 1:95–103
44. Bronte V, Wang M, Overwijk WW et al (1998) Apoptotic death of CD8+ T lymphocytes after immunization: induction of a suppressive population of Mac-1+/Gr-1+ cells. J Immunol 161:5313–5320
45. Dugast AS, Haudebourg T, Coulon F et al (2008) Myeloid-derived suppressor cells accumulate in kidney allograft tolerance and specifically suppress effector T cell expansion. J Immunol 180:7898–7906
46. Marigo I, Bosio E, Solito S et al (2010) Tumor-induced tolerance and immune suppression depend on the C/EBPbeta transcription factor. Immunity 32:790–802
47. Garcia MR, Ledgerwood L, Yang Y et al (2010) Monocytic suppressive cells mediate cardiovascular transplantation tolerance in mice. J Clin Invest 120:2486–2496
48. Hock BD, Mackenzie KA, Cross NB et al (2012) Renal transplant recipients have elevated frequencies of circulating myeloid-derived suppressor cells. Nephrol Dial Transplant 27:402–410
49. De Wilde V, Van Rompaey N, Hill M et al (2009) Endotoxin-induced myeloid-derived suppressor cells inhibit alloimmune responses via heme oxygenase-1. Am J Transplant 9:2034–2047
50. Casiraghi F, Azzollini N, Cassis P et al (2008) Pretransplant infusion of mesenchymal stem cells prolongs the survival of a semiallogeneic heart transplant through the generation of regulatory T cells. J Immunol 181:3933–3946
51. English K, Ryan JM, Tobin L et al (2009) Cell contact, prostaglandin E(2) and transforming growth factor beta 1 play non-redundant roles in human mesenchymal stem cell induction of CD4+CD25 (High) forkhead box P3+ regulatory T cells. Clin Exp Immunol 156:149–160
52. Wood KJ, Bushell A, Hester J (2012) Regulatory immune cells in transplantation. Nat Rev Immunol 12:417–430
53. Ding Y, Xu D, Feng G et al (2009) Mesenchymal stem cells prevent the rejection of fully allogenic islet grafts by the immunosuppressive activity of matrix metalloproteinase-2 and -9. Diabetes 58:1797–1806

54. Ge W, Jiang J, Baroja ML et al (2009) Infusion of mesenchymal stem cells and rapamycin synergize to attenuate alloimmune responses and promote cardiac allograft tolerance. Am J Transplant 9:1760–1772
55. Shlomchik MJ, Craft JE, Mamula MJ (2001) From T to B and back again: positive feedback in systemic autoimmune disease. Nat Rev Immunol 1:147–153
56. Mauri C (2010) Regulation of immunity and autoimmunity by B cells. Curr Opin Immunol 22:761–767
57. Mauri C, Bosma A (2012) Immune regulatory function of B cells. Annu Rev Immunol 30:221–241
58. Fillatreau S, Sweenie CH, McGeachy MJ et al (2002) B cells regulate autoimmunity by provision of IL-10. Nat Immunol 3:944–950
59. Mizoguchi A, Mizoguchi E, Takedatsu H et al (2002) Chronic intestinal inflammatory condition generates IL-10-producing regulatory B cell subset characterized by CD1d upregulation. Immunity 16:219–230
60. Mauri C, Gray D, Mushtaq N et al (2003) Prevention of arthritis by interleukin 10-producing B cells. J Exp Med 197:489–501
61. Tu W, Lau YL, Zheng J et al (2008) Efficient generation of human alloantigen-specific CD4+ regulatory T cells from naive precursors by CD40-activated B cells. Blood 112:2554–2562
62. Flores-Borja F, Bosma A, Ng D et al (2013) CD19+CD24hiCD38hi B cells maintain regulatory T cells while limiting TH1 and TH17 differentiation. Sci Transl Med 5:173ra123
63. Newell KA, Asare A, Kirk AD et al (2010) Identification of a B cell signature associated with renal transplant tolerance in humans. J Clin Invest 120:1836–1847
64. Heidt S, Hester J, Shankar S et al (2012) B cell repopulation after alemtuzumab induction-transient increase in transitional B cells and long-term dominance of naive B cells. Am J Transplant 12:1784–1792
65. Taylor PA, Lees CJ, Blazar BR (2002) The infusion of ex vivo activated and expanded CD4(+)CD25(+) immune regulatory cells inhibits graft-versus-host disease lethality. Blood 99:3493–3499
66. Wood KJ, Sakaguchi S (2003) Regulatory T cells in transplantation tolerance. Nat Rev Immunol 3:199–210
67. Sakaguchi S, Miyara M, Costantino CM et al (2010) FOXP3+ regulatory T cells in the human immune system. Nat Rev Immunol 10:490–500
68. Vlad G, Cortesini R, Suciu-Foca N (2008) CD8+ T suppressor cells and the ILT3 master switch. Hum Immunol 69:681–686
69. Li XL, Menoret S, Bezie S et al (2010) Mechanism and localization of CD8 regulatory T cells in a heart transplant model of tolerance. J Immunol 185:823–833
70. Thomson CW, Lee BP, Zhang L (2006) Double-negative regulatory T cells: non-conventional regulators. Immunol Res 35:163–178
71. Zeng D, Lewis D, Dejbakhsh-Jones S et al (1999) Bone marrow NK1.1(−) and NK1.1 (+) T cells reciprocally regulate acute graft versus host disease. J Exp Med 189:1073–1081
72. Monteiro M, Almeida CF, Caridade M et al (2010) Identification of regulatory Foxp3+ invariant NKT cells induced by TGF-beta. J Immunol 185:2157–2163
73. Hayday A, Tigelaar R (2003) Immunoregulation in the tissues by gammadelta T cells. Nat Rev Immunol 3:233–242
74. Josefowicz SZ, Rudensky A (2009) Control of regulatory T cell lineage commitment and maintenance. Immunity 30:616–625
75. Francis RS, Feng G, Tha-In T et al (2011) Induction of transplantation tolerance converts potential effector T cells into graft-protective regulatory T cells. Eur J Immunol 41:726–738
76. Wood KJ, Bushell A, Jones ND (2011) Immunologic unresponsiveness to alloantigen in vivo: a role for regulatory T cells. Immunol Rev 241:119–132
77. Graca L, Thompson S, Lin CY et al (2002) Both CD4(+)CD25(+) and CD4(+)CD25 (−) regulatory cells mediate dominant transplantation tolerance. J Immunol 168:5558–5565
78. Feng G, Wood KJ, Bushell A (2008) Interferon-gamma conditioning ex vivo generates CD25+CD62L+Foxp3+ regulatory T cells that prevent allograft rejection: potential avenues for cellular therapy. Transplantation 86:578–589
79. Hester J, Schiopu A, Nadig SN et al (2012) Low-dose rapamycin treatment increases the ability of human regulatory T cells to inhibit transplant arteriosclerosis in vivo. Am J Transplant 12:2008–2016
80. Grohmann U, Orabona C, Fallarino F et al (2002) CTLA-4-Ig regulates tryptophan catabolism in vivo. Nat Immunol 3:1097–1101
81. Kingsley CI, Karim M, Bushell AR et al (2002) CD25+CD4+ regulatory T cells

prevent graft rejection: CTLA-4- and IL-10-dependent immunoregulation of alloresponses. J Immunol 168:1080–1086

82. Wing K, Onishi Y, Prieto-Martin P et al (2008) CTLA-4 control over Foxp3+ regulatory T cell function. Science 322:271–275
83. Siegmund K, Feuerer M, Siewert C et al (2005) Migration matters: regulatory T-cell compartmentalization determines suppressive activity in vivo. Blood 106:3097–3104
84. Gandolfo MT, Jang HR, Bagnasco SM et al (2009) Foxp3+ regulatory T cells participate in repair of ischemic acute kidney injury. Kidney Int 76:717–729
85. Graca L, Cobbold SP, Waldmann H (2002) Identification of regulatory T cells in tolerated allografts. J Exp Med 195:1641–1646
86. Kendal AR, Chen Y, Regateiro FS et al (2011) Sustained suppression by Foxp3+ regulatory T cells is vital for infectious transplantation tolerance. J Exp Med 208:2043–2053
87. Hara M, Kingsley CI, Niimi M et al (2001) IL-10 is required for regulatory T cells to mediate tolerance to alloantigens in vivo. J Immunol 166:3789–3796
88. Bushell A, Wood K (2007) GITR ligation blocks allograft protection by induced CD25+CD4+ regulatory T cells without enhancing effector T-cell function. Am J Transplant 7:759–768
89. Issa F, Hester J, Goto R et al (2010) Ex vivo-expanded human regulatory T cells prevent the rejection of skin allografts in a humanized mouse model. Transplantation 90:1321–1327
90. Nadig SN, Wieckiewicz J, Wu DC et al (2010) In vivo prevention of transplant arteriosclerosis by ex vivo-expanded human regulatory T cells. Nat Med 16:809–813
91. Warnecke G, Bushell A, Nadig SN et al (2007) Regulation of transplant arteriosclerosis by CD25+CD4+ T cells generated to alloantigen in vivo. Transplantation 83:1459–1465
92. Liu Z, Tugulea S, Cortesini R et al (1999) Inhibition of CD40 signaling pathway in antigen presenting cells by T suppressor cells. Hum Immunol 60:568–574
93. Trzonkowski P, Zilvetti M, Chapman S et al (2008) Homeostatic repopulation by CD28−CD8+ T cells in alemtuzumab-depleted kidney transplant recipients treated with reduced immunosuppression. Am J Transplant 8:338–347
94. Gilliet M, Liu YJ (2002) Generation of human CD8 T regulatory cells by CD40 ligand-activated plasmacytoid dendritic cells. J Exp Med 195:695–704
95. Cai J, Lee J, Jankowska-Gan E et al (2004) Minor H antigen HA-1-specific regulator and effector CD8+ T cells, and HA-1 microchimerism, in allograft tolerance. J Exp Med 199:1017–1023
96. Zhang ZX, Yang L, Young KJ et al (2000) Identification of a previously unknown antigen-specific regulatory T cell and its mechanism of suppression. Nat Med 6:782–789
97. Ford MS, Young KJ, Zhang Z et al (2002) The immune regulatory function of lymphoproliferative double negative T cells in vitro and in vivo. J Exp Med 196:261–267
98. Hill M, Thebault P, Segovia M et al (2011) Cell therapy with autologous tolerogenic dendritic cells induces allograft tolerance through interferon-gamma and epstein-barr virus-induced gene 3. Am J Transplant 11:2036–2045
99. McIver Z, Serio B, Dunbar A et al (2008) Double-negative regulatory T cells induce allotolerance when expanded after allogeneic haematopoietic stem cell transplantation. Br J Haematol 141:170–178
100. Li Y, Koshiba T, Yoshizawa A et al (2004) Analyses of peripheral blood mononuclear cells in operational tolerance after pediatric living donor liver transplantation. Am J Transplant 4:2118–2125
101. Martinez-Llordella M, Lozano JJ, Puig-Pey I et al (2008) Using transcriptional profiling to develop a diagnostic test of operational tolerance in liver transplant recipients. J Clin Invest 118:2845–2857
102. Jukes JP, Wood KJ, Jones ND (2007) Natural killer T cells: a bridge to tolerance or a pathway to rejection? Transplantation 84:679–681
103. Leveson-Gower DB, Olson JA, Sega EI et al (2011) Low doses of natural killer T cells provide protection from acute graft-versus-host disease via an IL-4-dependent mechanism. Blood 117:3220–3229
104. Salomon B, Lenschow DJ, Rhee L et al (2000) B7/CD28 costimulation is essential for the homeostasis of the CD4+CD25+ immunoregulatory T cells that control autoimmune diabetes. Immunity 12:431–440
105. Tang Q, Henriksen KJ, Boden EK et al (2003) Cutting edge: CD28 controls peripheral homeostasis of CD4+CD25+ regulatory T cells. J Immunol 171:3348–3352

106. Lenschow DJ, Walunas TL, Bluestone JA (1996) CD28/B7 system of T cell costimulation. Annu Rev Immunol 14:233–258
107. Salomon B, Bluestone JA (2001) Complexities of CD28/B7: CTLA-4 costimulatory pathways in autoimmunity and transplantation. Annu Rev Immunol 19:225–252
108. Dai Z, Konieczny BT, Baddoura FK et al (1998) Impaired alloantigen-mediated T cell apoptosis and failure to induce long-term allograft survival in IL-2-deficient mice. J Immunol 161:1659–1663
109. Ozkaynak E, Gao W, Shemmeri N et al (2001) Importance of ICOS-B7RP-1 costimulation in acute and chronic allograft rejection. Nat Immunol 2:591–596
110. Guo L, Li XK, Funeshima N et al (2002) Prolonged survival in rat liver transplantation with mouse monoclonal antibody against an inducible costimulator (ICOS). Transplantation 73:1027–1032
111. Kosuge H, Suzuki J, Gotoh R et al (2003) Induction of immunologic tolerance to cardiac allograft by simultaneous blockade of inducible co-stimulator and cytotoxic T-lymphocyte antigen 4 pathway. Transplantation 75:1374–1379
112. Nakamura Y, Yasunami Y, Satoh M et al (2003) Acceptance of islet allografts in the liver of mice by blockade of an inducible costimulator. Transplantation 75:1115–1118
113. Nanji SA, Hancock WW, Anderson CC et al (2004) Multiple combination therapies involving blockade of ICOS/B7RP-1 costimulation facilitate long-term islet allograft survival. Am J Transplant 4:526–536
114. Guillonneau C, Aubry V, Renaudin K et al (2005) Inhibition of chronic rejection and development of tolerogenic T cells after ICOS-ICOSL and CD40-CD40L co-stimulation blockade. Transplantation 80:546–554
115. Harada H, Salama AD, Sho M et al (2003) The role of the ICOS-B7h T cell costimulatory pathway in transplantation immunity. J Clin Invest 112:234–243
116. Fallarino F, Grohmann U, Hwang KW et al (2003) Modulation of tryptophan catabolism by regulatory T cells. Nat Immunol 4:1206–1212
117. Bour-Jordan H, Esensten JH, Martinez-Llordella M et al (2011) Intrinsic and extrinsic control of peripheral T-cell tolerance by costimulatory molecules of the CD28/B7 family. Immunol Rev 241:180–205
118. Fife BT, Guleria I, Gubbels BM et al (2006) Insulin-induced remission in new-onset NOD mice is maintained by the PD-1-PD-L1 pathway. J Exp Med 203:2737–2747
119. Ozkaynak E, Wang L, Goodearl A et al (2002) Programmed death-1 targeting can promote allograft survival. J Immunol 169:6546–6553
120. Cai J, Terasaki PI (2010) Induction immunosuppression improves long-term graft and patient outcome in organ transplantation: an analysis of United Network for Organ Sharing registry data. Transplantation 90:1511–1515
121. Singh N, Pirsch J, Samaniego M (2009) Antibody-mediated rejection: treatment alternatives and outcomes. Transplant Rev (Orlando) 23:34–46
122. Famulski KS, Broderick G, Einecke G et al (2007) Transcriptome analysis reveals heterogeneity in the injury response of kidney transplants. Am J Transplant 7:2483–2495
123. Muhlberger I, Perco P, Fechete R et al (2009) Biomarkers in renal transplantation ischemia reperfusion injury. Transplantation 88: S14–S19
124. Pallet N, Fougeray S, Beaune P et al (2009) Endoplasmic reticulum stress: an unrecognized actor in solid organ transplantation. Transplantation 88:605–613
125. Kim IK, Bedi DS, Denecke C et al (2008) Impact of innate and adaptive immunity on rejection and tolerance. Transplantation 86:889–894
126. Carvalho-Gaspar M, Billing JS, Spriewald BM et al (2005) Chemokine gene expression during allograft rejection: comparison of two quantitative PCR techniques. J Immunol Methods 301:41–52
127. Larsen CP, Morris PJ, Austyn JM (1990) Donor dendritic leukocytes migrate from cardiac allografts into recipients' spleens. Transplant Proc 22:1943–1944
128. Hosgood SA, Nicholson ML (2010) The role of perfluorocarbon in organ preservation. Transplantation 89:1169–1175
129. Moers C, Varnav OC, van Heurn E et al (2010) The value of machine perfusion perfusate biomarkers for predicting kidney transplant outcome. Transplantation 90:966–973
130. Herrera OB, Golshayan D, Tibbott R et al (2004) A novel pathway of alloantigen presentation by dendritic cells. J Immunol 173:4828–4837
131. Wood KJ, Goto R (2012) Mechanisms of rejection: current perspectives. Transplantation 93:1–10
132. Anglicheau D, Suthanthiran M (2008) Noninvasive prediction of organ graft rejection

and outcome using gene expression patterns. Transplantation 86:192–199

133. Terasaki PI, Cai J (2008) Human leukocyte antigen antibodies and chronic rejection: from association to causation. Transplantation 86:377–383

134. Win TS, Pettigrew GJ (2010) Humoral autoimmunity and transplant vasculopathy: when allo is not enough. Transplantation 90:113–120

135. Colvin RB, Smith RN (2005) Antibody-mediated organ-allograft rejection. Nat Rev Immunol 5:807–817

136. Bloom DD, Chang Z, Fechner JH et al (2008) CD4+ CD25+ FOXP3+ regulatory T cells increase de novo in kidney transplant patients after immunodepletion with Campath-1H. Am J Transplant 8:793–802

137. Battaglia M, Stabilini A, Migliavacca B et al (2006) Rapamycin promotes expansion of functional CD4+CD25+FOXP3+ regulatory T cells of both healthy subjects and type 1 diabetic patients. J Immunol 177:8338–8347

138. McMurchy AN, Bushell A, Levings MK et al (2011) Moving to tolerance: clinical application of T regulatory cells. Semin Immunol 23:304–313

139. Sagoo P, Perucha E, Sawitzki B et al (2010) Development of a cross-platform biomarker signature to detect renal transplant tolerance in humans. J Clin Invest 120:1848–1861

140. Tan J, Wu W, Xu X et al (2012) Induction therapy with autologous mesenchymal stem cells in living-related kidney transplants: a randomized controlled trial. JAMA 307:1169–1177

Chapter 13

Method of Generating Tolerogenic Maturation-Resistant Dendritic Cells and Testing for Their Immune-Regulatory Functions In Vivo in the Context of Transplantation

Sherrie J. Divito and Adrian E. Morelli

Abstract

During that past two decades, advances in techniques for generating in vitro immune-suppressive dendritic cells (DCs) have heralded the use of these pro-tolerogenic DCs as therapeutics against transplant rejection and autoimmune diseases. In transplantation, previous dogma assumed that systemically administered therapeutic DCs bearing donor antigens (Ags) control the anti-donor response by directly interacting with anti-donor T cells in vivo. However, recent evidence indicates that the exogenously-administered therapeutic DCs instead function as Ag-transporting cells that transfer donor Ags to recipient's Ag-presenting cells (APCs) for presentation to T cells. In secondary lymphoid organs, presentation of acquired donor Ags by recipient's quiescent DCs triggers deficient activation and eventual apoptosis of donor-specific effector T cells, leading to a relative increase in the percentage of donor-specific regulatory T cells. This chapter describes the methodology to generate in vitro immune-suppressive DCs that are resistant to maturation, and to assess in vivo both their survival and their ability to regulate donor-specific T cells in a mouse model.

Key words Tolerogenic dendritic cells, Vitamin D_3, Cell therapy, Transplantation, Mouse

1 Introduction

Dendritic cells (DCs) are a heterogeneous population of hematopoietic-derived antigen (Ag)-presenting cells (APCs) that orchestrate the adaptive immune response to self and foreign Ags. DCs serve as a crucial link between innate and adaptive immunity as they are the only APCs capable of priming naïve T cells [1, 2]. DCs exist in three different stages of maturation in the periphery: immature, semi-mature or quiescent, and mature or activated. In the steady state, immature DCs have high phagocytic ability and low surface expression of MHC:peptide complexes, CD40, and the co-stimulatory molecules CD80 and CD86 [1–3]. Upon Ag uptake and exposure to pro-inflammatory stimuli, DCs mature, resulting in decreased phagocytic ability and increased surface

Ashleigh S. Boyd (ed.), *Immunological Tolerance: Methods and Protocols*, Methods in Molecular Biology, vol. 1899,
https://doi.org/10.1007/978-1-4939-8938-6_13, © Springer Science+Business Media, LLC, part of Springer Nature 2019

expression of peptide-loaded MHC class-I and -II molecules, CD40, CD80 and CD86, and the chemokine receptor CCR7 [3]. Immature/semi-mature DCs expressing MHC:peptide complexes (signal 1) with low levels of costimulatory molecules (signal 2) provide sub-threshold stimulation to T cells and defective T-cell activation [4–6]. Incomplete T-cell activation results in poor cellular proliferation followed by deletion, anergy, and likely differentiation/expansion of regulatory T (Treg) cells, all mechanisms leading to T-cell hypo-responsiveness [4, 5].

The ability of DCs to downregulate the T-cell response in an Ag-specific manner, coupled with the development of techniques to propagate large numbers of DCs in vitro, has heralded the use of immature or maturation-resistant (MR) DCs as therapeutics against transplant rejection or autoimmune disorders. A number of methods, including culture-conditioning with different cytokines or growth factors, treatment with pharmacologic agents, and genetic engineering [7], have been developed to increase DC immunosuppressive potential and/or render immunosuppressive/tolerogenic DC resistant to maturation (MR-DCs), the latter to prevent the risk of in vivo maturation/activation of the administered DCs and thus patient sensitization.

The active form of vitamin D_3 (VD_3) 1α,25-dihydroxyvitamin D_3 ($1\alpha,25(OH)_2D_3$), is a secosteroid hormone known for its importance in calcium, phosphorus, and bone metabolism, but also is now appreciated as a potent modulator of the immune system [8–10]. DCs treated with $1\alpha,25(OH)_2D_3$, VD_3-DCs, have decreased T-cell allostimulatory capacity [11, 12], and T cells stimulated by VD_3-DCs in primary mixed lymphocyte cultures (MLCs) become hypo-responsive [13], and have increased expression of CTLA-4 with decreased CD40 ligand (CD154) expression and IFN-γ production [11].

Whereas treatment of patients with $1\alpha,25(OH)_2D_3$ has the potentially deleterious side effects of hypercalcemia and nonspecific immunosuppression which could increase susceptibility to infection and malignancies, treating patients with in vitro generated VD_3-DCs is a promising alternative. Notably, VD_3-DCs have been shown to be pro-tolerogenic in vivo, as their adoptive transfer (i.v.) significantly prolongs skin and cardiac allograft survival in mice [12, 14, 15].

In this chapter, we describe a method of generating immunosuppressive/tolerogenic DCs in vitro from bone marrow (BM) cells via treatment with VD_3. We further discuss how to confirm that these immune-suppressive DCs are resistant to maturation, to semi-quantify their accumulation/survival in vivo, and to assess their ability to regulate Ag-specific T cells in vivo.

2 Animals and Materials

All solutions, plasticware, and dissecting instruments must be sterile.

1. C57Bl/6 (B6) mice and BALB/c/cByJ (BALB/c) mice, 8–12 weeks old, preferably male, are used for generating BM-DCs. These mice are also used as host/recipient mice for in vivo and ex vivo assays and as a source of naïve splenic T cells. 1H3.1 TCR transgenic Ragl$^{-/-}$ Thyl.1 congenic B6 mice (provided by C. Viret and C. Janeway, Yale University, New Heaven, CT) were bred at the University of Pittsburgh Animal Facility and were used as a source of Ag-specific CD4 T cells.
2. Phosphate-buffered saline (PBS 1×) without Ca and Mg.
3. Fine forceps and scissors.
4. Plasticware: Petri dishes (6 or 9 cm in diameter), 1 and 10 ml syringes, 27½ G needles, pipettes, 70 μm cell strainers, 15 and 50 ml conical tubes, tissue culture-grade flasks (75 cm^2), 24-well plates, and round-bottom 96-well plates.
5. Biosafety cabinet, pipette aids, refrigerated bench-top centrifuge. Freezer (−80 °C). Gamma-irradiator for cells, cell harvester and beta counter for 96-well plates.
6. RPMI-1640 culture medium: with sodium bicarbonate, without L-glutamine, sterile-filtered, endotoxin tested. To prepare complete RPMI medium, supplement the medium with 10% v/v heat-inactivated fetal calf serum (FCS), L-glutamine (2 mM), nonessential amino acid solution (1×), sodium pyruvate (0.11 mg/ml), HEPES (10 mM), 2-mercaptoethanol (0.55 mM), penicillin and streptomycin (100 U each), mouse GM-CSF (1000 U/ml), and mouse IL-4 (500 U/ml).
7. Red blood cell lysis buffer: dissolve 4.1 g NH_4Cl (150 mM), 0.5 g $KHCO_3$ (1 mM), and 18.6 mg Na_2EDTA (0.1 mM) in 400 ml of deionized distilled water. Adjust pH to 7.2–7.4 with HCl, if needed. Bring the solution to a final volume of 500 ml and filter it through 500 ml filter system (0.22 μm). Store the solution in the refrigerator and use it at room temperature (RT).
8. Monoclonal Abs against red blood cell precursors (clone TER-119), CD3 (clone 1782), B220 (clone RA3-6B2), NK-1.1 (clone PK136), Grl (clone RB6-8C5), and agonistic Ab against CD40 Ab (10 μg/ml, clone HM40-3) (eBioscience).
9. Low toxicity rabbit complement solution (Cedarlane).
10. FACS staining buffer: PBS containing 1% heat-inactivated FCS and 0.01% Na azide.

11. 1α,25$(OH)_2$ VD_3, LPS and polyriboinosinic acid/polyribocytidylic acid (poly I:C) (Sigma-Aldrich).
12. Mouse GM-CSF, IL-4, TNF-α, IFN-γ, and IL-1β (PeproTech).
13. DC_1-maturation cocktail: IFN-γ (20 ng/ml), IL-1β (20 ng/ml), TNF-α (50 ng/ml), and poly I:C (1 μM) final concentrations in RPMI-1640 complete medium.
14. Protease inhibitor cocktail for use with mammalian cell and tissue extracts, DMSO solution (Sigma).
15. Mouse CD3+ T Cell Enrichment Columns (R&D Systems).
16. CD4 Dynabeads® negative isolation kit (Dynal at Thermo Fisher).
17. Dynabeads® sheep anti-rat IgG (Dynal at Thermo Fisher).
18. Dynal magnet for 15 ml tubes (Dynal at Thermo Fisher).
19. Rocking or orbital shaker placed in cold room.
20. Vybrant CFDA SE Cell Tracer (CFSE) (Thermo Fisher).
21. CD11c microbeads mouse (Miltenyi).
22. CD40 (clone FGK45.5) and NK1.1 (clone PK136) antibodies (Abs) for in vivo administration (BioXCell).
23. DNeasy Tissue Kit (Qiagen Inc).
24. Illustra PuReTaq Ready-To-Go PCR beads (GE Healthcare).
25. $IE\alpha_{52-68}$ peptide (ASFEAQGALANIAVDKA) HPLC-purified.

3 Methods

3.1 Generation of MR-DCs

1. Dissect femurs and tibias from two mice with sterile fine forceps and scissors. Remove the surrounding soft tissues from the bones while they are still in place (*see* **Note 1**). Place the bones in a Petri dish containing sterile PBS on ice. Immerse the bones for 1 min in 70% ethanol in a Petri dish. Remove traces of ethanol by rinsing the bones twice in cold PBS. When removing the bones, do not cut the epiphyses (bone endings) as this could cause BM contamination and damage of the BM cells from the ethanol.
2. In a Petri dish, cut the epiphyses near to the end of the bones to reduce loss of BM cells. Transfer the bone shafts to a new Petri dish and remove the BM cells by flushing the BM cavity with cold RPMI-medium loaded in a 10 ml syringe with a 27½ G needle. With a transfer pipette, transfer the BM fragments and cells from the Petri dish to a 70 μm cell strainer placed on top of a 50 ml conical tube. Disaggregate the BM clumps retained on

the strainer by pressing gently with the flat end of a 1 ml syringe plunger and rinse the cell strainer with cold RPMI-medium.

3. Pellet the BM cells (650 × *g*, 5 min, 4 °C), and lyse the erythrocytes by incubating the cells (3 min, RT) with 3 ml of red blood cell lysis buffer.
4. Stop lysis by adding 25 ml of cold PBS followed by centrifugation. Remove the supernatant, and resuspend the BM cells isolated from two mice in 500 μl of cold culture medium in preparation for complement-mediated depletion.
5. For removal of erythroid precursors, T and B lymphocytes, NK cells, and granulocytes, BM cells are incubated (30 min, on ice) with Abs against red blood cell precursors (clone TER-119), CD3 (clone 1782), B220 (clone RA3-6B2), NK-1.1 (clone PK136), and Gr1 (clone RB6-8C5) (1 μg of each Ab per 100 μl of volume containing up to 10^8 cells/ml). After incubation, cells are rinsed with cold PBS, centrifuged and incubated (45 min, 37 °C) with 4 ml of low-toxicity rabbit complement solution. To stop cell lysis, wash the cells twice with ice-cold PBS.
6. Count viable cells.
7. Plate 15 × 10^6 BM cells per 75 cm^2 culture flask in a final volume of 22 ml of complete culture medium supplemented with mouse GM-CSF (1000 U/ml) and IL-4 (500 U/ml) (day 0).
8. On days 2, 4, and 6 of culture, 17 ml of culture medium (containing floating cells) are removed and centrifuged in 50 ml conical tubes (650 × *g*, 5 min, 4 °C). The cells are resuspended with a similar volume of fresh medium with GM-CSF plus IL-4 and placed back in the flasks. For generation of MR-DCs, cultures are also supplemented with 10 nM VD_3 on days 2, 4, and 6.
9. On day 7, the culture supernatants are harvested by gently pipetting the culture medium against the flat surface of the culture flask. Collect the culture medium with the floating and loosely adherent DCs in 50 ml conical tubes. Rinse the culture flasks with cold PBS several times and add the PBS to the 50 ml conical tubes containing the DCs. Pellet the cells by centrifugation (650 × *g*, 5 min, 4 °C) then resuspend in appropriate volume and medium per desired assay (see below).

3.2 Testing for Maturation-Resistance of BM-DCs In Vitro

MR-DCs generated in vitro with VD_3 are MHC class-$II^{low/int}$ $CD40^{neg}$ $CD80/86^{neg/low}$ by day 7. Following challenge with DC-maturation stimuli, MR-DCs fail to increase (1) surface expression of MHC class-II, CD40, and CD80/86 molecules; (2) IL-12p70 secretion; and (3) their ability to allo-stimulate T cells.

Immature BM-DCs not exposed to exogenous VD_3 are used as controls. This section explains how to analyze these variables.

1. Treat both control- and VD_3-treated BM-DCs (on day 6) for 48 h with DC_1-maturation cocktail; or with LPS (50 ng/ml); or agonistic CD40 Ab (10 μg/ml, clone HM40-3) (*see* **Note 2**).
2. After the 48 h stimulation, harvest the BM-DCs from culture flasks as described in **step 9** of Subheading 3.1.
3. To assess surface expression of DC maturation markers, resuspend 10^6 control- and VD_3-treated BM-DCs (treated or not with the DC-maturation stimuli) in 100 μl FACS staining buffer and incubate with anti-CD16/32 blocking Ab for 20 min on ice, then add fluorochrome-conjugated Abs against CD80 (clone 16.10A1), CD86 (clone PO3-1) CD40 (clone IC10), CD11c (clone N418) and IA^d (clone AMS-32.1, if BALB/c-derived) at the appropriate dilutions (30 min, on ice). Thereafter, wash cells twice with 1 ml FACS staining buffer and resuspend the stained cells in 200 μl of 4% paraformaldehyde (fixative). Analyze by flow cytometry the expression of surface markers within the $CD11c^+$ DC gate.
4. To quantify cytokine production, control- and VD_3-treated BM-DCs are incubated or not (control) with the DC-maturation stimuli as explained in **step 1** of this section. After 48–72 h, collect supernatants, remove cells by centrifugation, and add protease inhibitor cocktail to the cell-free supernatants. Aliquot supernatants in small volumes to prevent thawing and freezing. Keep supernatants at −80 °C until samples are assessed by ELISA for the detection of IL-10, IL-12p70, and IL-23 following the manufacturer's instructions.
5. The T-cell stimulatory function of control- and VD_3-treated BM-DCs, incubated or not (control) with the DC-maturation stimuli, is assessed in MLCs. Floating BM-DCs are collected (purity $\geq$ 85%, based on CD11c expression analyzed by FACS), centrifuged, resuspended in culture medium without cytokines (4×10^5 cells/ml), γ-irradiated (2000 rads), and used as stimulatory cells of allogeneic or syngeneic (control) splenic T cells purified by mouse CD3+ T Cell Enrichment Columns (R&D Systems), and resuspended in complete medium without cytokines (2×10^6 cells/ml).
6. In a round-bottom 96-well plate (*see* **Note 3**), add 200 μl of the DC suspension into three consecutive wells (triplicate), and 100 μl of medium alone in the following wells until completing two consecutive rows of wells. Two fold dilutions of the DC concentration are made with a multichannel pipettor loaded with three yellow tips. Make consecutive dilutions of the DCs

plated in the first three wells, by transferring 100 μl out of the original 200 μl into the following three wells loaded with 100 μl of medium alone. Pipet up and down to distribute evenly the transferred DCs and then transfer 100 μl to the next three wells. Continue the DC transfer until you reach the final three wells of the second row. Discard the excess 100 μl volume of the last three wells, so each well contains 100 μl of medium with the DCs. With a multichannel pipettor, add 100 μl of the T-cell suspension to each well, so the DC:T cell ratio will vary from 1:5 in the first three wells (4×10^4 DCs + 2×10^5 T cells in 200 μl of medium) to 1:640 (312 DCs + 2×10^5 T cells in 200 μl of medium) in the last three wells (*see* **Note 4**). Include as negative control wells loaded with T cells alone.

7. Three days later, T-cell proliferation is evaluated based on incorporation of [^{3}H] thymidine added 18 h before harvest (1 μCi per well in 10 μl of volume). The amount of radioisotope incorporated is determined with a beta counter.

3.3 MR-DC Semi-Quantification and Assessment of Immune-Regulatory Function of MR-DCs In Vivo

Intravenous (i.v.) administration of donor-derived (BALB/c) immature BM-DCs or MR-DCs (5×10^6 cells, 7 days before transplant) prolongs significantly survival of BALB/c heart allografts in B6 recipients (mean survival time 53.6 ± 15.1 days and 52.2 ± 33.4 days, respectively, compared to 14.5 ± 0.5 days in control recipients treated with syngeneic B6 MR-DCs) [15]. Accordingly, therapy with donor-derived immature or MR-DCs is associated with reduced intra-graft inflammation and decreased systemic anti-donor response through the direct and indirect pathways of allo-recognition, assessed by IFN-γ ELISPOTs in the recipient's spleen [15]. This section explains how to prepare MR-DCs for systemic administration, semi-quantify the amount of injected MR-DCs mobilized into the spleen at different time points, and analyze the effect of the injected donor-derived MR-DCs on the anti-donor CD4 T cell response in vivo.

3.3.1 Systemic Administration of MR-DCs

1. Collect VD_3-treated MR-DCs (day 7) into 50 ml conical tubes as described in **step 9** of Subheading 3.1. Pellet the MR-DCs (650 × *g*, 5 min, 4 °C) and pool all the cells in a 15 ml conical tube, to reduce cell loss. MR-DCs may contain a small percentage of $CD11c^+$ $CD86^+$ mature DCs that may sensitize the host/recipient mice. Therefore, $CD86^+$ cells are depleted by negative selection by incubating the MR-DCs with CD86 Ab (clone GL1, developed in rat) (30 min, on ice), followed by negative depletion with Dynabeads® sheep anti-rat IgG, according to the manufacturer's instructions (30 min incubation of cells with beads on slow motion on an orbital or rocking shaker in the cold room). Check the efficiency of $CD86^+$ cell

depletion by a quick staining of a small aliquot of cells with CD11c and CD86 Abs, followed by FACS analysis. If the purity of the CD11c$^+$ cells is <90%, MR-DCs are further purified by positive selection with CD11c microbeads (Miltenyi).

2. Count viable MR-DCs and rinse cells with cold PBS.
3. Pellet the MR-DCs (650 × *g*, 5 min, 4 °C), then resuspend the cells at 5 × 10^6 cells per 300 μl cold PBS, and keep cells in a tube on ice. Draw the cell suspension up into a 1 ml syringe and inject 5 × 10^6 BM-DCs (300 μl) into mouse tail vein using a 27½ G needle.

3.3.2 Semi-Quantification by PCR of Adoptively Transferred Donor-Derived (BALB/c) MR-DCs in Recipient's (B6) Spleen

Following i.v. injection of a therapeutic dose of donor-derived (BALB/c) MR-DCs (5 × 10^6 cells) into recipient (B6) mice, very few MR-DCs are usually detected in the spleen by immunofluorescence microscopy on tissue sections. This is because donor-derived MR-DCs also migrate to peripheral tissues, and have a short life-span (24–72 h) in vivo, at least in part due to killing by recipient's NK and CTLs due to their fully allogeneic origin. Therefore, the number of BALB/c MR-DCs mobilized into the spleen of B6 host mice is better estimated semi-quantitatively by genomic PCR analysis for the *IgG2a^a* allele, which is encoded in the BALB/c, but not B6, genome. Alternatively, detection of donor MHC class-I or -II genes absent in the host/recipient genome can also be used.

1. Inject i.v. donor-derived (BALB/c) VD_3-treated MR-DCs into host B6 mice (5 × 10^6 cells/mouse). At various time points post-injection (i.e., 1, 6, 24, and 72 h) harvest the spleens of the injected mice and disaggregate the tissue into single cell suspensions (*see* **Note 5**).
2. Isolate DNA with the DNeasy Tissue Kit following the manufacturer's instructions.
3. Perform genomic PCR using primers for IgG2a^a (BALB/c and B6 mice encode for the *IgG2a^a* and *IgG2a^b* alleles, respectively) [16]: F 5′ ACAAAGTCCCTGGTTTGGTGC; R 5′ GGCATTTGCATGGAGGACAG; 111 Kb product. Add 750 ng DNA to Illustra PuReTaq Ready-To-Go PCR beads and run at 94 °C 3 min; (94 °C 30 s, 67.7 °C 30 s, 72 °C 50 s) × 38 cycles, and 72 °C for 10 min.
4. Run PCR products on 2% agarose gels along with a DNA ladder for comparison.
5. To determine the limit of assay sensitivity, serially dilute BALB/c MR-DCs in single cell suspensions of a fixed number of B6 splenocytes at ratios 1:1, 1:10, 1:10^2, 1:10^3, 1:10^4, 1:10^5, and 1:10^6. Include B6 splenocytes alone, BALB/c MR-DCs alone, and no cells, as controls. Isolate DNA from

these cells and perform genomic PCR as explained in **steps 2** and **3** of this section. Run PCR products on 2% agarose gels. The detection limit of the assay should be at least 1 BALB/c MR-DC per 10^4 B6 splenocytes.

3.3.3 Assay for the Ability of Donor-Derived (BALB/c) MR-DCs to Regulate Donor-Specific T Cells in Recipient's (B6) Mice

We have previously demonstrated [15, 17] that donor-derived (BALB/c) MR-DCs administered systemically at the dose that prolongs cardiac allografts survival (5×10^6 cells), fail to downregulate the anti-donor response via direct contact with allo-reactive T cells in vivo. By contrast, the exogenous MR-DCs transfer donor Ags to recipient's conventional ($CD11c^{hi}$) DCs resident in secondary lymphoid organs [15, 17]. This Ag-transfer allows the relatively few donor-derived MR-DCs mobilized to the spleen to transfer donor allo-Ags to a much higher number of recipient's conventional DCs, therefore increasing the efficiency of donor-specific immune-regulation. Due to the brief lifespan of the donor-derived MR-DCs in vivo, the transferred donor-derived allo-Ag is presented by recipient's splenic quiescent conventional $CD11c^{hi}$ $CD8\alpha^{-\ or\ +}$ to T cells via the indirect pathway of allorecognition (donor peptide presented by recipient's MHC molecules) only briefly in vivo (less than 3 days after DC administration) [15, 17, 18]. Presentation of donor allo-peptides by recipient's quiescent ($CD80/86^{low}$) conventional DCs results in defective activation of the allo-reactive T cells followed by T-cell apoptosis and increased percentages of donor-specific CD4 FoxP3 Treg cells in the spleen [15, 17]. Interestingly, the absolute number of splenic donor-specific CD4 FoxP3 Treg cells did not change significantly compared to controls that did not receive MR-DCs, suggesting that Treg cells exhibit a survival advantage compared to effector T cells following donor MR-DC therapy [15, 17].

In the BALB/c (donor) > B6 (host/recipient) strain combination, it is possible to detect presentation of donor (BALB/c) MHC class-II derived peptides ($IE\alpha_{52-68}$) loaded in recipient's (B6) MHC class-II (IA^b) molecules by means of the 1H3.1 CD4 TCR transgenic T cells (Thy1.1 congenic) that are specific for the BALB/c $IE\alpha_{52-68}$ peptide presented by B6 IA^b molecules. In this system, the BALB/c MR-DCs delivered i.v. have to be reprocessed and presented by host (B6) APCs to 1H3.1 T cells. This section explains how to detect in vivo reprocessing and presentation of donor allo-Ags derived from therapeutically administered (BALB/c) MR-DCs by recipient's (B6) APCs.

1. Isolate spleen and lymph nodes of naïve $Thy1.1^+$ $Rag1^{-/-}$ 1H3.1 mice (*see* **Note 6**). Prepare single cell suspensions, pool the cells, and deplete red blood cells by adding 3 ml of red blood cell lysis buffer (3 min, RT). Stop the cell lysis by adding 25 ml cold PBS and centrifuge ($650 \times g$, 5 min, 4 °C). Add 25 ml of PBS, pass the cells through a 70 μm cell strainer to eliminate cell debris resulting from the lysis.

2. Optional: purify CD4 T cells with the CD4 Dynabeads® negative isolation kit according to the manufacturer's instructions.
3. After purification, CD4 T cells are CFSE-labeled. To do this, resuspend T cells (10^7 cells/ml) in warmed (37 °C) PBS with 10% FCS. Add 7.5 μM CFSE, distribute the dye evenly by pipetting, and incubate for 30 min at 37 °C. Wash cells with warmed PBS + 10% FCS. Resuspend cells in warmed PBS + 10% FCS, and incubate for another 30 min at 37 °C. Wash cells twice with cold PBS. Count viable cells. Resuspend cells (3×10^6 cells/300 μl) in cold PBS. Keep the tube with the cells on ice until injection.
4. Inject in the tail vein the CFSE-labeled 1H3.1 CD4 T cells (Thy1.1$^+$) in recipient naïve B6 (Thy1.2$^+$) mice (3×10^6 cells in 300 μl of PBS per mouse).
5. One day later, inject (tail vein) the BALB/c MR-DCs (5×10^6 cells/mouse) into the naïve B6 mice injected with the CFSE-labeled 1H3.1 CD4 T cells. As negative control, include B6 mice injected only with CFSE-labeled 1H3.1 CD4 T cells (no DCs), and B6 mice injected with CFSE-labeled 1H3.1 CD4 T cells plus syngeneic (B6) MR-DCs. As positive control of full 1H3.1 CD4 T cell activation, add B6 mice injected with CFSE-labeled 1H3.1 CD4 T cells (on day −1) and BALB/c MR-DCs (on day 0), plus agonistic CD40 antibody (clone FGK45.5, 150 μg/dose, i.p., on days 0, 1 and 2).
6. Three and 14 days after DC injection, T-cell proliferation, activation and apoptosis, and generation/expansion of FoxP3 Treg cells are analyzed in the adoptively transferred CFSE-labeled 1H3.1 CD4 T cells in the spleen. To do this, harvest spleens and prepare single cell suspensions. Deplete red blood cells with lysis buffer and count the absolute number of splenocytes per mouse, which will be necessary later on to calculate the absolute number of 1H3.1 T cells per spleen based on the percentage of 1H3.1 cells detected by flow cytometry. Splenocytes are distributed into FACS tubes, FcR-blocked with CD16/32 Ab and then labeled with fluorochrome-conjugated Abs against Thy1.1 (clone HIS51), CD4 (GK1.5), CD69 (clone H1.2F3), CD127 (clone A7R34), and CD62L (clone MEL-14) (30 min, on ice). Wash cells with FACS staining buffer, pellet the cells ($650 \times g$, 5 min, 4 °C), and resuspend the pellet in 200 μl 4% paraformaldehyde as fixative. In parallel, splenocytes are (a) labeled with PE-conjugated annexin-V plus fluorochrome-conjugated Thy1.1 and CD4 Abs, for assessment of 1H3.1 T cell apoptosis; and (b) surface labeled with fluorochome-coupled Thy1.1 and CD4 Abs, incubated with FoxP3 Fixation/Permeabilization working solution (eBioscience), and labeled with PE-coupled FoxP3 Ab (clone

FJK-16s, eBioscience) according to the eBioscience protocol. Analyze the samples by flow cytometry (*see* **Note 7**).

7. For detection of ex vivo secretion of IL-2 and Th1 (IFN-γ), Th2 (IL-5, IL-13), Th17 (IL-17) and Treg (IL-10, TGFβ) cytokines by splenic 1H3.1 T cells in response to donor Ag-specific stimulation, harvest spleens 3 and 14 days after BALB/c MR-DC administration. Incubate the splenocytes in 24 well-plates (5×10^6 splenocytes/well) in complete medium with $IE\alpha_{52-68}$ peptide (10 μg/well). After 24 h, collect supernatants, remove cells by centrifugation, and add to the cell-free supernatants protease inhibitor cocktail. Aliquot supernatants in small volumes to avoid repeat thawing and freezing. Keep supernatants at −80 °C until samples are assessed by ELISA.

4 Notes

1. Male C57Bl/6 mice (8–12 weeks) provide nearly twice as many BM cells as BALB/c mice. The recovery of BM cells decreases with older mice. Two B6 mice will generate approximately six 75 cm^2 flasks of BMDCs. It is easier to clean the bones from the soft tissues when the bones are still in place at the hip joint than when they are free in the Petri dish.
2. For those experiments that require BM-DCs for the assessment of their surface phenotype, cytokine secretion, or T-cell allostimulatory function, control and VD_3-treated BM-DCs can be generated in 6-well plates instead of 75 cm^2 flasks, to minimize the amount of expensive reagents needed to generate the DCs (i.e., DC1-maturation cocktail, CD40 Ab). We recommend plating 10^6 BM cells in 4 ml of complete medium with GM-CSF + IL-4 per well of a 6-well plate on day 0. On days 2, 4, and 6 replace 3 ml of medium with fresh cytokines $\pm$ VD_3. Do not transfer floating BM-DCs generated in a 75 cm^2 flask into 6-well plates, since this mechanical procedure alters the stage of maturation of the BM-DCs.
3. MLCs require close contact between stimulatory and responder cells, which is achieved in round-bottom (or V bottom) wells. For that reason, flat-bottom wells are not recommended.
4. Alternatively, the T-cell allostimulatory function of the DCs can be assessed in CFSE-MLCs, using as responders CFSE-labeled (7.5 μM) splenic T cells in 96-well round-bottom plates.

   For CFSE-labeling of T cells refer to **step 3** of Subheading 3.3.3. For CFSE-MLCs, the stimulator and responders are in general mixed at a single APC:T cell ratio, that in this case is

1 DC:10 T cells per well. Prepare 1–2 rows of wells per condition tested, so you will end up with sufficient cells for labeling with Abs and analysis by FACS. Include as a control, a row of wells with CFSE-labeled T cells alone in medium supplemented with 2 U/ml of IL-2 (to keep T cells alive). In general, mouse CFSE-MLCs are harvested after *5 days*. The cells from the replicate wells of each condition tested are pooled in FACS tubes, rinsed with ice-cold PBS + 10 mM EDTA to disaggregate cell clusters, and labeled with fluorochrome-conjugated CD3 Ab alone, or in combination with CD4 or CD8 Abs. Dead cells are excluded by labeling with annexin-V and/or by their FSC^{low} vs. SSC^{high} profile by flow cytometric analysis. CFSE dilution in $CD3^{+}$ T cells is analyzed by flow cytometry.

5. A percentage of the injected donor-derived (BALB/c) MR-DCs are killed by recipient's (B6) NK cells. Thus, treatment of the host animal with the NK-depleting antibody NK1.1 (clone PK136, 200 μg, i.p, 1 day before DC administration) augments the quantity of BALB/c DNA detected by PCR and demonstrates whether the injected DCs are targeted by NK cells when using a different donor-host/recipient strain combination.
6. The yield of lymphocytes obtained from $Rag1^{-/-}$ mice is much lower than that from $Rag1^{+}$ animals. After the CD4 purification and CFSE-labeling, approximately 3×10^{6} CFSE-labeled 1H3.1 splenocytes are obtained per $Rag1^{-/-}$ 1H3.1 mouse (8–12 weeks old).
7. After the FACS-analysis, the absolute number of 1H3.1 T cells per spleen is calculated by multiplying the percentage of $Thy1.1^{+}$ $CD4^{+}$ cells in the sample by the absolute number of splenocytes. The rest of the variables of the 1H3.1 T cells are analyzed on the cells within the $Thy1.1^{+}$ $CD4^{+}$ gate (at least collect $2–3 \times 10^{3}$ cells in the $Thy1.1^{+}$ $CD4^{+}$ gate).

Acknowledgments

We thank the comments of the Research Specialist William J. Shufesky (Univ. of Pittsburgh, Pittsburgh, PA, USA).

References

1. Banchereau J, Briere F, Caux C et al (2000) Immunobiology of dendritic cells. Annu Rev Immunol 18:767–811
2. Banchereau J, Steinman RM (1998) Dendritic cells and the control of immunity. Nature 392:245–252
3. Cella M, Sallusto F, Lanzavecchia A (1997) Origin, maturation and antigen presenting function of dendritic cells. Curr Opin Immunol 9:10–16
4. Steinman RM, Hawiger D, Nussenzweig MC (2003) Tolerogenic dendritic cells. Annu Rev Immunol 21:685–711

5. Steinman RM, Nussenzweig MC (2002) Avoiding horror autotoxicus: the importance of dendritic cells in peripheral T cell tolerance. Proc Natl Acad Sci U S A 99:351–358
6. Schwartz RH (1990) A cell culture model for T lymphocyte clonal anergy. Science 248:1349–1356
7. Morelli AE, Thomson AW (2007) Tolerogenic dendritic cells and the quest for transplant tolerance. Nat Rev Immunol 7:610–621
8. Griffin MD, Xing N, Kumar R (2003) Vitamin D and its analogs as regulators of immune activation and antigen presentation. Annu Rev Nutr 23:117–145
9. Lemire JM (1995) Immunomodulatory actions of 1,25-dihydroxyvitamin D3. J Steroid Biochem Mol Biol 53:599–602
10. Rigby WF (1988) The immunobiology of vitamin D. Immunol Today 9:54–58
11. Penna G, Adorini L (2000) 1 Alpha,25-dihydroxyvitamin D3 inhibits differentiation, maturation, activation, and survival of dendritic cell leading to impaired alloreactive T cell activation. J Immunol 164:2405–2411
12. Yates SF, Paterson AM, Nolan KF et al (2007) Induction of regulatory T cells and dominant tolerance by dendritic cells incapable of full activation. J Immunol 179:967–976
13. Piemonti L, Monti P, Sironi M et al (2000) Vitamin D3 affects differentiation, maturation, and function of human monocyte-derived dendritic cells. J Immunol 164:4443–4451
14. Griffin MD, Lutz W, Phan VA et al (2001) Dendritic cell modulation by 1alpha,25 dihydroxyvitamin D3 and its analogs: a vitamin D receptor-dependent pathway that promotes a persistent state of immaturity in vitro and in vivo. Proc Natl Acad Sci U S A 98:6800–6805
15. Divito SJ, Wang Z, Shufesky WJ et al (2010) Endogenous dendritic cells mediate the effects of intravenously injected therapeutic immunosuppressive dendritic cells in transplantation. Blood 116:2694–2705
16. Tiffany LJ, Garcia-Ojeda PA, Stein KE (1999) Determination of the IgG2a allotype of CXB recombinant inbred mouse strains by a PCR-based method. Immunogenetics 50:71–73
17. Wang Z, Larregina AT, Shufesky WJ et al (2006) Use of the inhibitory effect of apoptotic cells on dendritic cells for graft survival via T-cell deletion and regulatory T cells. Am J Transplant 6:1297–1311
18. Wang Z, Divito SJ, Shufesky WJ et al (2012) Dendritic cell therapies in transplantation revisited: deletion of recipient DCs deters the effect of therapeutic DCs. Am J Transplant 12:1398–1408

Part V

The Breakdown of Immunological Tolerance in Disease

Chapter 14

Luminex-Coupled EliFACS: A Multiparametric Method to Enumerate and Functionally Characterize Antigen-Specific T cells in Human Peripheral Blood

HuiJuan Lv, Khadir Raddassi, and Myra A. Lipes

Abstract

We describe a Luminex-coupled EliFACS assay that integrates multiplexing technology, enzyme-linked immunospot (ELISPOT), and intracellular cytokine FACS staining for the detection of multiple parameters of antigen-specific T-cell activation in human peripheral blood. Although our protocol is for measuring T-cell responses against cardiac myosin heavy chain and myelin basic protein, the major autoantigens in myocarditis and multiple sclerosis, respectively, these methods could be used for the detection of T-cell responses to other antigens, including foreign antigens.

Key words Human T-cell assay, Peripheral blood mononuclear cells, Autoimmune disease, ELISPOT assay

1 Introduction

Although T cells are the primary mediators of numerous human autoimmune diseases, the presence of autoreactive T cells in peripheral blood is not routinely assessed. Challenges include the lack of knowledge regarding pathologically relevant T-cell autoantigens, the lack of robust assays to detect low-frequency autoreactive T cells in peripheral blood, and the need for relatively large sample volumes [1]. In addition, traditional T-cell proliferation assays based on [^{3}H]thymidine incorporation are limited in the ability to detect specific autoreactive T cells. Although ELISPOT assays are more sensitive, they provide limited information regarding individual cell subsets.

Here, we describe a Luminex-coupled EliFACS assay that integrates xMAP® (Multi-Analyte Panel) technology, ELISPOT, and intracellular cytokine FACS staining for the detection of multiple parameters of antigen-specific T-cell activation. Integrating advanced technologies including microspheres, Luminex has

Ashleigh S. Boyd (ed.), *Immunological Tolerance: Methods and Protocols*, Methods in Molecular Biology, vol. 1899,
https://doi.org/10.1007/978-1-4939-8938-6_14,

greatly expanded the capabilities of the traditional enzyme-linked immunosorbent assay (ELISA) in identifying and quantifying cytokines and chemokines produced by human blood mononuclear cells (PMBCs). Because the Luminex technology is capable of simultaneously measuring as many as 100 analytes in a single sample, it can offer a comprehensive view of cytokine responses of antigen-specific T cells. On the other hand, the ELISPOT assay allows the detection of the frequencies of cells secreting a given cytokine; while the FACS-based assay couples the phenotypical and functional detection of activated T cells by simultaneously staining for surface markers and intracellularly localized cytokines. Furthermore, labeling PBMCs with 5,6-carboxyfluorescein diacetate succinimidyl ester (CFSE) enables the visualization of antigen-specific proliferation of T cells.

Although our protocol is for measuring autoreactive T-cell responses against cardiac myosin heavy chain (MyHC) and myelin basic protein (MBP), the major autoantigens in myocarditis [2, 3] and multiple sclerosis (MS) [4], respectively, these methods could be used for the detection of T-cell responses to other antigens, including foreign antigens. In the protocol described here, we have chosen IFN-γ as the cytokine marker of T-cell activation in the ELISPOT assay because our previous studies have shown the predominant T helper 1 pro-inflammatory phenotype of CD4 T cell responses in myocarditis [3], but these assays could be modified for the detection of other cytokines.

2 Materials

2.1 Materials for Purifying Cardiac Myosin

1. Solutions: All reagents are available from Sigma-Aldrich. All solutions are sterilized by filtering through a 0.22 μm filter.
   (a) Solution I: 0.3 M KCl, 0.15 M K_2HPO_4, 0.01 M $Na_4P_2O_7$, 1 mM $MgCl_2$, pH 6.8.
   (b) Solution II: 0.3 M KCl, 0.01 M Imidazole, 5 mM $MgCl_2$, 5 mM Adenosine 5′-triphosphate disodium salt (Na_2ATP), pH 6.8.
   (c) Solution III: 0.3 M KCl, 0.01 M Imidazole, pH 6.8.
   (d) Solution IV: 50 mM $Na_4P_2O_7$, pH 7.4.
2. Water: Milli-Q water, autoclaved, stored at 4 °C.
3. 1,4-Dithiothreitol (DTT): Roche Diagnostics Cat# 10197777001.

   Make 1 M stock in water and store small aliquots at −20 °C.
4. Glycerol: Invitrogen, Cat# 15514-011.

5. Tubes for ultra-centrifugation: Beckman Coulter.

Polypropylene centrifuge tubes, Cat# 355642, 25 × 89 mm, 32 ml.
Polyallomer centrifuge tubes, Cat# 326819, 13 × 51 mm, 5 ml.

6. Homogenizers.
   (a) Electric: KINEMATICA, POLYTRON PT 1200 E.
   (b) Glass: Teflon glass homogenizer.
7. Bradford assay reagent: Bio-Rad, Cat# 500-0006.

2.2 Materials for Isolating and Handling Human PBMCs

1. Anticoagulant tubes: BD Vacutainer, green-top, Cat# 367880.
2. Dulbecco's Phosphate-Buffered Saline (DPBS), calcium- and magnesium-free: Corning Cellgro, Cat# 21-031.
3. Phosphate-Buffered Saline (PBS): Corning Cellgro, Cat# 21-040.
4. Lymphoprep: STEMCELL technologies, Cat# 07811.
5. Human AB serum: Gemini, Cat# 100-512.
6. Dimethyl Sulphoxide (DMSO): Sigma-Aldrich, Cat# D2650.
7. Cryovials: Thermo Scientific, Cat# 377267.
8. Cryo freezing container: Thermo Scientific, Cat# 5100-0001.

2.3 Materials for Human EliFACS Assay

1. Complete HL-1 medium (cHL-1) containing:

   HL-1 medium: Lonza, Cat# 77201.

   L-Glutamine (200 mM), diluted at 1/100: Life Technologies, Cat# 25030.

   Penicillin-Streptomysin (10,000 U/ml), diluted at 1/100: Life Technologies, Cat# 15140.

   MEM Non-Essential Amino Acids Solution (100×), diluted at 1/100: Life Technologies, Cat# 11140-050.

   HEPES (1 M), diluted at 1/100: Life Technologies, Cat# 15630.

   Sodium Pyruvate (100 mM), diluted at 1/100: Life Technologies, Cat# 11360.

2. CFSE: Life Technologies, Cat# C34554.

   Make CFSE stock at 25 μM by first dissolving 50 μg of CFSE in 36 μl of DMSO to obtain a 2.5 mM solution, which is further diluted for 100 times in HBSS. The 25 μM stock solution should be aliquoted and stored at −20 °C until use.
3. Recombinant human IL-7: R&D systems, Cat# 207-IL/CF.
4. MultiScreen filter plates: EMD Millipore, Cat# S2EM004M99.
5. Anti-human IFN-γ antibodies: BD ELISPOT human IFN-γ pair, BD Cat# 551873.

6. Anti-human CD3 (NA/LE): BD Pharmingen, Cat# 555329.
7. Anti-human CD28 (NA/LE): BD Pharmingen, Cat# 555725.
8. Tetanus Toxoid: Akorn, Cat# 17478-131-01 (stored at −80 °C).
9. Human myelin basic protein (MBP): Abcam, Cambridge, UK.
10. Multiple sclerosis peptides: Anaspec, Fremont, CA.
11. BSA: Sigma-Aldrich, Cat# 7906.
12. PBST: PBS containing 0.05% Tween-20.
13. 1% BSA/PBS: PBS containing 1% (w/v) BSA.
14. 1% BSA/PBST: PBS containing 1% (w/v) BSA and 0.05% Tween-20.
15. ExtrAvidin® Alkaline Phosphatase (ExtrAvidin® AP): Sigma-Aldrich, Cat# E2636.
16. BCIP/NBT Alkaline Phosphatase Substrate (BCIP/NBT): Sigma-Aldrich, Cat# B5655.
17. Plate Washer for 96-well plates or multichannel pipettes.
18. Incubator capable of 37 °C, 5% CO_2, and ≥90% humidity.
19. Luminex system: EMD Millipore Luminex® 200 or equivalent.
20. ELISPOT plate reader: C.T.L., ImmunoSpot® Analyzers.
21. Round bottom 96-well plates for cell culture: Corning Life Sciences, Cat# 3799.
22. Stimulation reagents for intracellular cytokine staining:

    Phorbol 12-myristate 13-acetate (PMA): Sigma-Aldrich, Cat# P8139.

    Make stock solution at 20 mM in DMSO, store at −20 °C.

    Ionomycin: Sigma-Aldrich, Cat# I0634.

    Make stock solution at 10 mg/ml in DMSO, store at −20 °C.
23. Protein transport inhibitor for intracellular cytokine staining:

    Monensin solution (GolgiStop): BD Pharmingen, Cat# 554724 or.

    Brefeldin A solution (GolgiPlug): BD Pharmingen, Cat# 555029.
24. Fixation/permeabilization solution for intracellular cytokine staining:

    BD Pharmingen, Cat# 554714.
25. FACS staining buffer: 1% BSA/PBS.
26. Human Fc Block: BD Pharmingen, Cat# 564220.

27. Fixable viability dye: Life Technologies, Cat# L-23102.

    Make the stock solution by adding 50 μl of DMSO to one vial of dye and mixing well by vortex. Aliquot this stock and store at −20 °C.

28. Antibodies for surface markers:

    Anti-human CD3/ APC-H7: Clone SK7, BD Pharmingen Cat# 560176.

    Anti-human CD4/BV650: Clone SK3, BD Pharmingen Cat# 563876.

    Anti-human CD25/PE: Clone M-A251, BD Pharmingen Cat# 555432.

29. Antibodies for intracellular cytokines.

    Anti-human IL-2 /AF700: Clone MQ1-17H12, Biolegend Cat# 500320.

    Anti-human IFN-γ/V500: Clone B27, BD Pharmingen Cat# 561980.

    Anti-human TNF-α/V450: Clone MAb11, BD Pharmingen Cat# 561311.

    Anti-human IL-17A/PerCP-Cy5.5: Clone N49-653, BD Pharmingen Cat# 560799.

    Anti-human IL-10/PE-Cy7: Clone JES3-9D7, Biolegend Cat# 501420.

    Anti-human IL-4/APC: Clone MP4-25D2, BD Pharmingen Cat# 554486.

30. Flow cytometer: BD LSRII or equivalent.
31. Software for data analysis: FlowJo or equivalent.

3 Methods

3.1 Antigen Preparation

Full-length human myelin basic protein is commercially available and MS peptides are custom-made. Because it is not feasible to efficiently produce recombinant full-length human MyHC in *E. coli*, we provide a method we commonly use to purify MyHC from human heart tissues [2, 3, 5]. This protocol is based on modification of the classic method of Shiverick and colleagues [6] which involves homogenization of heart tissue and successive rounds of precipitation-dissolution, and does not require chromatography. We typically obtain ~3 mg myosin/g human atrial tissue, and ~8 mg myosin/g human ventricle or human skeletal (soleus) muscle tissues.

1. Grind snap-frozen heart tissues (*see* **Notes 1** and **2**) to fine powder in a mortal precooled on dry ice. Transfer tissue powder into a 50 ml conical tube and weigh.
2. Add 10 ml/g tissue of ice-cold Solution I (*see* **Note 3**) containing 2 mM DTT to the tissue powder. Homogenize the tissue/Solution I mixture with an electric homogenizer for 30 s with 5-s intervals. Extract homogenate by stirring the mixture continuously on a magnetic stirrer for 1.5 h at 4 °C.
3. Transfer Solution I/tissue mixture to a 32 ml tube for ultracentrifugation (*see* Subheading 2) and remove the tissue debris by centrifuging at 12,000 × *g*. The supernatant is further centrifuged for 4 h at 140,000 × *g*, followed by diluting the second supernatant with 20 volumes of water and keeping it at 4 °C overnight to precipitate myosin. *This first precipitation-redissolution cycle removes sarcoplasmic proteins and MyHC becomes the major contractile protein component.*
4. The myosin containing fraction is collected by centrifuging at 12,000 × *g* and the pellets are redissolved in Solution II by homogenizing in a glass homogenizer. The homogenate is centrifuged at 43,000 × *g* for 30 min to remove actin. Myosin is precipitated again by diluting the supernatant with 8 volumes of water and settling at 4 °C for 3 h. *This second cycle removes troponin-tropomyosin.*
5. The enriched myosin containing fraction is collected by centrifuging at 12,000 × *g* and the pellets are redissolved in Solution III as in **step 4**. The homogenate is centrifuged at 43,000 × *g* for 30 min to remove actomyosin and smaller proteins. The supernatant is diluted with 6.5 volumes of water and allowed to stand at 4 °C for 1 h. The purified myosin pellet is collected by centrifugation at 12,000 × *g* for 10 min. Decant the supernatant and add 300–400 μl of Solution IV to dissolve the pellet (*see* **Note 4**).
6. Determine the concentration of myosin by Bradford assay and confirm the purity of myosin by electrophoresis with 10% SDS gels. Staining the SDS gels with Coomassie Blue should reveal a major ~220 kDa band corresponding to MyHC (Fig. 1, arrows).

3.2 Isolation of Human Peripheral Blood Mononuclear Cells (PBMCs)

PBMCs are isolated from whole blood (*see* **Note 5**) by Ficoll-density gradient centrifugation. Procedures in Subheadings 2.2 and 2.3 are performed in a sterile laminar flow hood at room temperature (RT) observing biosafety regulations and observing sterile techniques. All reagents are warmed to RT or 37 °C as indicated.

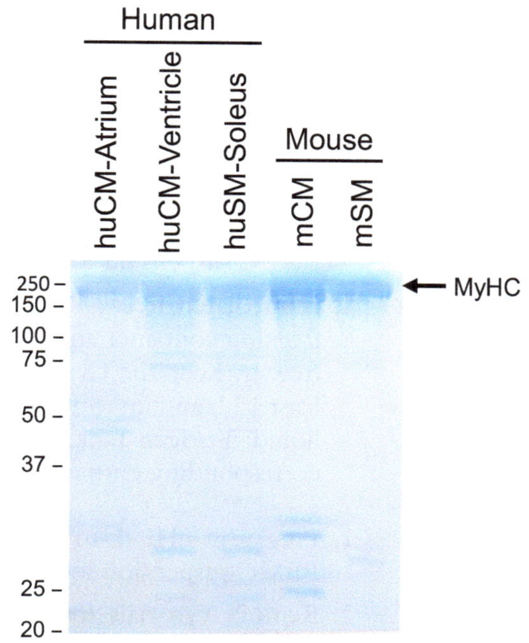

Fig. 1 Purified cardiac and skeletal myosin from human and control mouse tissues. Ten microgram of purified myosin was loaded on a 10% SDS-polyacrylamide gel and stained with Coomassie G-250. Myosin heavy chain (MyHC) is as indicated (arrow)

1. Collect human blood in anticoagulant tubes coated with lithium heparin. Dilute whole blood with an equal volume of DPBS.
2. Add up to 4 ml of Lymphoprep® to a 15 ml conical tube pretreated with serum (*see* **Note 6**). Gently overlay up to 8 ml of diluted blood onto the Lymphoprep® using a sterile serological pipette tilted at ~45 °C.
3. Centrifuge at 400 × *g* for 30 min at RT with the *brake off* to ensure that deceleration does not disrupt the density gradient.
4. Remove the upper layer without disturbing the interface. Harvest PBMCs residing on the interface in as little volume as possible into a fresh 15 ml conical tube.
5. Fill the tube with DPBS and gently invert the tube three times. Centrifuge at 200 × *g* for 15 min with the brake on. Resuspend PBMCs in 10 ml of DPBS and centrifuge as above.
6. Resuspend the washed PBMC pellet in 1–3 ml of DPBS and determine the cell count with a hemocytometer. If the T-cell assay is set up on the same day, aliquot the amount of cells needed and proceed to Subheading 3.4. Freeze down PBMCs that are not immediately used according to the procedures in Subheading 3.3.

3.3 Handling Frozen Human PBMCs

3.3.1 Cryopreserving PBMCs

1. Bring human AB serum to RT (*see* **Note 7**).
2. Pre-label cryovials with donor ID, total number of viable cells per vial, and date of cryopreservation. Create an entry for each PBMC sample with full information in an electronic log.
3. Resuspend each ten million PBMCs in 0.5 ml of 100% serum, followed by adding 0.5 ml of serum containing 20% DMSO drop-by-drop with gentle agitation of the tube. Aliquot 1 ml of PBMC suspension to a cryovial (*see* **Note 8**).
4. Immediately freeze PBMCs by placing cryovials into the Cryo freezing container and transferring the container to a −80 °C freezer. Keep the Cyro freezing container in the freezer for at least 12 h and up to 14 days before transferring cryovials to the liquid nitrogen tank. Record the location of samples to the corresponding entries in the electronic log.

3.3.2 Thawing PBMCs

1. Pre-warm cHL-1 to RT and aliquot 5 ml for each 1 ml of PBMC suspension into a conical centrifuge tube.
2. Remove cyrovials from liquid nitrogen tank to dry ice and quickly transfer vials to a 37 °C water bath (handle no more than two vials at a time). Gently shake floating vials until cells have just started to thaw but frozen cores can still be seen in vials (this should take not more than 2 min).
3. Immediately transfer cells by decanting the contents of the vials into 10% serum-containing cHL-1 medium and rinsing vials with 1 ml of medium. Gently shake the conical tube to completely thaw the frozen core.
4. Centrifuge at 200 × *g* for 10 min at RT. Resuspend cells in 1 ml of pre-warmed cHL-1 medium containing 5% human AB serum and perform a cell count.

3.4 Luminex-Coupled EliFACS Assay for a Three-Dimensional Detection of Cardiac Myosin-Specific Autoreactive T Cells

1. On day 1, prepare PBMCs either from fresh blood or by thawing a frozen batch as in Subheading 2.3, **item 2** (*see* **Note 9**). Resuspend the PBMC pellet in cHL-1 containing 5% human AB serum and count the cells.
2. Wash the aliquot of PBMCs that will be CFSE-labeled with HBSS once and resuspend the cell pellet at 5 × 10^6/ml in DPBS. All the steps afterward should be performed with minimal exposure to bright light.
3. Add 40 μl of CFSE stock solution to every 1 ml of PBMC suspension in DPBS. Incubate at 37 °C for 7 min.
4. Immediately add 0.1 ml/ml PBMC suspension of human AB serum at the end of the 7 min incubation. Spin down the cells at 200 × *g* for 10 min.
5. Resuspend the cell pellet in cHL-1 containing 5% human AB serum and adjust the cell density to 4 × 10^6 ml^{-1}. Aliquot 0.25 ml of PBMC suspension to a 15 ml conical tube.

6. Prepare twofold myosin solutions in cHL-1 containing 5% human AB serum to reach final concentrations ranging from 0 to 100 μg/ml. Human IL-7 is also added to reach the final concentration of 5 ng/ml. Dispense 0.25 ml of each myosin solution to the corresponding conical tube containing 1×10^6 PBMCs (**step 2**). Gently shake the tube and carefully loosen the cap. Place all the tubes up-straight in a rack and incubate the PBMC cultures in a 37 °C incubator supplied with 5% CO_2 and 98% humidity for 48 h. It is important to include the proper negative and positive controls in the experimental design (*see* **Note 10**).
7. On day 2, coat each MultiScreen filter well with 100 μl of 4–10 μg/ml anti-human IFN-γ capture antibody diluted in PBS. Place the plates at 4 °C overnight.
8. On day 3, wash antibody-coated plates with PBS for three times and block the plates with 1% BSA/PBS (200 μl per well) at 37 °C for 1 h.
9. Meanwhile, remove the PBMC cultures from the incubator. For Luminex assay, carefully transfer 400 μl of culture supernatant to a pre-labeled Eppendorf tube without disturbing cells settled at the bottom of the conical tube (*see* **Note 11**). Add 1 ml of cHL-1 pre-warmed in 37 °C incubator to each conical tube and spin down cells at $200 \times g$ for 15 min. Carefully remove the supernatant with a pipette and gently resuspend the cell pellet in 300 μl of pre-warmed cHL-1 containing 5% human AB serum.
10. Remove the blocking buffer from the MultiScreen filter plates by flicking vigorously. Dispense a triplicate for each condition by adding 100 μl of PBMC suspension to each well.
11. Place the plates back to the incubator for another 16 h.
12. On day 4, carefully collect the cells from each well without touching the PVDF filter at the bottom of the well. Pool the cells from a triplicate for each condition into one round-bottomed well of a 96-well cell culture plate.
13. Centrifuge the plate at $200 \times g$ for 10 min. Remove the supernatant and add 200 μl of fresh cHL-1 containing 5% human AB serum. Place the plate in an incubator of 37 °C, >90% humidity, 5% CO_2 for 5 more days.
14. For the MultiScreen filter plate (*see* **Note 12**), lyse the residual PBMCs by washing each well with 250 μl of ice-cold water twice and keeping the plates on ice for 10 min after the second addition of water. Flick out the liquid and dry the plates on a stack of paper towels.
15. Wash the plates by filling the filter well with PBST and flicking out the liquid. Repeat for four times and dry the plate well on the paper towel after the last wash.

16. Dilute biotin-conjugated anti-human IFN-γ antibody (detection antibody) in 1% BSA/PBST at 2 μg/ml and dispense 100 μl to each well. Place the plates in a humidified 37 °C incubator for 2 h.
17. Wash the plates as in **step 15**.
18. Dilute ExtrAvidin® AP in 1% BSA/PBS at a volume ratio of 1:1000. Add 100 μl to each well and incubate the plates in a humidified 37 °C incubator for 2 h.
19. Wash the plates with PBST three times, followed by three washes with PBS. Meanwhile, dissolve the BCIP/NBT tablet in water (10 ml/tablet) by vigorous shaking. After the last wash, dry the plates well and add 100 μl of BCIP/NBT solution to each well. Incubate the plates at RT for 1–2 min and immediately rinse the plates with running tap water. After dry the plates on paper towel, leave them on bench overnight.
20. On day 5, enumerate spots of MultiScreen filter plates on ELISPOT plate reader (*see* **Note 13** for assay standardization).
21. One day 7, to each well of the cell culture plate, add PMA and ionomycin at 250 ng/ml (400 μM) and 50 ng/ml, respectively, together with GolgiStop (0.8 μl/well). Mix well by gently pipetting up-and-down. Place cells in the humidified 37 °C incubator for 4 h.
22. Centrifuge the plate at 200 × *g* for 10 min. Remove the supernatant and wash cells with 200 μl of DPBS (Note for V-shape plate).
23. Prepare the working solution of the fixable viability dye by adding 1 μl of DMSO stock solution to 4 ml of DPBS. Resuspend the cells from **step 22** with 150 μl of this working solution. Incubate the plate in the dark at RT for 20 min.
24. Add 100 μl of FACS staining buffer to each well and centrifuge at 200 × *g* for 10 min. Remove the supernatant by flicking out the liquid and briefly tapping wells on a stack of paper towel.
25. Prepare the antibody mix for surface markers at the pre-titrated dilution times, including Fc block, anti-CD3, anti-CD4, and anti-CD25. Resuspend the cells from **step 24** in 50 μl/well of the antibody mix. Incubate the plate in the dark at RT for 20 min.
26. Wash cells as in **step 24**.
27. Resuspend cells with 150 μl/well of fixation buffer (prepared as the manufacturer's instruction). Incubate the plate in the dark at RT for 20 min (alternatively, at 4 °C overnight).
28. Prepare the permeabilization buffer as the manufacturer's instruction. Add 100 μl/well of permeabilization buffer and centrifuge the plate at 500 × *g* for 4 min. Remove the

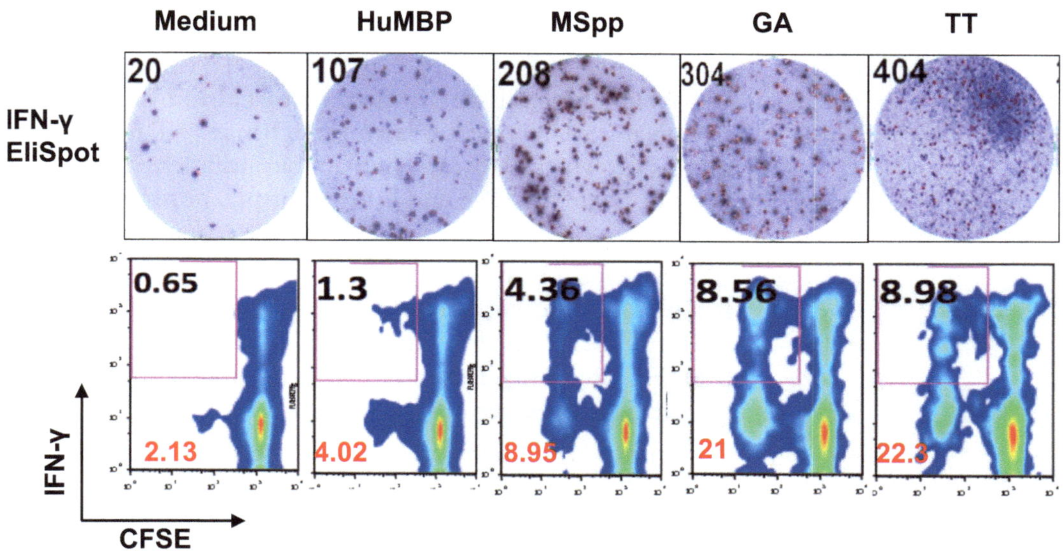

Fig. 2 EliFACS assay on a patient with multiple sclerosis. PBMCs were isolated from peripheral blood of a multiple sclerosis patient, counted, and labeled with CFSE. After washing, PBMCs were cultured for 42 h with medium alone, 1 μg/ml of whole human myelin basic protein (huMBP), 1 μg/ml of myelin peptides (MSpp = MBP14-33 + MBP111-129 + MBP145-164 + MOG1-20 + MOG35-55 + PLP139-154), 50 μg/ml of glatiramer acetate (GA) or 0.1 U/ml of tenanus toxoid (TT). After 42 h, cells were transferred to an ELISPOT plate to measure the secretion of IFN-γ. The cells were for 5 more days before staining them for viability, CD3 and CD4. After fixation and permeabilization, they were stained for IFN-γ (shown) and IL-10 and analyzed by flow cytometry for proliferation and cytokine production. *Top panel*: data represent the number of spots/ 300,000 cells. *Bottom panel:* gating was done on lymphocytes (with doublet discrimination), then CD3+CD4+. The graphs represent percent of dividing CD3+CD4+ (red numbers in bottom), the top numbers in the flow cytometry plots represent the percent of dividing CD3+CD4+ T cells producing IFN-γ

supernatant and wash the cell pellets with 200 μl/well permeabilization buffer.

29. Prepare the antibody mix for intracellular staining in the permeabilization buffer at the pre-titrated dilution times (1/400–1/100 depending on the antibody and the fluorochrome). Resuspend the washed cells in 50 μl/well of the antibody mix. Incubate the plate in the dark at RT for 20 min.
30. Wash cells with permeabilization buffer as **step 28**.
31. Resuspend each cell pellet in 200 μl (for 96-well plate format) or 500 μl (for tube format) of FACS staining buffer. Acquire events on a flow cytometer (*see* **Note 14**). At least 50,000 $CD3^{+}CD4^{+}$-gated events should be acquired for each sample.
32. Analysis is performed using FlowJo. *See* **Note 15** for data interpretation. Representative results are shown in Fig. 2.

4 Notes

1. We obtain human tissues, including heart atrium and ventricle, from National Disease Research Interchange (NDRI, Philadelphia, PA) which provides human biospecimens to research laboratories in the USA and Europe (http://ndriresource.org).
2. The human heart expresses two closely related isoforms of cardiac myosin heavy chain (MyHC)—alpha (α) and beta (β). β-MyHC is the major isoform expressed in ventricle and α-MyHC is restricted to atrial tissue. Therefore, α-MyHC and β-MyHC are purified from human atrial and ventricular heart muscle tissue, respectively.
3. The entire myosin purification procedure should be performed on ice.
4. The myosin pellet is gel-like and can be soaked in Solution IV overnight. On the next day, gently pipette up and down the softened pellets in order to completely dissolve myosin. For long term storage, add an equal volume of 100% glycerol to the myosin solution and store at −80 °C.
5. Human PBMCs are obtained after informed consent under Institutional Review Board (IRB) or Ethics Committee-approved protocols. Written informed consent should be received prior to inclusion in these studies. Biorepositories of PBMCs from clinically well-characterized subjects obtained during clinical trials are also becoming available.
6. The height ratio of Lympoprep®: blood should be maintained at approximate 4:5. 50-ml conical tubes can be used for larger volumes of blood. We find that pre-treating polypropylene tubes with serum can minimize the disturbance of the gradient interface when layering discontinuous gradients. Add 2 ml of serum to 15 ml conical tubes and swirl to coat the inner surface of the tube. Recycle the serum and aspirate the residual.
7. For freezing human PBMCs, the use of serum at RT can increase the recovery rate and the functionality of the thawed cells [7].
8. To save costs, PBMCs can be cryopreserved at up to 30 million cells/ml and aliquoted at 5–10 million cells/cryovial. On the other hand, using fetal bovine serum (FBS) (instead of human AB serum) to cryopreserve human PBMCs often results in high background of cell signals, reducing the sensitivity of the assay. However a particular "lot" of FBS could be used if it is pre-tested and found to be equivalent to human AB serum.
9. Cryopreservation does not noticeably compromise the ability of human PBMCs to function in ELISPOT assays [8].

10. It is important to include in the experimental design a negative control, e.g., cells stimulated with stimulus diluents (e.g., DMSO); and a positive control, e.g., cells stimulated with plate-bound anti-CD3/anti-CD28. Tetanus toxoid can be used as positive control for antigen processing and presenting.
11. Luminex assays are normally performed on specialized instruments by trained technicians. The cytokine/chemokine panels can either be pre-made or customized by companies such as EMD Millipore, Bio-Rad, Affymetrix, etc., with which the Luminex company (www.luminexcorp.com) has partnered to manufacture their xMAP® technology-based immunoassay products. We have had successful experience with the 41-analyte cytokine/chemokine panel (EMD Millipore) using as little as 25 μl of supernatants from human PBMC cultures. Besides offering the advantages of simultaneous measurement of multiple cytokines/chemokines, high-throughput (96- and 384-well formats) and low sample volume, Luminex assays are capable of measuring cytokine concentrations in a much wider range than ELISA, with excellent accuracy.
12. For Methods Subheading 2.3, **items 1–14** and **22** should be carried out aseptically in a laminar flow hood, while **items 15–21** and **23–32** can be moved to bench area.
13. Standardization and validation of ELISPOT assays:

    To standardize ELISPOT assay for all experiments, there should be at least two types of controls. (a) For each run, a blank ELISPOT well should be set up with medium and reagents (especially serum) but without PBMCs. Another control should be PBMCs from healthy donors stimulated with anti-CD3/anti-CD28. This will serve to monitor and correct the performance of the tested samples against known standards. Whenever possible the PBMCs should be prepared from a leukopak and cryopreserved in five million or ten million aliquots. For each run, one aliquot is thawed and treated the same way as the other samples to serve as an internal control. (b) Before or at the first run, an ELISPOT calibration plate should be either purchased or prepared with blank wells and reference cells stimulated with various doses of anti-CD3/anti-CD28. This plate after development should be kept in a box in the dark, dry, and dust-free environment. This plate will serve to calibrate the reader before and at the end of each use to check for an eventual drift of the initial calibration values. The reader should be set at 0 spots for blank well and the original number of spots for the reference wells. This setting should be kept as much as possible unchanged along the duration of the study.

14. The flow cytometer should be calibrated using CS&T beads (BD Bioscience) every day or every time it is turned on. Optimization of the noise to signal should be performed using the application setting. Compensation should be performed using OneComp eBeads® (eBioscience) with the same antibody lot and concentration used to stain the samples, except for autofluorescence, CFSE and the fixable viability dye where respectively, unstained cells, cells stained with CFSE alone and cells stained with viability dye alone are used.
15. Since distinct human leukocyte antigen (HLA) class II alleles can determine the presence or absence as well as the magnitude of T-cell responses to a given autoantigen, we routinely perform HLA genotyping of all study subjects and controls on DR and DQ loci [2], and healthy controls are selected for expression of at least one matched HLA allele. HLA typing can be performed with kits (e.g., Invitrogen) [2], but this procedure can also be outsourced [e.g., Proimmune (Oxford, UK), Quest Diagnostics (Madison, NJ, USA) or for type 1 diabetes or celiac disease-related studies, HLA Core Laboratory (Barbara Davis Center for Childhood Diabetes, Aurora, CO, USA)].

References

1. Roep BO et al (2012) The problems and promises of research into human immunology and autoimmune disease. Nat Med 18(1):48–53
2. Gottumukkala RV et al (2012) Myocardial infarction triggers chronic cardiac autoimmunity in type 1 diabetes. Sci Transl Med 4 (138):138ra80
3. Lv H et al (2011) Impaired thymic tolerance to alpha-myosin directs autoimmunity to the heart in mice and humans. J Clin Invest 121 (4):1561–1573
4. Wucherpfennig KW et al (1997) Recognition of the immunodominant myelin basic protein peptide by autoantibodies and HLA-DR2-restricted T cell clones from multiple sclerosis patients. Identity of key contact residues in the B-cell and T-cell epitopes. J Clin Invest 100 (5):1114–1122
5. Taylor JA et al (2004) A spontaneous model for autoimmune myocarditis using the human MHC molecule HLA-DQ8. J Immunol 172 (4):2651–2658
6. Shiverick KT, Thomas LL, Alpert NR (1975) Purification of cardiac myosin. Application to hypertrophied myocardium. Biochim Biophys Acta 393(1):124–133
7. Kreher CR et al (2003) CD4+ and CD8+ cells in cryopreserved human PBMC maintain full functionality in cytokine ELISPOT assays. J Immunol Methods 278(1–2):79–93
8. Janetzki S et al (2005) Standardization and validation issues of the ELISPOT assay. Methods Mol Biol 302:51–86

Chapter 15

Clinical and Functional Evaluation of Ocular Inflammatory Disease Using the Model of Experimental Autoimmune Uveitis

Jun Chen and Rachel R. Caspi

Abstract

Non-infections uveitis in humans is an autoimmune disease of the retina and uvea that can be blinding if untreated. Its laboratory equivalent is experimental autoimmune uveitis (EAU) induced in susceptible rodents by immunization with retinal antigens and described elsewhere in this series (Agarwal et al., Methods Mol Biol, 900:443–469, 2012). Evaluation and quantitation of the disease is usually performed by fundus examination and/or histopathology, which provide limited information on structural and no information on functional changes as disease progresses. Here, we describe methods for systematic evaluation of disease using noninvasive clinical assessments by fundus examination and photography, optical coherence tomography, and functional evaluation by electroretinography, which are then compared to histopathology. Using these methodologies, we demonstrate that clinical variants of disease can be accurately evaluated both clinically and functionally, facilitating longitudinal follow-up and providing information that cannot be obtained by fundoscopy and histology alone. These methodologies can be useful to obtain additional information and to evaluate effects of therapeutic modalities under investigation.

Key words Uveitis, EAU, Autoimmunity, T cells, Tolerance, IRBP, S-Ag, Mouse, Optical coherence tomography, Fundoscopy, Histology, Electroretinography

1 Introduction

The eye is known as an immunologically privileged organ. Immune privilege protects the delicate ocular structures from damage resulting from exposure to environmental inflammatory insults [1]. Research into the nature of immune privilege has revealed its highly complex character, which is still not fully understood and continues to be studied. Multiple mechanisms are involved: (1) physical barriers: an efficient blood-retinal barrier and lack of efferent lymphatics prevent free movement of cells and even larger molecules into and out of the globe [1]; (2) the expression of immunosuppressive factors in ocular fluids and on ocular resident cells can be inhibitory to activation and function of inflammatory

Ashleigh S. Boyd (ed.), *Immunological Tolerance: Methods and Protocols*, Methods in Molecular Biology, vol. 1899, https://doi.org/10.1007/978-1-4939-8938-6_15,

leukocytes and can promote induction of T regulatory cells in the ocular microenvironment [2–6]; (3) induction of regulatory immunity to retinal antigens at the systemic levels, including the phenomenon known as anterior chamber immune deviation (ACAID) and post-recover tolerance [3, 7, 8]. However, separation from the immune system also impedes efficient induction of peripheral tolerance to eye-specific antigens. In addition, we recently found that retina-specific cells activated outside the eye are relatively resistant to the inhibitory effects of the ocular microenvironment, which may help to explain why, despite immune privilege, the eye is subject to destructive autoimmunity manifesting as uveitis [5, 6, 9].

Uveitis is a group of potentially blinding inflammatory diseases that result in the destruction of the light-sensitive photoreceptor cells of the retina [10]. Patients have responses to unique retinal antigens, and these responses are felt to be involved in driving their disease. To better understand disease mechanisms, animal models of uveitis have been developed (reviewed in ref. 11). The model of experimental autoimmune uveitis (EAU) has been described in an earlier issue of this series [12]. The murine model of EAU has been particularly useful, permitting to dissect basic mechanisms as well as serving as a template for translational therapies. The B10.RIII mouse strain is the most susceptible strain known. Briefly, disease is induced in these mice by immunization with IRBP or its peptides in the absence of pertussis toxin, of which the most frequently used is $IRBP_{161-180}$, sequence SGIPYIISYLHPGNTILHVD [12]. Less than 10 μg of this peptide induces severe uveitis in B10.RIII mice. The typical histological appearance of EAU resembles that of human uveitis, with inflammatory infiltrates in the vitreous, retina, and choroid and damage to the photoreceptor cell layer (Fig. 1).

To better use the EAU model for clinical studies, an accurate and convenient method of longitudinal evaluation is needed which must, moreover, be noninvasive, so as not to affect disease development and progression. The approaches routinely used in most laboratories consist of clinical scoring by standard fundoscopy and digital fundus imaging, with occasional confirmation by histopathology. Although fundus examination provides an in vivo way to clinically assess the disease severity, the information obtained is incomplete as to cellular infiltrates in the vitreous cavity, retinal thickness, the anatomic location of the lesions in the retina, which are all important quantitative indicators of disease severity, and gives no information on visual function. In addition, comparison of results from different laboratories can be difficult, since clinical grading is subjective and scoring criteria can vary among research groups. To close these gaps, we describe here additional methods that can be used to document and evaluate and quantitate clinical disease using objective measurements.

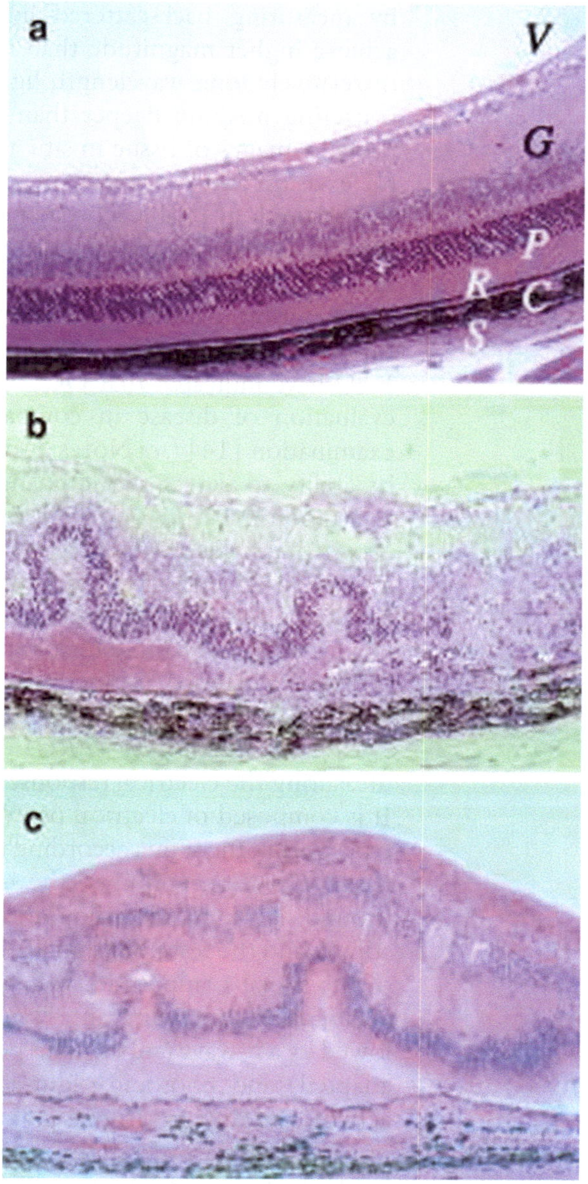

Fig. 1 Histopathology of mouse EAU compared with human uveitis. Eyes were collected from B10.RIII mice before (**a**) and 21 days after uveitogenic immunization with IRBP (**b**). Note disorganized retinal architecture and damage to ganglion and photoreceptor cell layers, retinal folds, subretinal hemorrhage, vasculitis, focal damage to the retinal pigment epithelium, and choroiditis. Uveitis in the patient with ocular sarcoidosis (**c**). Note gross similarity in pathological picture between **b** and **c** (Photographs provided by Dr. Chi-Chao Chan, Laboratory of Immunology, National Eye Institute) (Reprinted from ref. 9)

Optical coherence tomography (OCT) is a relatively new method of biomedical optical imaging. It performs micrometer-resolution, three-dimensional imaging of microstructure in biological systems by measuring backscattered light. Image resolutions of OCT achieve higher magnitude than conventional ultrasound. The use of relatively long wavelength light allows it to penetrate into the scattering medium deeper than confocal microscope [13]. OCT provide images of tissue in situ and in real time, without the need for excision and processing of specimens. The unique features of this technology enable a broad range of research and clinical applications. Up to now, OCT has been useful for serial observation of different retinal diseases in patients, e.g., age-related macular degeneration, glaucoma, posterior uveitis, and birdshot chorioretinopathy [14–21]. Our previous studies in the mouse model of EAU have indicated that OCT has distinct advantages for clinical evaluation of disease in comparison with conventional fundus examination [14] (*see* **Notes 1–6**). *First*, OCT is more sensitive in its ability to detect subtle changes (such as initiation of cellular infiltration from the optic nerve cup) during the onset of disease. *Second*, it is able to accurately measure retinal thickness, thus adding a valuable dimension to assessments of disease activity and retinal function. *Third*, it can discern retinal lesions. The cross-sectional images almost resemble histological images and assist in the diagnosis of posterior segment pathology at various time points [22, 23].

Electroretinography (ERG) is a well-accepted technology for measuring the electrical responses of various cell types in the retina. It is composed of electrical potentials contributed by different cell types within the retina according to the stimulus conditions, such as flash or pattern stimulus, the colors of the stimulus and background. During a recording, the eyes are exposed to standardized stimuli and the resulting signal is displayed showing the time course of the signal's amplitude (voltage). Sufficiently bright flashes will elicit ERGs containing an a-wave (initial negative deflection) followed by a b-wave (subsequent positive deflection). Scotopic (dark-adapted) and photopic (light-adapted) ERGs reflect retinal cell activities of different signal pathways. The dark-adapted response of ERG is primarily from the rod system, and ERGs performed on a light adapted eye reflect the activity of the cone system. Clinically, ERG is widely used by ophthalmologists for the diagnosis of various retinal diseases [24, 25].

2 Materials

2.1 Mice and Immunization for EAU

1. 6–8 weeks old B10.RIII mice (Jackson Laboratories, Bar Harbor, ME).
2. Emulsion of human $IRBP_{161-180}$ peptides in complete Freund's adjuvant (CFA; 1:1 v/v) (Difco, Detroit, MI) by sonication to provide 6–20 μg peptide in 0.2 ml emulsion per mouse.

3. EAU is induced in B10.RIII mice by subcutaneous injection of $IRBP_{161-180}$ peptides emulsified in CFA (Sigma, St. Louis, MO) as described in detail in another chapter in this series [12].

2.2 Anesthetics

1. Ketamine-Xylazine mixture (100 mg/kg body weight ketamine; 10 mg/kg body weight xylazine; i.p.) for systemic anesthesia.
2. Hypodermic needles (29 G).
3. 1 mL syringes.
4. 0.5% Alcaine drops for local anesthesia.
5. Ophthalmic dilating solutions: 1% Tropicamide (Alcon Laboratories, Inc., Fort Worth, TX) and 0.5% phenylephrine hydrochloride (Bausch & Lomb).

2.3 Fundoscopy

1. An optics fundus microscope using epi-illumination (reflective) light sources.
2. Glass coverslip.
3. Artificial tears (Systane Ultra, Alcon).

2.4 Fundus Photography

1. Micron II small animal in vivo retinal imaging system (Phoenix Research Laboratories, INC) (Fig. 2).
2. Phoenix StreamPix 5-Single Camera.

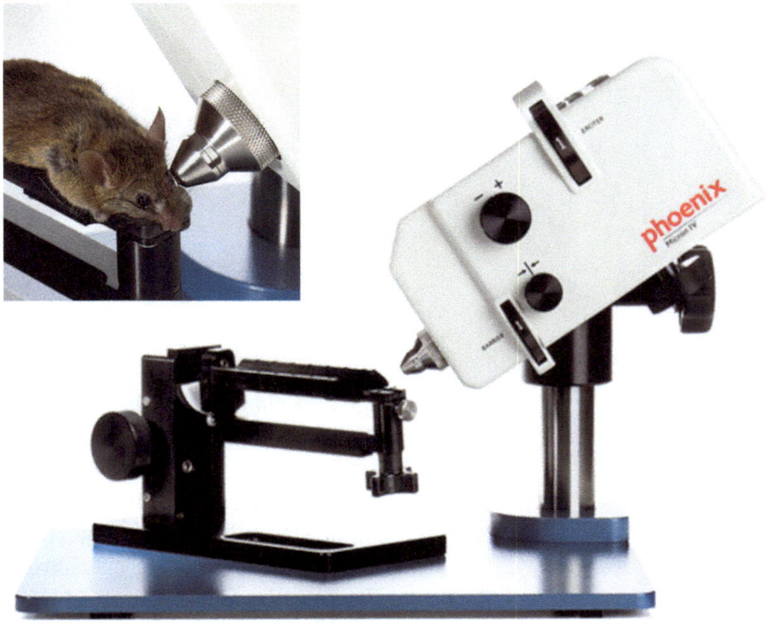

Fig. 2 Phoenix Micron II small animal retinal imaging system (Phoenix Research Laboratories, Inc). The apparatus is comprised of a base system that incorporates a host computer as well as a Phoenix StreamPix 5-Single camera and rodent imaging holder. Photographs are reproduced from the website of www.kellogg.umich.edu with permission

3. Phoenix StreamPix imaging program.
4. A host computer.
5. Rodent imaging table to adjust mouse posture for scanning.
6. Foot pad control.
7. Artificial tears (Systane Ultra, Alcon).

2.5 Spectral Domain Optical Coherence Tomography (SD-OCT)

1. Bioptigen Spectral Domain Ophthalmic Imaging System (Bioptigen Envisu R2200, North Carolina) (Fig. 3).
2. A host computer system.
3. 840 nm OCT engine with reference arm attachment.

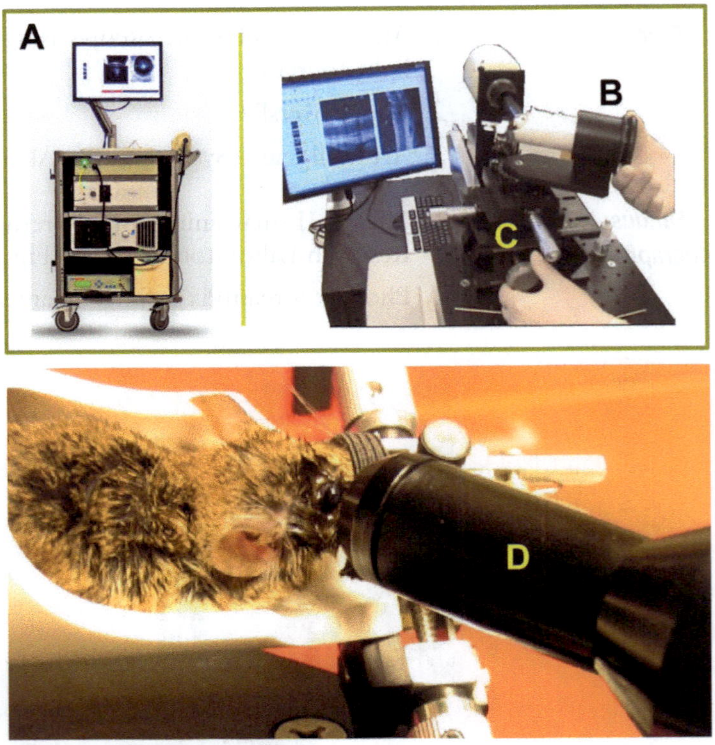

Fig. 3 Bioptigen Spectral Domain Ophthalmic Imaging System (Bioptigen, Inc., Durham, NC). The apparatus consists of a base system (**A**), an animal imaging mount (**B**), and rodent alignment stage (**C**), which houses a SD-OCT probe (**D**). The base system incorporates a host computer, 840 nm OCT engine with reference arm attachment, and the probe. The SD-OCT scanner is encased in the animal imaging mount, which allows forward and backward adjustment of the probe. The InVivoVue Clinic software enables the creation, display, loading, and saving of OCT image files. The rodent alignment system contains an X- (micrometer), Y- (scissor jack), and Z-translators along with stereotactic rotational cassette (for holding the mouse) within a bushing and platform base. The entire device is attached to a slit-lamp base. Photographs are reproduced from Bioptigen, Inc., with permission

4. SD-OCT probe (for cornea and retina).
5. Bioptigen InVivoVue Clinic software.
6. Bioptigen animal imaging mount.
7. Rodent alignment stage apparatus.
8. Aiming tip.
9. Cotton-tip applicator (Rush Dental & Medical Supply; Santa Monica, CA).
10. Surgical gauze pad (Allegro Medical).
11. Artificial tears.

2.6 Electroretinography (ERG)

1. Espion E2 ERG system (Diagnosys LLC) (Fig. 4).
2. A mouse table with animal temperature control (Diagnosys LLC).

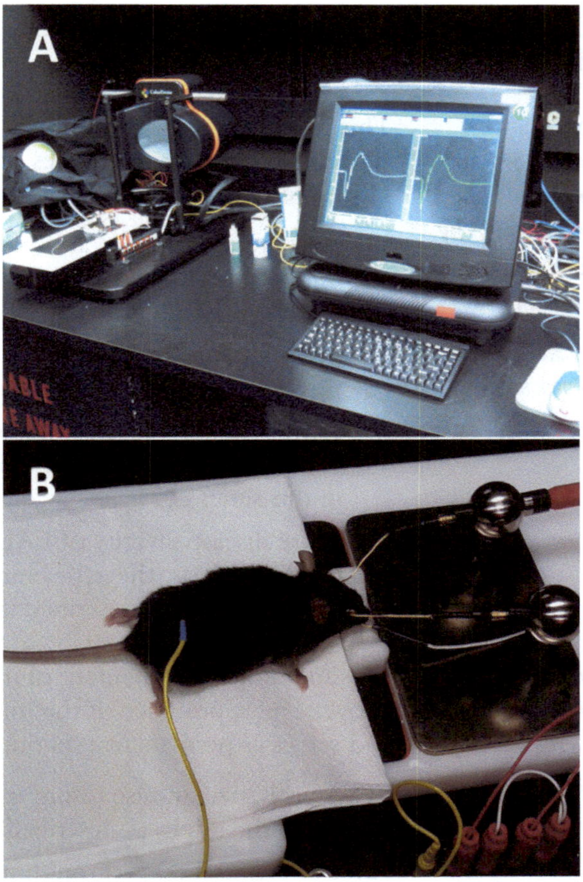

Fig. 4 Espion E2 ERG recording system (Diagnosys LLC). The device is composed of a base system that incorporates a touchscreen PC configuration as well as an ERG dome and mouse Table (**A**). Mouse is placed on an animal table and connected to electrodes for ERG recording (**B**)

3. Touchscreen PC configurations.
4. Espion software for protocol design and data analysis.
5. ERG dome.
6. ERG-electrodes.
7. Cotton-tip applicator (Rush Dental & Medical Supply; Santa Monica, CA).
8. Surgical gauze pad (AllegroMedical).
9. Artificial tears.

2.7 Histology

1. 4% glutaraldehyde in phosphate-buffered saline (PBS) (Fisher Scientific, Fair Lawn, NJ).
2. 10% neutral-buffered formalin (Sigma-Aldrich).
3. Methacrylate embedding compound.
4. Hematoxylin and eosin stain.

3 Methods

3.1 Clinical Manifestation of EAU in Mouse Models of Uveitis as Revealed by Fundus Examination and OCT Imaging

3.1.1 Clinical Evaluation of EAU by Fundoscopy

This method consists of visual inspection of the fundus. The observer assigns disease scores according to the number, size, and type of lesions observed through a binocular microscope.

1. Anesthetize mouse and dilate the pupils as described in Subheading 2.
2. Use artificial tears throughout the procedure to maintain corneal moisture and clarity.
3. Press cornea of the eye gently with a glass coverslip and perform the fundus examination using a fundus microscope. Details of the fundoscopy procedure are described elsewhere in this series [12].
4. Score disease severity of EAU semi-quantitatively on a scale of 0–4, based on the type, number, and size of retinal lesions using the criteria described in Table 1 and depicted in Fig. 5.

3.1.2 Clinical Evaluation of EAU by Fundus Photography

This method is a refinement of the visual inspection of the fundus, above. The appearance of the fundus is recorded photographically and serves as permanent experimental record (Fig. 5).

1. Anesthetize mouse using a ketamine/xylazine cocktail and dilate the pupils as described in Subheading 2.
2. Use artificial tears throughout the procedure to maintain corneal moisture and clarity.
3. Set up computer program.

Table 1
Clinical scoring criteria of EAU

Grade	Criteria for fundoscopy
0	Normal retina
0.5/ trace	Few (<3), small and focal lesions; minimal vasculitis and vitritis
1	Mild vasculitis; multiple, peripheral and focal lesions
2	Retinal edema; severe vasculitis (large size, thick wall, infiltrations); diffuse chorioretinal lesions and/or infiltrations; linear lesions
3	Retinal edema; pattern of linear lesions; large confluent chorioretinal lesions; subretinal hemorrhages
4	Large retinal detachment

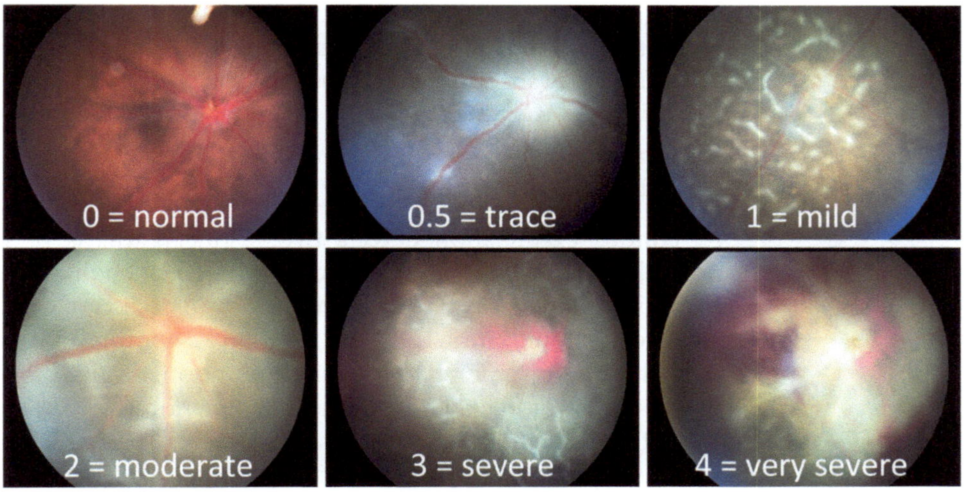

Fig. 5 Fundus images of EAU in B10.RIII mice. Eyes were photographed with a Micron II fundus imaging system during the acute phase of disease (day 13–21), showing a range of disease severity scores that parallel the histology scores in Fig. 7

4. Place mouse on an animal imaging table and position the eye toward camera lens to ensure the imaging is on the retina.
5. Visualize the retina through a digital camera during alignment, and obtain the image acquisition using the Micron II in vivo retinal imaging microscope (Phoenix Research Laboratories, INC).

3.1.3 SD-OCT Imaging for Evaluation of EAU

OCT provides visualization of lesions in the retina and choroid, as well as measurement of retinal edema (retinal thickness). These are important complements to photographic documentation of the retinal lesions.

1. Computer programing: set up reference arm as "1180" and SD-OCT probe for mouse retina.
2. Anesthetize mouse and dilate the pupils as described in Subheading 2.
3. Use artificial tears throughout the procedure to maintain corneal moisture and clarity.
4. Place mouse into an animal imaging mount, adjust the probe toward the eye.
5. Use the aiming tip, with cassette tongue, and aiming target for determining geometrical working distance for the optical lens bore to the mouse eye.
6. Use the rodent alignment system to position the eye to ensure that the incident OCT beam is perpendicular to the cornea of eye.
7. During alignment and centering, visualize the retina through a digital camera and obtain the image acquisition in line and rectangular scanning modes using the Bioptigen InVivoVue Clinic software that enables the creation, display, loading, and saving of OCT image files.
8. Analyze images of the retina using proprietary Bioptigen software.

Fundus examination detects two distinct patterns of EAU: monophasic and chronic (Fig. 6 and **Note** 7 [27]). Higher intensity immunization typically results in an acute form of disease with early onset post immunization (p.i.) and widespread photoreceptor damage, whereas lower intensity of immunization results in milder disease with prolonged and chronic inflammation [27, 28]. At the peak of disease (14 days p.i.), posterior uveitis (perivascular exudates, subretinal hemorrhage, and retinal folds) was associated with

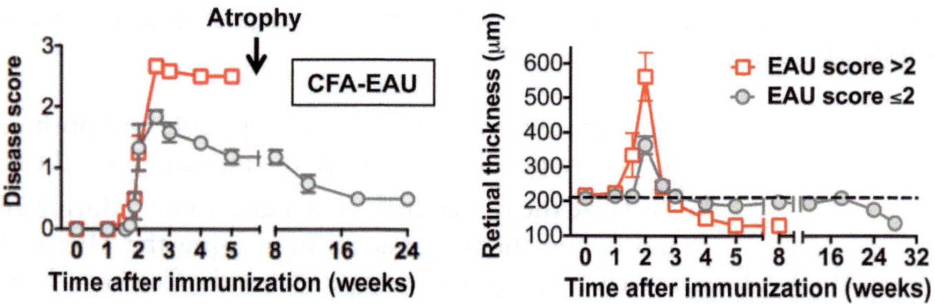

Fig. 6 Comparison of the clinical course and disease severity in monophasic vs. chronic EAU by fundus examination and OCT imaging. EAU was induced in B10.RIII mice by active immunization with $IRBP_{161-180}$ in adjuvant. Left panel, disease scores of EAU at different stages of disease were evaluated using an adapted fundus microscope. Right panel, B-scan OCT of the retina was evaluated at the indicated time points using a Bioptigen SD-OCT imaging system. Retinal thickness was measured and averaged from OCT images of the retina (adapted from ref. 27) (*See* **Note 7**)

a transient severe anterior uveitis (including signs of an irregular pupil, deposition of fibrin, opacification of the anterior chamber, as well as hemorrhages). The subsequent disease progression pattern of individual animals depended on the severity of the initial acute phase of retinal inflammation, with mice that developed severe disease (scores >2) manifesting a monophasic course followed by a rapid resolution of active inflammation around week 3 and retinal thinning (atrophy) around 4–5 weeks p.i. In contrast, animals that developed milder scores (<2) continued to show low-grade disease lasting for 5–6 months until retinal atrophy set in (Fig. 6). Thus, together with visual fundus examination and fundus photography, OCT provides an additional parameter of clinical course of EAU by measuring retinal thickness from cross-sectional OCT images. Retinal thickness that reflects disease activity correlated well with the course of disease in monophasic and chronic forms of EAU. Direct comparison of retinal and choroidal lesions seen by visual and OCT fundus examination is described ahead and compared to histology.

3.2 Anatomical Evaluation of EAU by Histopathology

1. Euthanize mice and confirm death by lack of heartbeat and respiration. Immediately enucleate and fix eyes, as post mortem deterioration of retinal tissue occurs rapidly. To enucleate, stretch the skin on the head by holding the ears so that the eyes bulge. Carefully pluck the eye out of its socket with a curved forceps.
2. Briefly, pre-fix enucleated globes in 4% glutaraldehyde (Fisher Scientific, Fair Lawn, NJ) for 1 h, then transfer to 10% neutral-buffered formalin (Sigma-Aldrich) for at least 12 h. Eyes can be kept in formalin for a long time.
3. The eyes are then dehydrated, embedded in methacrylate, sectioned through the pupillary-optic nerve axis, and stained with hematoxylin and eosin. Additional details on histology protocol are described elsewhere in this series [12].
4. The histology score of EAU is evaluated in a masked fashion on a scale of 0–4 based on the number, type, and size of lesions using the criteria described in Fig. 7 and Table 2 [12].

3.3 Side-by-Side Comparison of the Various Methods of Clinical Disease Evaluation and Histological Disease Evaluation in the Same Eye

Eye pathology in mouse models of uveitis was evaluated using noninvasive fundus imaging and SD-OCT imaging systems in comparison with histopathology examination (Fig. 8). As we reported previously [14] (*see* **Notes 1–6**), OCT imaging is a noninvasive reliable tool to distinguish retinal pathology in 3D view. In keeping with the fundus images of the same eye in mouse developing severe monophasic form of EAU (day 18 p.i.), horizontal-sections of OCT volume scan images captured eye lesions in multiple layers of the retina. Engorged blood vessels and peri-vascular exudates (green arrow) were visualized in ganglion cell and inner

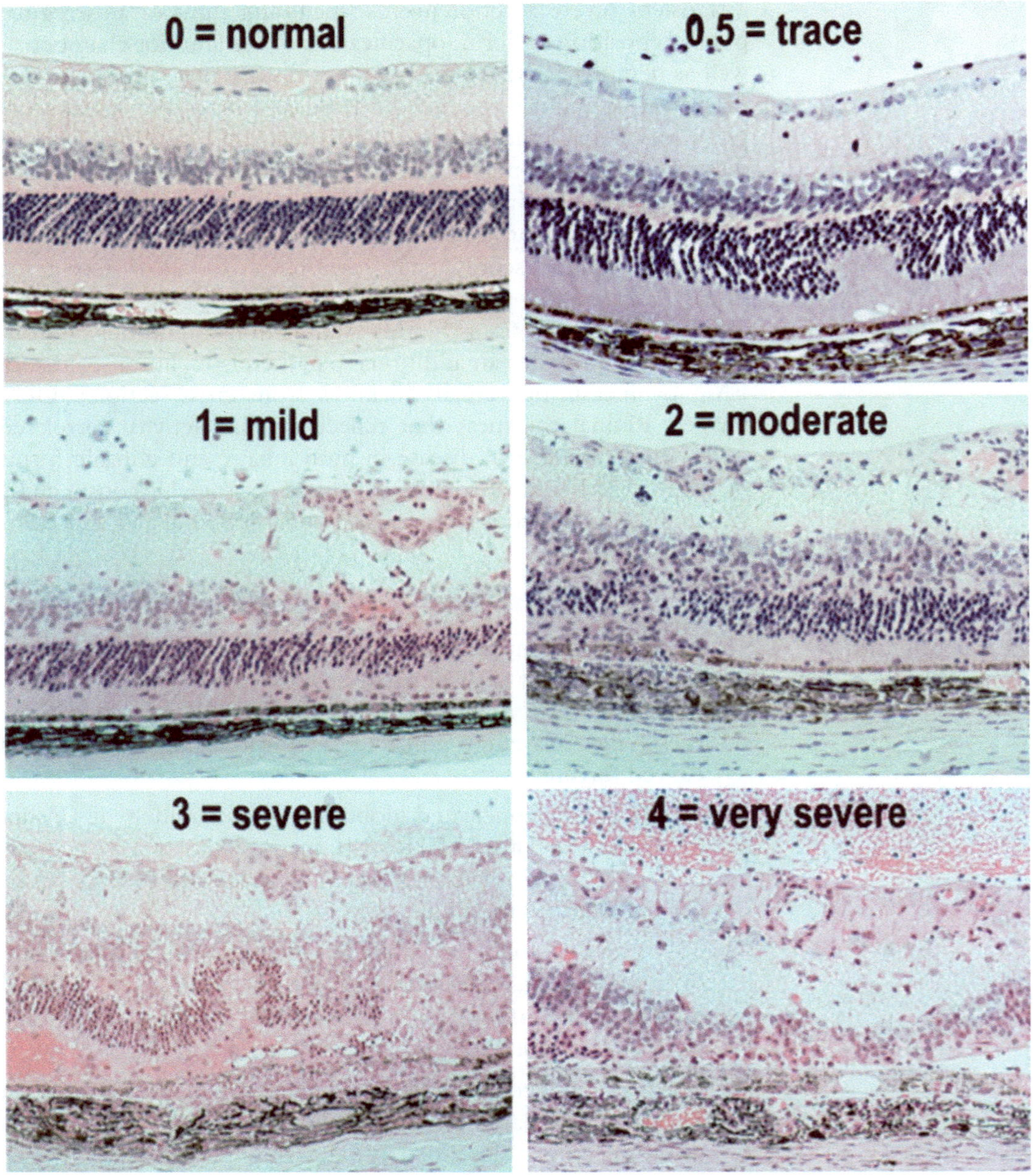

Fig. 7 Histopathology of EAU in the B10.RIII mouse. Eyes were collected from B10.RIII mice 21 days after uveitogenic immunization with IRBP, representing a range of disease scores (Figure is reprinted from ref. 26)

plexiform layers. Severe vitreal and subretinal hemorrhages (red arrow, dark area) in ganglion cell/inner plexiform layer as well as in inner/outer nuclear and IS/OS of photoreceptor layer recapitulated the pattern seen in the fundus image. Inflammation (yellow arrow) was also noted in RPE and choroid layers. Cross-sections of OCT B-scan images were parallel to histopathological findings, resolved the vitreal hemorrhage (red arrow) and cellular infiltrates (green arrow) observed by fundus imaging in the retina, and

Table 2
Histology scoring of EAU in the mouse

Grade	Criteria for histopathology
0	Normal retina structure
0.5/trace	Mild inflammatory cell infiltration. No tissue damage
1	Infiltration; retinal folds and focal retinal detachments; few small granulomas in choroid and retina, perivasculitis
2	Moderate infiltration; retinal folds, detachments and focal photoreceptor cell damage; small to medium sized granulomas, perivasculitis and vasculitis
3	Medium to heavy infiltration; extensive retinal folding with detachments, moderate photoreceptor cell damage; medium sized granulomatous lesions; subretinal neovascularization
4	Heavy infiltration; diffuse retinal detachment with serous exudate and subretinal bleeding; extensive photoreceptor cell damage; large granulomatous lesions; subretinal neovascularization

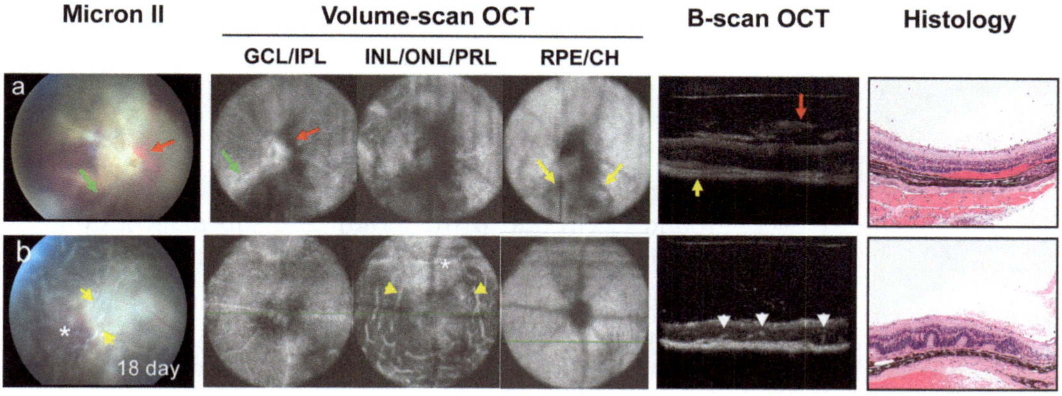

Fig. 8 Comparison of fundus photography, OCT, and histology for the evaluation of the acute/monophasic and the chronic forms of EAU. Retinal lesions were visualized using Micron-II fundus imaging and Bioptigen SD-OCT imaging systems, and followed by histological examination of (**a**) monophasic, and (**b**) chronic forms of EAU. Note all images are of the same eye. Note engorged blood vessels and peri-vascular exudates (green arrow) in ganglion cell layer (GCL) and inner plexiform layer (IPL), vitreal and subretinal hemorrhages (red arrow, dark area) visible in all retinal layers and corresponding to the same lesions in the fundus image and in OCT B-scan cross-sections and choroidal inflammation (yellow arrow) in retinal pigment epithelium (RPE) and choroid (CH) (Figure is modified from refs. 14, 27) (*See* **Notes 1–7**)

choroiditis (yellow arrow). In mice that developed a chronic form of EAU, OCT visualize focal lesions of the retina. Disease is characterized by multi-focal retinal folding (yellow arrow) in inner/outer nuclear and IS/OS of photoreceptor layer with less damage to PRL as compared to monophasic EAU. Thus, OCT imaging provided additional information that correlated well with the fundus and histological evaluation of EAU.

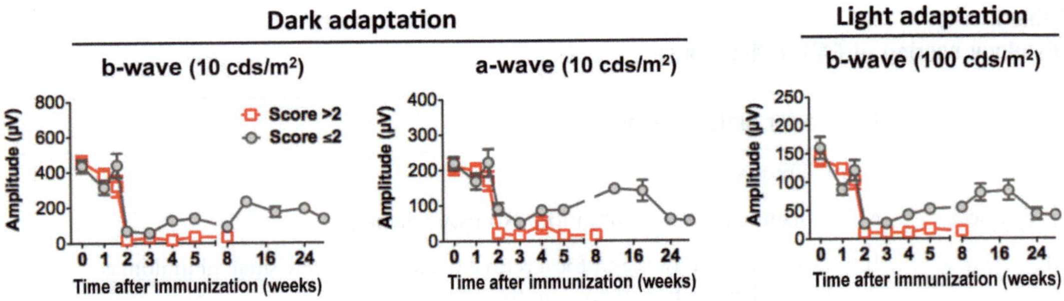

Fig. 9 Kinetics of dark- and light-adapted ERG responses in mouse model of EAU. Mice were monitored and followed up at the indicative time points by ERG. Amplitude of dark- and light-adapted ERGs was recorded and analyzed (adapted from ref. 27) (*See* **Note 7**)

3.4 Electroretinography for Evaluation of Retinal Function

Unlike all the procedures described above, which deal with various morphological and anatomical aspects of lesions characteristic of EAU, electroretinography (ERG) provides an evaluation of visual function by quantitating the response of the retina to the light signal.

1. Keep mouse in a dark room overnight (>12 h) for dark adaptation.
2. After anesthesia with a ketamine/xylazine cocktail (100/10 mg/kg), place mouse on a mouse table with animal temperature control inside an ERG dome of Espion E2 System (Diagnosys LLC).
3. Place electrodes on the central cornea, and attach reference and ground electrodes to the mouth and subcutaneously in the posterior neck-back region.
4. Record the dark-adapted ERG followed by the light-adapted ERG using Espion E2 System (Diagnosys LLC). Measure amplitude of ERG waveforms at a series of flash intensities.
5. Perform all procedures under dim red light.

Retinal function of mice with the different forms of EAU was evaluated using an ERG recording system in the same mice (depicted in Fig. 9), in which retinal lesions were measured by OCT imaging and fundus examination. We followed both scotopic (dark-adapted) and photopic (light-adapted) ERG responses during the course of disease. Although scotopic and photopic ERGs reflect retinal cell activities of different signal pathways, representing rod- and cone-mediated visual signals, reduction of ERGs in response to either dark or light adaptation exhibited in a similar pattern during inflammation. However, the pattern of ERG reduction differed between the monophasic and chronic forms of EAU.

The a-wave is produced by the photoreceptors, while the b-wave is produced by a mixture of cells including photoreceptors, bipolar, amacrine, and Müller retinal glial cells. During EAU, a sharp decline in both b-wave and a-wave amplitudes is measured in mice in both dark- and light-adapted conditions during the peak of inflammation (14 days p.i.). However, in the chronic form of EAU, disease resolution is followed by partial recovery of retinal function with ERGs that last 5–6 months and followed by a decline when retinal degeneration occurs. The pattern of ERG reduction seen in the chronic forms of uveitis correlates well with the reduction of the retinal thickness obtained by OCT (depicted in Fig. 6). Thus, retinal thickness using noninvasive OCT imaging appears to predict the change of retinal function during the course of EAU.

4 Notes

1. Good anesthesia, which completely prevents ocular movements and breathing artifacts, is key for performing noninvasive assessment such as fundus imaging and OCT in animals. Systemic as well as local anesthesia must be used.
2. Systemic anesthesia by injection of a ketamine/xylazine cocktail leads to cataract formation in mice within 20 min. This should be sufficient time to perform imaging, however, Avertin, which does not lead to cataract formation, may be a better substitute if prolonged imaging is required.
3. Adequate dilation of the pupil is important to obtain good quality imaging (such as fundoscopy, fundus photography, and OCT imaging). Sufficient time should be allowed for dilation to at least 6 mm.
4. Artificial tears must be applied both to the cornea through the procedure of fundoscopy and fundus imaging. Mice do not close their eyes when anesthetized. Application of artificial tears prevents corneal dehydration and opacification of the cornea due to keratitis, which could compromise subsequent imaging sessions.
5. It is also important to keep a clear and undisturbed cornea for OCT imaging. Prior to OCT scanning, additional artificial tears should be wrapped off gently from surface of the cornea using cotton-tip applicator.
6. During the peak of uveitis (around day 14 p.i.), opacification of visual media occurs due to heavy proteinaceous exudation and cellular infiltration in the anterior and posterior segments of the eye. This interferes with the OCT signal and its ability to clearly resolve retinal layers. OCT therefore shares the limitation of fundus imaging during this phase of disease.
7. For ERG recording, electrodes placed in the center of the cornea are held in place and conductivity ensured by application of artificial gels. Gels should be washed off from electrodes after the imaging session.

References

1. Streilein JW (2003) Ocular immune privilege: the eye takes a dim but practical view of immunity and inflammation. J Leukoc Biol 74:179–185
2. Caspi RR, Roberge FG, Nussenblatt RB (1987) Organ-resident, nonlymphoid cells suppress proliferation of autoimmune T-helper lymphocytes. Science 237:1029–1032
3. Stein-Streilein J (2008) Immune regulation and the eye. Trends Immunol 29:548–554
4. Taylor AW (2007) Ocular immunosuppressive microenvironment. Chem Immunol Allergy 92:71–85
5. Zhou R, Horai R, Silver PB, Mattapallil MJ, Zarate-Blades CR, Chong WP, Chen J, Rigden RC, Villasmil R, Caspi RR (2012) The living eye "disarms" uncommitted autoreactive T cells by converting them to Foxp3(+) regulatory cells following local antigen recognition. J Immunol 188:1742–1750
6. Zhou R, Horai R, Mattapallil MJ, Caspi RR (2011) A new look at immune privilege of the eye: dual role for the vision-related molecule retinoic acid. J Immunol 187:4170–4177
7. Stein-Streilein J, Streilein JW (2002) Anterior chamber associated immune deviation (ACAID): regulation, biological relevance, and implications for therapy. Int Rev Immunol 21:123–152
8. Kitaichi N, Namba K, Taylor AW (2005) Inducible immune regulation following autoimmune disease in the immune-privileged eye. J Leukoc Biol 77:496–502
9. Caspi RR (2006) Ocular autoimmunity: the price of privilege? Immunol Rev 213:23–35
10. Nussenblatt Rb WS (2004) Uveitis: fundamentals and clinical practice. Mosby (Elsevier), Philadelphia, PA
11. Caspi RR (2010) A look at autoimmunity and inflammation in the eye. J Clin Invest 120:3073–3083
12. Agarwal RK, Silver PB, Caspi RR (2012) Rodent models of experimental autoimmune uveitis. Methods Mol Biol 900:443–469
13. Fujimoto JG (2003) Optical coherence tomography for ultrahigh resolution in vivo imaging. Nat Biotechnol 21:1361–1367
14. Chen J, Qian H, Horai R, Chan CC, Caspi RR (2013) Use of optical coherence tomography and electroretinography to evaluate retinal pathology in a mouse model of autoimmune uveitis. PLoS One 8:e63904
15. Huang D, Swanson EA, Lin CP, Schuman JS, Stinson WG, Chang W, Hee MR, Flotte T, Gregory K, Puliafito CA, Et A (1991) Optical coherence tomography. Science 254:1178–1181
16. Toth CA, Narayan DG, Boppart SA, Hee MR, Fujimoto JG, Birngruber R, Cain CP, Dicarlo CD, Roach WP (1997) A comparison of retinal morphology viewed by optical coherence tomography and by light microscopy. Arch Ophthalmol 115:1425–1428
17. Drexler W, Morgner U, Ghanta RK, Kartner FX, Schuman JS, Fujimoto JG (2001) Ultrahigh-resolution ophthalmic optical coherence tomography. Nat Med 7:502–507
18. Gallagher MJ, Yilmaz T, Cervantes-Castaneda RA, Foster CS (2007) The characteristic features of optical coherence tomography in posterior uveitis. Br J Ophthalmol 91:1680–1685
19. Markomichelakis NN, Halkiadakis I, Pantelia E, Peponis V, Patelis A, Theodossiadis P, Theodossiadis G (2004) Patterns of macular edema in patients with uveitis: qualitative and quantitative assessment using optical coherence tomography. Ophthalmology 111:946–953
20. Van Velthoven ME, Ongkosuwito JV, Verbraak FD, Schlingemann RO, De Smet MD (2006) Combined en-face optical coherence tomography and confocal ophthalmoscopy findings in active multifocal and serpiginous chorioretinitis. Am J Ophthalmol 141:972–975
21. Chong GT, Lee RK (2012) Glaucoma versus red disease: imaging and glaucoma diagnosis. Curr Opin Ophthalmol 23:79–88
22. Alam S, Zawadzki RJ, Choi S, Gerth C, Park SS, Morse L, Werner JS (2006) Clinical application of rapid serial fourier-domain optical coherence tomography for macular imaging. Ophthalmology 113:1425–1431
23. Wojtkowski M, Srinivasan V, Fujimoto JG, Ko T, Schuman JS, Kowalczyk A, Duker JS (2005) Three-dimensional retinal imaging with high-speed ultrahigh-resolution optical coherence tomography. Ophthalmology 112:1734–1746
24. Vincent A, Robson AG, Holder GE (2013) Pathognomonic (diagnostic) ERGs. A review and update. Retina 33:5–12
25. Young B, Eggenberger E, Kaufman D (2012) Current electrophysiology in ophthalmology: a review. Curr Opin Ophthalmol 23:497–505
26. Cortes LM, Avichezer D, Silver PB, Luger D, Mattapallil MJ, Chan CC, Caspi RR (2008) Inhibitory peptide analogs derived from a

major uveitogenic epitope protect from anti-retinal autoimmunity by inducing type 2 and regulatory T cells. J Leukoc Biol 84:577–585

27. Chen J, Qian H, Horai R, Chan CC, Falick Y, Caspi RR (2013) Comparative analysis of induced vs. spontaneous models of autoimmune uveitis targeting the interphotoreceptor retinoid binding protein. PLoS One 8:e72161

28. Silver PB, Chan CC, Wiggert B, Caspi RR (1999) The requirement for pertussis to induce EAU is strain-dependent: B10.RIII, but not B10.A mice, develop EAU and Th1 responses to IRBP without pertussis treatment. Invest Ophthalmol Vis Sci 40:2898–2905

Chapter 16

Methods of Isolation and Analysis of TREG Immune Infiltrates from Injured and Dystrophic Skeletal Muscle

Dalia Burzyn, Amy Wagers, Diane Mathis, and Massimiliano Cerletti

Abstract

The immune infiltrate present in acutely injured or dystrophic skeletal muscle has been shown to play an important role in the process of muscle regeneration. Our work has described, for the first time, muscle regulatory T cells (Tregs), a unique population in phenotype and function capable of promoting skeletal muscle repair. Herein, we describe the methods we have optimized to study muscle Tregs, including their isolation from injured muscle, immuno-labeling for analysis/separation by flow cytometry, and measurement of their proliferation status.

Key words Regulatory T cell, Skeletal muscle infiltrate, Tissue-resident leukocytes, Treg proliferation, Skeletal muscle injury, Muscular dystrophy

1 Introduction

In addition to primary and secondary lymphoid tissues, numerous immune cell populations can be found residing in nonlymphoid tissues. Growing evidence indicates that these tissue-resident leukocytes are important players in the maintenance of tissue homeostasis and immune tolerance. Resident innate and adaptive immune cells must keep a fine balance that allows efficient immune responses without causing detrimental effects on the tissue. Interestingly, CD4+ regulatory T cells expressing the transcription factor Foxp3 (Tregs) have been shown to be part of the nonlymphoid tissue-resident immune system in several organs. Because of their strong immunosuppressive capacity, Tregs have a key role in controlling immune over-reactivity in autoimmunity, allergies, infectious diseases, and cancer. Tregs residing in peripheral nonlymphoid tissues have a distinctive phenotype, and are essential for keeping tissue homeostasis and immune tolerance in place [1–3].

The repair of skeletal muscle injuries resulting from trauma, neuromuscular diseases, or other insults, depends essentially on the activity of satellite cells, a pool of skeletal muscle precursors with

Ashleigh S. Boyd (ed.), *Immunological Tolerance: Methods and Protocols*, Methods in Molecular Biology, vol. 1899,
https://doi.org/10.1007/978-1-4939-8938-6_16,

regenerative potential [4–11]. However, successful regeneration can only be achieved with the support of other cellular and molecular systems present at the site of injury. The immune infiltrate that accompanies the repair process has been shown to play an important role in the resolution of the injury, through complex interactions with muscle precursors, dead and nascent fibers, and stroma cells [12, 13]. In particular, our work has shown that a phenotypically and functionally distinct population Foxp3$^+$ regulatory T cells (Tregs) accumulates at the injury site in high frequency and number, and that these cells are required for proper recovery of an acute injury and stabilization of dystrophic disease. Muscle Tregs are important to control the inflammatory response and myofiber regeneration. Muscle Tregs express Amphiregulin, a growth factor that acts directly on satellite cells in vitro and improves muscle repair in vivo [14].

In this chapter we describe the methods for isolation and characterization of immune cells from mouse skeletal muscle, in particular muscle Tregs. The isolation protocol combines enzymatic digestion and density separation, allowing an excellent recovery of infiltrating leukocytes in terms of quality and cell numbers. To analyze the isolated infiltrates, flow cytometry is the main method of choice, given its versatility to study several surface and intracellular markers simultaneously. Success in using this technique will depend on the careful selection of antibody panels and an appropriate gating strategy.

2 Materials

2.1 Immune Cell Isolation Reagents

1. *Processing buffer*: DMEM without phenol red complemented with 2% fetal bovine serum (FBS) and HEPES 10 mM.
2. 2× *Digestion buffer*: 0.4% collagenase II (Invitrogen) and 300 μg/ml DNAse I (Sigma) in processing buffer.
3. *Percoll*: Before preparing the different density solutions, osmolality needs to be adjusted by mixing 9 parts of Percoll with 1 part of 10× PBS. Then, 40 and 80% Percoll solutions are prepared by diluting adjusted Percoll with 1× PBS to the desired concentration.

2.2 Immunostaining Reagents

1. *Staining buffer*: DMEM without phenol red (or PBS) complemented with 2% FBS and HEPES 10 mM.
2. *Antibodies*. Unless noted, all antibodies are from Biolegend, *Treg staining panel*: Pacific Blue anti-mouse CD45 (clone 30-F11), FITC anti-mouse TCRβ (clone H5-7597), PerCP-Cy5.5 anti-mouse CD4 (clone GK1.5 or RM4-5), PE anti-mouse CD25 (clone PC61), APC anti-mouse Foxp3 (clone FJK-16s), biotin anti-mouse amphiregulin (polyclonal,

R&D), streptavidin-PE, anti-KI-67 (clone B56, BD Biosciences). *Myeloid cell staining panel*: Pacific Blue anti-mouse CD45 (clone 30-F11), APC-Cy7 anti-mouse Ly6G (clone 1A8), PerCP-Cy5.5 anti-mouse CD11b (clone M1/70), PE anti-mouse I-A/I-E (clone M5/114.15.2), APC anti-mouse F4/80 (clone BM8), PE-efluor610 anti-mouse CD11c (clone N418), FITC anti-mouse Ly6c (clone HK1.4). For proliferation analysis: PE anti-mouse Ki67 (clone B56, BD Biosciences).

3. *FcBlock*: Commercial (such as anti-CD16/CD32) or supernatant from 2.4G2 hybridoma at a concentration of 1:5–1:10 of final staining volume.
4. *PFA Fixation buffer*: 2% paraformaldehyde in PBS. The solution can be stored for long time at 4 °C, protected from light.
5. *Fixation/permeabilization buffers for intracellular staining*: For nuclear antigens such as Foxp3, we use eBioscience Foxp3/Transcription Factor Staining Buffer Set. To prepare Fix/perm buffer: mix 1 volume of Fix/perm with 3 volumes of Fix/Perm diluent. Prepare only the amount needed each time, typically, 200 μl/well. To prepare permeabilization (Perm) buffer: mix 1 volume of 10× Perm buffer with 9 volumes of filtered water. Prepare only the amount needed each time.
6. *Click-iT EdU kit (Molecular Probes)*: EdU reconstitution, 5 mg/ml in PBS. Aliquot and store at −20 °C.

3 Methods

3.1 Muscle Dissection

1. Euthanize the mouse with CO_2.
2. Open skin and peritoneum to expose peritoneal cavity.
3. Cut the diaphragm to expose the heart, cut the cava vein, and immediately perfuse the mouse by injecting 30 ml of PBS into the left ventricle (slowly).
4. Dissect muscles. We usually use three hind limb muscles: tibialis anterior, gastrocnemius, and quadriceps (*see* **Note 1**). Avoid taking popliteal lymph nodes, tendons, and fat.
5. Place the muscles in an Eppendorf tube with 0.8–1 ml of buffer on ice.
6. Weigh tissue to allow calculation of cell numbers per gram of muscle.

3.2 Digesting the Tissue

1. With straight scissors, chop muscles into 0.1 in. pieces.
2. Using a plastic transfer pipette (with the tip cut) transfer tissue and buffer to a 50 ml tube containing 4 ml of processing buffer and add 5 ml of 2× digestion buffer (prepared the same day).

Final digestion volume will be 10 ml. If digesting muscles from two hind limbs (six muscles total), increase the digestion volume to 15 ml.

3. Place the tube horizontally in a 37 °C water bath with gentle shaking and digest for 30 min.
4. Filter through a 70 μm cell strainer, mashing the rest of the tissue with a syringe plunge. Add 20–30 ml of fresh buffer during the process to neutralize collagenase and clean the mesh. Centrifuge 400 × *g*, for 10 min at 4 °C. Carefully discard the supernatant, vortex the pellet, and add 15 ml of processing buffer. Centrifuge 5 min at 400 × *g* and carefully discard the supernatant.

3.3 Leukocyte Isolation by Density Gradient

1. Resuspend pellet in 6 ml of 40% Percoll and transfer to a 15 ml tube. Carefully underlay 6 ml of 80% Percoll. Spin for 25 min at 400 × *g*, at room temperature, with the brake off.
2. After centrifugation, leukocytes will band at the 40–80% interface. With a plastic transfer pipette, take the top layer of fat and dead cells and discard. With a clean pipette then carefully take all the white interface and transfer to a clean tube. Fill the tube with processing buffer, mix by inverting the tube 2–3 times, and centrifuge 400 × *g*, for 10 min at 4 °C. Repeat the washing step. Cells are now ready for use (*see* **Note 2**).

3.4 Immunolabeling of Muscle Infiltrate for Cytofluorometric Analysis of Surface and Intracellular Markers

We routinely stain using two antibody panels, one for analysis of Tregs and other T cells, and one for analysis of myeloid populations. Both panels require staining of surface markers, and the Treg panel requires a second step of permeabilization and intracellular staining for the transcription factor Foxp3. Inclusion of an anti-CD45 antibody in both panels is helpful to set the gating strategy. Although the Percoll separation step produces a clean leukocyte population, some debris is still present which might interfere with the analysis (Fig. 1). The basic panel for Tregs includes, in addition to Foxp3, CD25 (IL-2 receptor alpha), expressed by the majority of Tregs, which will facilitate gating during analysis (Fig. 1). Other markers can be added to both panels if the available flow cytometer allows for detection of more colors. Alternatively, some of the basic markers can be replaced by new markers of interest.

3.4.1 Surface Staining

(a) Aliquot cells for staining. In general, 0.1–2 × 10^6 cells are acceptable numbers for a good staining. If looking for rare populations (e.g., a subset of muscle Tregs), it is recommendable to use the whole cell suspension obtained from one mouse for one staining, as many events will need to be recorded in order to get significant results (*see* **Note 3**). For myeloid cell staining, set apart one fifth to one tenth of the whole cell suspension.

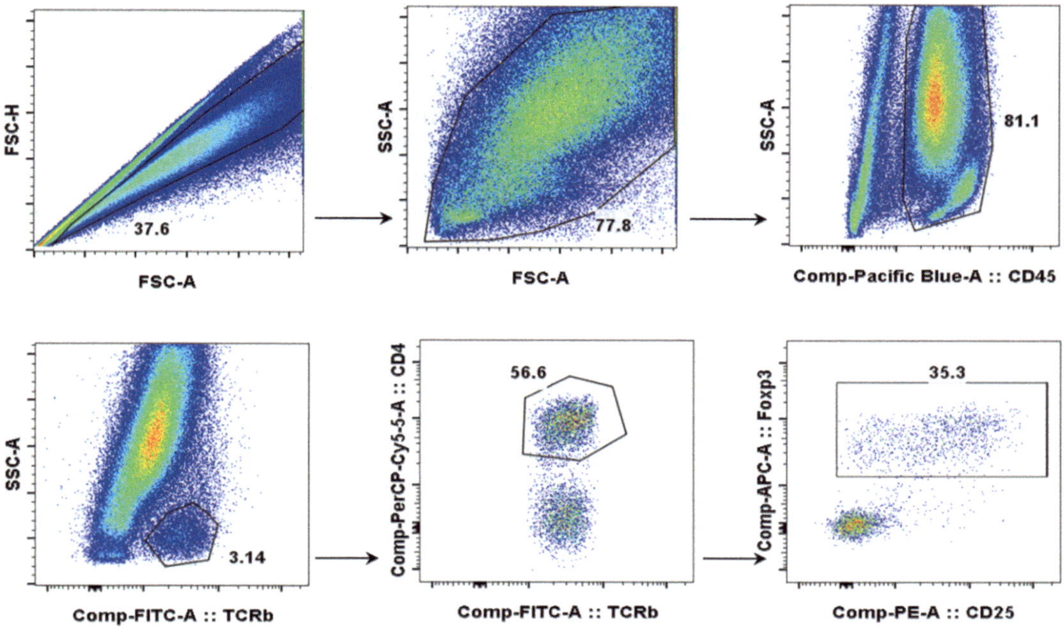

Fig. 1 Gating strategy for analysis of muscle Tregs. Careful exclusion of debris and cell doublets, gating on CD45 positive cells and gating on the TCR beta^{+}/side-scatter^{low} population are key steps to obtain a clean separation of Foxp3 vs. CD25 staining

(b) Set apart some cells for staining controls and isotype controls (*see* **Notes 4** and **5**). All the compensation controls and isotype controls should be treated as the samples of interest (fixation, permeabilization, etc.).

(c) Centrifuge cells 400 × *g*, for 3 min at 4 °C and resuspend the pellet in 50 μl of staining buffer containing FcBlock and the antibodies of interest (*see* **Notes 6–8**) to stain surface markers at the concentrations indicated by the manufacturer or by titration of the reagents. Skip APC-Cy7 conjugated antibodies in this step if doing a fix/perm step later (*see* **Note 9**). Incubate for 20–25 min on ice or at 4 °C, protected from light.

(d) Wash twice by adding staining buffer (0.2 ml if staining in plates, 0.5–1 ml if using tubes) and centrifuging at 4 °C.

(e) If a secondary step is needed, resuspend the cells in 50 μl of staining buffer containing the appropriate secondary reagent (fluorochrome-conjugated streptavidin or secondary antibody). Incubate for 15 min on ice or at 4 °C, protected from light.

(f) Wash twice by adding staining buffer and centrifuging at 4 °C.

(g) If intracellular staining will follow, proceed to Subheading 3.4.2.

(h) If no intracellular staining is required, cells are ready to run in the flow cytometer. If running samples immediately, resuspend the cells in 200 μl of staining buffer and keep at 4 °C until the moment of running. If samples are analyzed the following day/s, fix in 200 μl of PFA fixation buffer and store at 4 °C until the moment of running. Before running, spin down the cells and resuspend in 200 μl of staining buffer or PBS.

3.4.2 Intracellular Staining

(a) *Fixation*: After surface staining and washing, fix cells with 200 μl 1× Fix/perm buffer (eBioscience). Vortex or resuspend very well immediately. Incubate at 4 °C for at least 1.5 h and up to 16 h.

(b) *Wash step*: Centrifuge at 500 × *g*, 4 °C, discard the supernatant, and resuspend in 200 μl of staining buffer or PBS. Centrifuge again. Discard the supernatant.

The following permeabilization and staining steps should be done on the same day the samples will be run in the flow cytometer. If acquisition will not happen on the same day than the fixation step, the protocol can be put on hold by resuspending the cells in 200 μl of staining buffer or PBS and storing them at 4 °C (up to a couple of days). The day of acquisition, centrifuge at 500 × *g*, 4 °C, discard the supernatant and proceed with **step c**.

(c) *Permeabilization*: Resuspend cell pellets in 200 μl of 1× Perm buffer. Centrifuge at 500 × *g*, 4 °C. Discard the supernatant.

(d) *Staining*: The staining should be done in 1× Perm Buffer. Block Fc receptors and unspecific binding by resuspending the cells in 50 μl of 1× Perm Buffer with FcBlock in the appropriate concentration. Incubate 5–10′ at room temperature. Then add the antibodies for intracellular staining and APC-Cy7 conjugated antibody if applicable (*see* Subheading 3.4.1, **step c** and **Note 9**). Incubate for 45 minutes at room temperature, protected from light.

(e) *Wash step*: Add 100 ml of 1× Perm Buffer. Centrifuge at 500 × *g*, 4 °C, discard the supernatant, and resuspend in 200 μl of 1× Perm Buffer. Centrifuge again. Discard the supernatant.

(f) Resuspend the cells in 200 μl of staining buffer and keep at 4 °C until the moment of running.

3.5 Analysis of Treg Cell Proliferation in Skeletal Muscle Infiltrates

In this section we describe two methods to study proliferation in skeletal muscle infiltrates by flow cytometry. The first one is detection of the Ki67 antigen, which is expressed intracellularly by cycling cells (only undetectable during G_0 phase). The second protocol, measurement of EdU (5-ethynyl-2′-deoxyuridine) incorporation, allows the detection of cells that were in S phase at the time of EdU exposure. EdU is a nucleoside analog that can be used in replacement of the classical BrdU (bromo-deoxyuridine). As with BrdU, EdU is administered to mice to allow in vivo labeling of cycling cells, followed by staining of isolated cells to detect the presence of EdU-containing DNA. With the EdU detection method, mild fixation and detergent permeabilization are sufficient for the small molecule-based detection reagent to gain access to the DNA, as opposed to the BrdU detection method, which uses anti-BrdU antibodies following DNA denaturation by harsh methods (HCl, heat, or enzymes) to expose the BrdU molecules, affecting sample integrity and quality. We successfully combined Foxp3 intracellular staining with EdU detection protocol to study Treg proliferation.

3.5.1 Staining Protocol for Analysis of Ki-67 Expression

(a) Stain surface markers following instructions in Subheading 3.4.1.

(b) Follow instructions for intracellular staining in Subheading 3.4.2, including the anti-Ki67 clone 56. Titration and use of an isotype control are highly recommendable (*see* **Note 10**).

3.5.2 EdU Incorporation

(a) Inject intra vein 1 mg EdU per adult mouse, 4 or 24 h before collecting tissues (*see* **Note 11**).

(b) Isolate muscle infiltrate as described above and stain for cell surface and intracellular markers as usual. Important: avoid using PE, PE-TXRD, APC-Cy7, or other tandem colors, which are incompatible with EdU detection reagents.

(c) After the last wash with Perm buffer of the intracellular staining protocol, add 100 μl EdU mix (prepared following the manufacturer's protocol) and incubate for 30 min at room temperature.

(d) Wash twice with Foxp3 Perm buffer by centrifuging at $500 \times g$, 4 °C.

(e) If necessary, stain with APC-Cy7-conjugated antibody in staining buffer (include FcBlock).

4 Notes

1. Diaphragm from dystrophin-deficient mice (mdx) can also be dissected and processed with this protocol. For perfusion, make an incision between ribs instead of cutting the diaphragm. Reduce digestion volume to 5 ml, the wash volumes by half, and the Percoll band volume to 4 ml.

2. Cell counting is advisable at this point, since the Percoll procedure yields a very clean population of leukocytes with little fiber debris and dead cells that facilitates the counting.
3. The number of cells to stain depends on the abundance of the cell population of interest. In an acute injury model, total leukocyte numbers infiltrating the muscle vary with time, peaking between days 2 and 4 after injury [14]. If working at these time points, injuring three muscles of one hind limb will yield enough cells for running 0.5–1.5 $\times$ 10^6 events in the flow cytometer. Staining can be done in round-bottom 96-well plates or FACS tubes.
4. Single color staining controls are needed for compensation to correct for spectral overlap during multicolor flow cytometry. Although it is always recommended to use an aliquot of the sample cells to make these controls, we routinely use cells from mouse lymph node or spleen without any complication.
5. Isotype controls (i.e., samples in which a particular antibody is replaced by a nonspecific antibody of the same immunoglobulin isotype as the antibody of interest) are particularly important for antigens that do not stain a clear cell population or have low expression, in order to be able to set the gates during sample acquisition in the flow cytometer, and later for analysis. Unlike single color controls (*see* **Note 4**), isotype controls must be prepared from the same cells that are being analyzed. The use of isotype controls is highly recommended when a new antibody is being used for the first time, and every time if a particular antigen gives a dim, low, or unclear staining pattern.
6. When staining immune cells isolated from non-immune tissues, it is important to include an anti-CD45 antibody to facilitate the analysis (Fig. 1).
7. Fluorochrome conjugates suggested in this protocol can be modified according to user preference. However, it is advisable to test new color combinations since occasionally different conjugates of the same clone can give variable levels of staining and/or trouble with compensation.
8. Percoll separation allows enrichment of live cells. However, a viability dye, actively excluded from live cells, can be included in the protocol. For unfixed cells, propidium iodide (2 μg/ml final) or DAPI (0.1 μg/ml final) can be added right before running the sample in the flow cytometer. For fixed cells (with or without permeabilization step) alternative methods exist that are compatible with fixation, in which the dye (such as LIVE/DEAD Fixable Aqua Dead Cell Stain Kit, Molecular Probes) is added and washed before fixation and it remains stable after the fixative is added.

9. APC-Cy7 conjugates can be affected by the fix/perm step. To overcome this issue, we add the APC-Cy7-conjugated antibodies at the intracellular staining step. We have successfully tested this with several markers (TCRβ, CD8, CD4, CD25, CD45). If using an APC-Cy7 conjugate to a different antigen, take into account that some epitopes can be modified after fixation, affecting antibody binding.
10. Clone B56 is sold as anti-human Ki-67 but cross-reactivity with mouse Ki67 has been shown, and this clone has been widely used in mouse assays. Please note that the antibody is sold in a low concentration solution, so a higher volume needs to be used (typically 10–20 μl/sample). Titration and use of isotype control are highly recommendable.
11. For analysis of proliferation in muscle infiltrates, we found that intra vein injection delivers higher levels of EdU to the muscle than intraperitoneal injection.

References

1. Josefowicz SZ, Lu LF, Rudensky AY (2012) Regulatory T cells: mechanisms of differentiation and function. Annu Rev Immunol 30:531–564
2. Burzyn D, Benoist C, Mathis D (2013) Regulatory T cells in nonlymphoid tissues. Nat Immunol 14:1007–1013
3. Feuerer M, Herrero L, Cipolletta D, Naaz A, Wong J, Nayer A, Lee J, Goldfine AB, Benoist C, Shoelson S, Mathis D (2009) Lean, but not obese, fat is enriched for a unique population of regulatory T cells that affect metabolic parameters. Nat Med 15:930–939
4. Shi X, Garry DJ (2006) Muscle stem cells in development, regeneration, and disease. Genes Dev 20:1692–1708
5. McKinnell IW, Parise G, Rudnicki MA (2005) Muscle stem cells and regenerative myogenesis. Curr Top Dev Biol 71:113–130
6. Seale P, Asakura A, Rudnicki MA (2001) The potential of muscle stem cells. Dev Cell 1:333–342
7. Sherwood RI, Christensen JL, Conboy IM, Conboy MJ, Rando TA, Weissman IL, Wagers AJ (2004) Isolation of adult mouse myogenic progenitors: functional heterogeneity of cells within and engrafting skeletal muscle. Cell 119:543–554
8. Montarras D, Morgan J, Collins C, Relaix F, Zaffran S, Cumano A, Partridge TA, Buckingham M (2005) Direct isolation of satellite cells for skeletal muscle regeneration. Science 309:2064–2067
9. Collins CA, Olsen I, Zammit PS, Heslop L, Petrie A, Partridge TA, Morgan JE (2005) Stem cell function, self-renewal, and behavioral heterogeneity of cells from the adult muscle satellite cell niche. Cell 122:289–301
10. Cerletti M, Jurga S, Witczak CA, Hirshman MF, Shadrach JL, Goodyear LJ, Wagers AJ (2008) Highly efficient, functional engraftment of skeletal muscle stem cells in dystrophic muscles. Cell 134:37–47
11. Sacco A, Doyonnas R, Kraft P, Vitorovic S, Blau HM (2008) Self-renewal and expansion of single transplanted muscle stem cells. Nature 456:502–506
12. Tidball JG, Villalta SA (2010) Regulatory interactions between muscle and the immune system during muscle regeneration. Am J Physiol Regul Integr Comp Physiol 298:1173–1187
13. Arnold L, Henry A, Poron F, Baba-Amer Y, Van Rooijen N, Plonquet A, Gherardi RK, Chazaud B (2007) Inflammatory monocytes recruited after skeletal muscle injury switch into anti-inflammatory macrophages to support myogenesis. J Exp Med 204:1057–1069
14. Burzyn D, Kuswanto W, Kolodin D, Shadrach JL, Cerletti M, Jang Y, Sefik E, Tan TG, Wagers AJ, Benoist C, Mathis D (2013) A special population of regulatory T cells potentiates muscle repair. Cell 155:12821895

INDEX

Ashleigh S. Boyd (ed.), *Immunological Tolerance: Methods and Protocols*, Methods in Molecular Biology, vol. 1899, https://doi.org/10.1007/978-1-4939-8938-6, © Springer Science+Business Media, LLC, part of Springer Nature 2019

MIX
Papier aus verantwortungsvollen Quellen
Paper from responsible sources
FSC® C105338

If you have any concerns about our products,
you can contact us on
ProductSafety@springernature.com

In case Publisher is established outside the EU,
the EU authorized representative is:
Springer Nature Customer Service Center GmbH
Europaplatz 3, 69115 Heidelberg, Germany

Printed by Libri Plureos GmbH
in Hamburg, Germany